W9-DDQ-349

American
Medical
Association

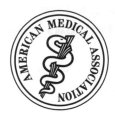

Complete
Guide to
Men's Health

Other books by the American Medical Association

American Medical Association
Family Medical Guide

American Medical Association
Complete Guide to Women's Health

American Medical Association
Complete Guide to Your Children's Health

American Medical Association
Handbook of First Aid and Emergency Care

American Medical Association
Family Health Cookbook

American Medical Association
Guide to Your Family's Symptoms

American Medical Association
Essential Guide to Asthma

American Medical Association
Essential Guide to Depression

American Medical Association
Essential Guide to Hypertension

American Medical Association
Essential Guide to Menopause

American Medical Association

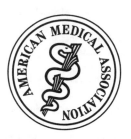

Complete Guide to Men's Health

Angela Perry, MD
Internal Medicine
Medical Editor

Mark Schacht, MD
Urology
Contributing Medical Editor

John Wiley & Sons, Inc.

New York • Chichester • Weinheim • Brisbane • Singapore • Toronto

This book is printed on acid-free paper. ∞

Copyright © 2001 by the American Medical Association. All rights reserved

Published by John Wiley & Sons, Inc.
Published simultaneously in Canada

Design and production by Navta Associates, Inc.

No part of this publication may be reproduced, stored in a retrieval system, or transmitted in any form or by any means, electronic, mechanical, photocopying, recording, scanning, or otherwise, except as permitted under Section 107 or 108 of the 1976 United States Copyright Act, without either the prior written permission of the Publisher, or authorization through payment of the appropriate per-copy fee to the Copyright Clearance Center, 222 Rosewood Drive, Danvers, MA 01923, (978) 750-8400, fax (978) 750-4744. Requests to the Publisher for permission should be addressed to the Permissions Department, John Wiley & Sons, Inc., 605 Third Avenue, New York, NY 10158-0012, (212) 850-6011, fax (212) 850-6008, email: PERMREQ@WILEY.COM

The recommendations and information in this book are appropriate in most cases; however, they are not a substitute for medical diagnosis. For specific information concerning a medical condition, the AMA suggests that you consult a physician. The names of organizations, products, or alternative therapies appearing in the book are given for informational purposes only. Their inclusion does not imply AMA endorsement, nor does the omission of any organization, product, or alternative therapy indicate AMA disapproval.

This publication is designed to provide accurate and authoritative information in regard to the subject matter covered. It is sold with the understanding that the publisher is not engaged in rendering professional services. If professional advice or other expert assistance is required, the services of a competent professional person should be sought.

Photograph of man playing tennis, on page 13, copyright PhotoDisc
Table, "Body Mass Index," on page 19, from the National Heart, Lung, and Blood Institute
Chart, "Comparing Types of Physical Activity," on page 21, adapted from "Physical Activity and Health: A Report of the Surgeon General Executive Summary," US Department of Health and Human Services, 1996
Photograph of man on scale, on page 68, copyright PhotoDisc
Table, "Healthy Weight Ranges for Men," on page 69, adapted from "Report of the Dietary Guidelines Advisory Committee on Dietary Guidelines for Americans," 1995
Photograph of warning signs of skin cancer, on page 92, reprinted with permission from the American Academy of Dermatology. All rights reserved.
Photograph of couple, on page 140, copyright PhotoDisc
Photograph of couple hugging, on page 144, copyright PhotoDisc
Chart, "Blood Pressure Classifications for People Age 18 and Older," on page 218, adapted from guidelines of the Joint National Committee on Detection, Evaluation, and Treatment of High Blood Pressure
Photograph of man reading a book, on page 330, copyright PhotoDisc
Photograph of laser surgery, on page 441, copyright PhotoTake

Library of Congress Cataloging-in-Publication Data

American Medical Association complete guide to men's health / American Medical Association.
     p. cm.
   Includes bibliographical references and index.
   ISBN 0-471-41411-5
   1. Men—Health and hygiene. 2. Self-care, Health. I. American Medical Association.
  RA777.8 . A46 2001
  613'.04234—dc21   2001017905

Printed in the United States of America

10 9 8 7 6 5 4 3 2 1

FOREWORD

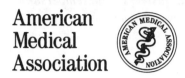

American
Medical
Association

Men have access to more information about healthcare than ever before, and they are more interested in learning how to live healthier, longer lives. Medicine has made great strides in understanding how to prevent some of the most serious diseases that many men face—including heart disease (the number-one killer), diabetes, and some forms of cancer. Advances in molecular biology and technology have given us new, more effective treatments that have improved the outcome of many disorders.

The *American Medical Association Complete Guide to Men's Health* can help you determine the steps to take to be healthy today and avoid the chronic disorders that many men face as they age. You will find discussions about complicated subjects such as cancer and difficult issues such as domestic violence and drug abuse as well as detailed information about a wide variety of diseases and disorders. We at the American Medical Association feel that the more knowledge you have about an illness that affects you or a loved one, the more effectively you will be able to work with your doctors to make informed decisions about treatments.

We feel sure that the *American Medical Association Complete Guide to Men's Health* will become a useful reference for you and your family when you are seeking medical information or are faced with important medical decisions.

American Medical Association

American Medical Association

| | Robert A. Musacchio | *Senior Vice President, Business and Membership* |
| | Anthony J. Frankos | *Vice President, Business Products* |

AMA Press
	Mary Lou S. White	*Editorial Director*
	Patricia Dragisic	*Senior Managing Editor*
	Donna Kotulak	*Managing Editor*
	Steven Michaels	*Senior Editor*
	Robin Husayko	*Contributing Editor*
	Claudia Appeldorn	*Copy Editor*
	Mary Ann Albanese	*Image Coordinator*
	Reuben Rios	*Editorial Assistant*
	Roger Banther	*Editorial Assistant*

Medical Editors
| | Angela Perry, MD | *Medical Editor* |
| | Mark Schacht, MD | *Contributing Medical Editor* |

Writers
Pam Brick
Michelle Kienholz
Donald Phillips

Illustration
Rolin Graphics Inc.

Medical Consultants
	Paul Chaiken, DDS	*Dentistry*
	Bruce Cohen, MD	*Neurology*
	David Cugell, MD	*Pulmonary Medicine*
	Arthur W. Curtis, MD	*Otolaryngology*
	Andrew Lazar, MD	*Dermatology*
	Gary S. Lissner, MD	*Ophthalmology*
	Domeena C. Renshaw, MD	*Psychiatry/Sexual Dysfunction*
	David Ross, MD	*Plastic Surgery*
	Irwin Siegel, MD	*Orthopedics*
	Mathew Sorrentino, MD	*Cardiology*
	Emanuel Steindler, PhD	*Addiction Medicine*
	Mark Stolar, MD	*Endocrinology*

Contents

ABOUT THIS BOOK

The *American Medical Association Complete Guide to Men's Health* provides up-to-date information that will enable you to adopt healthy habits that you can follow throughout your life. The book emphasizes the basics of a healthy lifestyle and the steps you can take to prevent illness.

In clear, easy-to-understand language, this book describes how different body systems work, answers many questions you may have about common diseases and disorders, and explains how many of these conditions can be prevented. The book guides you in making important decisions about your health based on the latest medical information. You will learn how to work effectively with your doctor and become a more active participant in your healthcare. The information in this book can benefit men of any age.

Take some time to familiarize yourself with the book. To get the most out of it, follow the cross-references to other parts of the book. To look up a specific disorder or to look for information about a specific topic, consult the index at the back of the book. The index contains many cross-references to other terms that will help you find the information you need.

"The Healthy Man" at the beginning of the book contains information about preventing illness and staying healthy and safe. Part II, "Staying Healthy," expands on the many things you can do—including eating a nutritious diet and exercising regularly—to stay healthy and reduce your risk of developing chronic disorders such as heart disease and cancer. This part will answer your questions about nutrition, fitness, body weight, and stress management. It also covers preventive health care, including the examinations and tests most helpful to you at every stage of life. You will also learn how to change behaviors such as smoking that put your health at risk.

Part III, "The Reproductive System," covers sexual and reproductive health, sexually transmitted diseases, and birth control. Part IV, "Common Health Concerns," covers major disorders of every system of the body. Included are the most common serious disorders that affect men. Each article answers the following questions about a disease or disorder: What is it? What are its symptoms? What are the risks? How is it treated? Information about self-care also is included whenever appropriate.

The glossary contains useful supplemental information and will help answer general questions about health.

PART ONE

The Healthy Man

INTRODUCTION

Men are staying healthier and living longer now than in decades past. This gain in life expectancy can be credited in part to better nutrition, improved public health and sanitation, and the advent of vaccines and antibiotics. But medical science has also made great strides in understanding and treating debilitating, chronic conditions such as heart disease and stroke. The stereotype of frailty in old age no longer applies as men take control of their own health by becoming better informed about health issues and their personal health risks. Men today are also making better lifestyle choices—eating more healthfully, not smoking, and exercising regularly. Such healthy lifestyle choices have been shown to help prevent the development of heart disease and some cancers—the top two causes of death in the United States. These good health habits, along with regular medical checkups, can greatly increase your chances of living longer and healthier.

Another way to reduce your risk of illness and early death is to avoid risky behaviors that could jeopardize your health. Males experience four out of five of all injuries from accidents involving motor vehicles or firearms, drownings, and fires. A large proportion of such accidents are caused by excessive alcohol consumption. Younger men are especially likely to die accidentally. You can reduce your risk of accidental injury by taking some simple and commonsense measures to protect yourself. For example, always wear a seat belt when you drive and a helmet when riding a bicycle or a motorcycle. Never drink alcohol and drive.

Drinking alcohol excessively carries many other health risks. It can lead to alcohol abuse and dependence, liver disease, and heart failure. If you choose to drink alcohol, do so only in moderation (two drinks a day or less). A typical drink is 5 ounces of wine, 1½ ounces of 80-proof distilled spirits, 12 ounces of wine cooler, or 12 ounces of beer (see page 24). Use of other recreational drugs also can cause dependence and impair your judgment and reflexes. Smoking cigarettes can have significant adverse effects on your health. Quitting smoking may be the best thing you can do to improve your overall health because, even if you eat right and exercise, the unhealthful effects of smoking will shorten your life. Practicing unsafe sex is another risky behavior that can have serious— sometimes fatal—health consequences.

Doctors know that early detection of disease often leads to more effective treatment. That's why it's important to see your doctor for checkups regularly. During the checkup, your doctor can order the appropriate medical tests to detect any health problems you might have, based on your family health history and other personal risk factors. Seeing your doctor regularly also can help you develop an effective patient-doctor relationship so you can become an active, informed consumer and take control of your health and medical care. Note that it is your responsibility to provide your doctor with specific information about your health, such as details about symptoms, so that he or she can perform needed tests, make an accurate diagnosis, and provide effective treatment.

Use this section of the book to find out how to stay healthy longer by adopting good health habits. The best disease-preventing measures include consuming a healthy diet, exercising regularly, maintaining an appropriate weight for your height, drinking alcohol only in moderation, not using tobacco, becoming more safety-conscious in your daily life, and seeing your doctor for periodic checkups. These measures may sound daunting at first, but they are effective ways to help you stay healthy.

A HEALTHY DIET

Good nutrition can help you achieve good health without having to sacrifice great-tasting food. Eating healthfully can help you work more productively, perform better athletically, maintain or reduce your weight, and dramatically lower your risk for heart disease and certain forms of cancer. A healthy diet is one that is well balanced, low in fat, high in fiber, and rich in whole grains, vegetables, and fruits. To consume a healthy diet, you need to choose foods that provide all the nutrients your body needs without an excess of fat, sugar, or calories.

No matter what your lifestyle, the Food Guide Pyramid is your best guide to making healthy food choices. Developed by the US Department of Agriculture, the Food Guide Pyramid is meant to be a general outline for healthy eating, not a rigid dietary prescription. It helps you choose the most nutritious foods in the correct proportions. The Food Guide Pyramid arranges all foods into five food groups—grains; vegetables and fruits; dairy; meat, poultry, and other protein foods; and fats, oils, and sweets. The grains group is at the base of the pyramid because it is the foundation of good nutrition.

The Food Guide Pyramid conveys three concepts about healthful eating: balance, variety, and moderation. To eat a balanced diet, consume more foods from the groups at the bottom of the pyramid and fewer from those near the top. Achieve variety in your diet by sampling an assortment of foods from the different pyramid groups and a variety of foods within each food group. Practice moderation by eating neither too much nor too little of any food.

The Food Guide Pyramid contains four levels that symbolize the importance of certain foods in your overall diet. At the bottom lies the bread, cereal, rice, and pasta group—all foods made from grains. This group is the largest of the food groups in the pyramid because grain-based foods should make up the largest proportion of the food in your diet. You should consume six to 11 servings of bread, cereal, rice, and pasta each day. A serving is one slice of bread, 1 ounce of ready-to-eat cereal, or half a cup of cooked cereal, rice, or pasta. Grain foods contain complex carbohydrates, which are an excellent source of energy, and many grain products are enriched with B vitamins and iron. Most grain foods are also low in fat and cholesterol. Whole-grain foods, such as brown rice, whole wheat or multigrain breads, and bran cereal, also supply fiber (see page 11), which has been shown to help lower blood cholesterol (see page 89) and which may reduce your risk for certain forms of cancer, such as colon cancer. Try to obtain at least half of your daily grain servings (at least three servings) from whole-grain foods.

The second level (from the bottom) of the pyramid contains the vegetable and fruit groups. The Food Guide Pyramid recommends that you eat three to five servings of vegetables and two to four servings of fruits each day—more vegetables than fruits because vegetables contain a wider variety of vitamins and minerals than do fruits. A serving is a cup of raw, leafy vegetables; half a cup of other vegetables, either cooked or chopped raw; one medium apple, orange, or banana; half a cup of chopped, cooked, or canned fruit; or ¾ cup of vegetable or fruit juice. The nutrients in vegetables and fruits vary considerably, so it is important to include a wide variety of these foods in your diet. However, many vegetables and fruits are rich in the antioxidant vitamins, E, C, and beta carotene (which converts to vitamin A in your body). Antioxidants (see page 9) may have the potential to lower your risk for heart disease.

The milk, yogurt, and cheese group appears on the same level of the Food Guide Pyramid as the meat, poultry, fish, dry beans, eggs, and nuts group. Two to three daily servings of both dairy products and protein foods are suggested for good health. Dairy foods are an important source of calcium but can be high in fat, especially saturated fat, so you need to choose low-fat or fat-free varieties of milk, yogurt, and cheese. You may be surprised that dried beans and nuts are grouped together with meat and poultry, but all these foods supply protein and the same kinds of nutrients, such as iron, zinc, and the B vitamins. A serving is 1 cup of milk or yogurt; 1½ to 2 ounces of cheese; or 2 to 3 ounces of cooked lean meat,

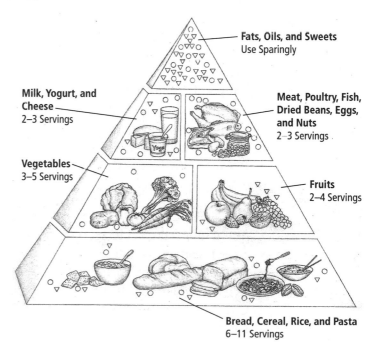

Fats, Oils, and Sweets
Use Sparingly

Milk, Yogurt, and Cheese
2–3 Servings

Meat, Poultry, Fish, Dried Beans, Eggs, and Nuts
2–3 Servings

Vegetables
3–5 Servings

Fruits
2–4 Servings

Bread, Cereal, Rice, and Pasta
6–11 Servings

poultry, or fish. (Half a cup of cooked dry beans, one egg, or 2 tablespoons of peanut butter count as 1 ounce of lean meat.) It is important for middle-aged or older men to become accustomed to the idea of eating a small portion (2 to 3 ounces) of meat or poultry.

At the top of the pyramid sits the smallest food group, made up of fats, oils, and sweets. It is best to consume foods high in fat and sugar only sparingly. High-fat foods contribute to the development of heart disease, and sugar contains many nutritionally empty calories. Overindulgence in foods from this group may lead to excess weight gain.

The bottom line is that a healthy diet can keep you healthy. But don't worry if you eat a high-fat cheeseburger or a sugary dessert once in a while. The important thing is to balance your diet over weeks or months so your overall diet is healthy. To make sure you are consuming a wide variety of foods, be adventurous. Try bok choy or bulgur if you've never had it before. Experiment with exotic herbs and spices to enliven the flavor of foods, both new and familiar. And be sure to balance what you eat with physical activity to maintain your proper body weight.

Dietary Guidelines for Americans

The US Department of Agriculture (USDA) and the US Department of Health and Human Services periodically publish Dietary Guidelines for Americans. These guidelines are designed to help people not only get the nutrients they need, but also lead more active lives so they can reduce their risk of chronic diseases such as heart disease and certain forms of cancer. The most current dietary guidelines provide sound, no-nonsense advice to help you build a healthy diet:

- Eat a variety of foods.
- Balance the food you eat with physical activity to maintain or improve your weight.
- Eat plenty of grain products, vegetables, and fruits.
- Limit your intake of fat, saturated fat, and cholesterol.
- Eat only moderate amounts of sugar.
- Limit the amount of salt (sodium) in your diet.
- If you drink alcoholic beverages, do so in moderation.

It's not difficult to incorporate these guidelines into your daily life. Just try these healthy-eating tips:

- Make grains the centerpiece of your meal; let meats be the garnish.
- Select lean meats and low-fat or fat-free dairy foods.
- Increase your fiber intake; eat a variety of whole grains, dry beans, and fiber-rich vegetables and fruits such as carrots, peas, pears, and berries.
- Choose dishes that contain servings from more than one food group, such as soups and stews.

- Maintain your weight in a healthy range. The guidelines no longer allow for gaining weight as you get older.
- Become more active: walk instead of drive, use the stairs, swim, bike, or do yard work. Better yet, start a regular exercise program.
- Have fresh fruit or yogurt for dessert. Sugar contains lots of calories but few nutrients.
- Snack on reduced-fat and low-salt multigrain crackers, cut-up fresh vegetables and fruits, rice cakes, raisins, low-salt pretzels, unbuttered popcorn, low-fat cheeses, and low-fat whole-grain breakfast cereal.
- Drink no more than two alcoholic beverages per day, if you drink at all.

Breakfast Jump-Starts Your Day

What's the big deal about breakfast? It's the most important meal of the day, just as your mother probably said. Breakfast literally means breaking the overnight fast. After not eating for 12 hours or more, your blood sugar level is low and your body needs fuel. Don't deprive your body of its first meal of the day just because you don't have much time. Instead, keep breakfast simple. Have a bowl of hot or cold cereal, yogurt, fresh fruit, toast, a smoothie (mix equal portions of fresh or frozen fruit, fat-free milk, and low-fat flavored yogurt in a blender; adding a few ice cubes will make your drink thicker), or eat leftovers from the night before. Take breakfast with you in the car or on the train. Still unconvinced about the benefits of a good breakfast? Consider these facts about breakfast eaters: they control their weight better and consume fewer calories throughout the day. Their blood cholesterol levels are lower, potentially reducing heart disease risk. They also concentrate better and perform better on work tasks. So put out a bagel or a muffin tonight for tomorrow morning and let breakfast help you boost your intake of grains.

How to Read Food Labels

Food labels contain many useful facts about the contents of packaged food and can help you select healthy foods when shopping for groceries. Nutrition labeling provides information about ingredients (in descending order of weight), serving size, number of calories, nutrient content, and how a food fits into your overall diet. The most informative part of any food label is the nutrition facts panel, because it shows not only the number of servings in a package but also the amount and percent of daily values of nutrients such as total fat, saturated fat, cholesterol, sodium, and carbohydrates. This label also indicates the fiber and sugar content of the food inside the package.

The bottom of the nutrition facts panel lists the percent of daily values for vitamins A and C, and for calcium and iron. This portion of the panel tells you that the food inside the package

Nutrition Facts

Serving Size 1/2 cup (114g)
Servings Per Container 4

Amount Per Serving	
Calories 90	Calories from Fat 30

	% Daily Value*
Total Fat 3g	5%
Saturated Fat 0g	0%
Cholesterol 0mg	0%
Sodium 300 mg	13%
Total Carbohydrate 13g	4%
Dietary Fiber 3g	12%
Sugars 3g	
Protein 3g	

Vitamin A 80%	•	Vitamin C 60%
Calcium 4%	•	Iron 4%

* Percent Daily Values are based on a 2,000 calorie diet. Your daily values may be higher or lower depending on your calorie needs.

contains a certain percentage of your recommended daily allowance of these nutrients. This area of the panel also shows the daily recommended values of such nutrients as total fat and cholesterol in a 2,000-calorie-per-day diet. You need to pay special attention to the listed nutrients that pertain to your particular health status and family health history (see page 80). For example, if you have a family history of heart disease, you will probably be most interested in the percent of daily value of fat listed on the label.

When reading food labels, look carefully at the health and nutrient-content claims on the package. For example, some labels claim that a food is "light" or "low-fat." The US government allows food manufacturers to make such claims only if the food meets the following strict guidelines:

Nutrient Content Claim	Guideline
Low fat	3 grams or less per serving
Low cholesterol	20 milligrams or less per serving
Reduced/less/lower	At least 25 percent less than that in a comparable unmodified food
Light	Must state percent reduction in fat or calories
No added sugars	Sugars not added during processing
High/rich in/excellent source of	Supplies at least 20 percent of daily value
Good source/contains/provides	Supplies 10 to 19 percent of daily value

Do You Need Vitamin and Mineral Supplements?

Many men take nutritional supplements because they believe that certain vitamins or minerals provide health benefits or help them increase athletic performance or endurance. But if you are otherwise healthy, you probably don't need to take a supplement as long as you follow the Food Guide Pyramid recommendations for a balanced diet. It's best to obtain nutrients from a wide variety of foods rather than from a vitamin or mineral supplement because your body may not absorb the vitamins from supplements as effectively as those obtained from food. Also, most people can obtain the suggested recommended dietary allowance (RDA) of vitamins and minerals by consuming a varied diet. For example, the RDA of vitamin C, which is 60 milligrams, can be obtained by eating five servings of fruits and vegetables each day. Smoking increases the need for vitamin C, however. If you smoke, you should be getting 100 milligrams of vitamin C per day.

It's especially unwise to take in large amounts of vitamins and minerals in excess of the recommended daily allowances over prolonged periods of time. There is no convincing evidence that taking megadoses of a particular vitamin will make you healthier. In fact, consuming huge amounts of certain vitamins can actually harm your health. For example, doses of vitamin C above 1,000 milligrams per day can cause nausea, stomach cramps, diarrhea, and even kidney stones.

However, certain people do need to take supplements. You may need to take a vitamin and mineral supplement if you:

- regularly skip meals
- are on a very low-calorie or low-carbohydrate diet for long periods
- are an older person who finds it hard to eat as much as you should
- eat a vegan diet (a vegetarian diet that omits dairy products and eggs)
- take medication that interferes with vitamin or mineral absorption
- are lactose intolerant and have been decreasing your calcium intake

If you fall into one of these categories, talk to your doctor about taking a daily multivitamin and mineral supplement. Even if you eat a balanced diet, a daily multivitamin won't harm you. But remember that taking a vitamin and mineral supplement is no substitute for eating a balanced, high-fiber, low-fat diet containing plenty of grains, vegetables, and fruits.

What Are Antioxidants?

Much interest has focused on the potential of antioxidants to fight disease and slow the aging process. But how reliable are these claims? How do antioxidants work?

Free radicals are unstable molecules that have an unpaired electron. They cause oxidation (a process whereby oxygen changes, damages, or breaks down cells) in your body, similar to the oxidation that occurs when metal rusts, as they seek stability by taking an electron from a surrounding molecule in a cell for themselves. The attacked molecule then has an unpaired electron, becoming a new free radical. The chain reaction continues indefinitely. Free radicals destroy DNA, and DNA destruction is thought to be one of the processes that triggers aging. Free radicals also can interfere with other processes in cells, causing cell changes that eventually can lead to cancer.

Antioxidants are compounds in foods that inhibit the oxidation caused by free radicals. The vitamins C and E and beta carotene (which converts to vitamin A in your body) and the minerals magnesium, copper, and zinc are antioxidants in foods that have shown promise in slowing down or preventing the chronic health problems, such as heart disease and cancer, that often accompany aging. Antioxidants also may help the body fight infection.

Vitamin E is found in nuts, seeds, and oils such as olive, peanut, and canola oil. You can increase your intake of beta carotene by eating more orange and deep yellow vegetables and fruits such as carrots, sweet potatoes, pumpkin, cantaloupe, apricots, and winter squash. Boost your vitamin C intake by consuming citrus fruits (oranges, grapefruit, lemons, or limes), berries, bell peppers, potatoes, broccoli, and cabbage.

The scientific evidence is strongest for the healthful effects of vitamin E and weakest for vitamin C. Experts stress that it is best to obtain antioxidant vitamins naturally, from your diet, rather than by taking supplements, especially in large amounts, until large-scale, long-term studies prove otherwise. As with vitamin and mineral supplements in general, taking antioxidant supplements cannot make up for the inadequacies of a poor diet. If you already have a health problem such as heart disease, taking antioxidants should never replace the goals of maintaining normal blood pressure, improving your cholesterol profile, or stopping smoking.

Good Sources of Antioxidants

The best way to take in antioxidants is to eat a varied, balanced diet that includes plenty of fruits, vegetables, and whole grains. The foods listed below are good sources of antioxidants. It is important to note that the fruits, vegetables, and whole grains that contain antioxidants also provide fiber. When you include these foods in your diet, you get the benefits of fiber along with the benefits of antioxidants.

Vitamins	Sources
A	Fortified milk and dairy products, eggs, cantaloupe, apricots, carrots, and dark green leafy vegetables such as spinach and kale
C	Citrus fruits, strawberries, tomatoes, bell peppers, broccoli, cauliflower, cabbage, potatoes, and leafy green vegetables
E	Vegetable oils, margarine, eggs, fish, whole grains, wheat germ, nuts, dried peas and beans, and leafy green vegetables
Beta carotene	Orange and deep yellow vegetables and fruits such as carrots, sweet potatoes, winter squash, cantaloupe, pumpkin, and mangoes, and dark green leafy vegetables such as spinach and broccoli

Minerals	Sources
Copper	Whole grains, mushrooms, dried fruits, grapes, nuts, liver, and shellfish
Magnesium	Dark green leafy vegetables, nuts, whole grains, dried peas and beans, dairy products, dried fruits, fish, shellfish, red meat, and poultry
Zinc	Red meat, poultry, oysters, eggs, dried peas and beans, nuts, milk, yogurt, and whole grains

Fiber

Most nutrients are absorbed and used by your body, but fiber passes through your digestive system without being absorbed. Still, it remains an important nutrient because it provides the bulk that helps your digestive system function properly and can protect against certain serious diseases.

There are two types of fiber: soluble and insoluble. Both types help prevent constipation, and soluble fiber has been shown to reduce the risk of colon cancer, diabetes, digestive disorders, and heart disease. Foods rich in soluble fiber include oat bran, oatmeal, beans, peas, rice bran, barley, and citrus fruits. Foods high in insoluble fiber are whole-wheat breads and cereals, wheat bran, rye, whole-grain rice, cabbage, carrots, and brussels sprouts. A diet rich in whole grains, vegetables, and fruits can easily provide the recommended 25 grams of fiber each day.

A Wake-up Call for Caffeine

Caffeine, an addictive chemical found in coffee, tea, colas, chocolate, and some pain relievers, acts as a stimulant in your body, increasing heart rate, blood pressure, and alertness. While moderate caffeine consumption—two or three cups of coffee per day—is not harmful, extremely high amounts can cause heart palpitations, insomnia, and anxiety. Even moderate amounts of caffeine can cause dehydration, so it's best to avoid caffeine-containing liquids on hot days or when exercising vigorously.

Many studies have been done to see if any link exists between caffeine and heart disease, but results have been inconclusive. Moderate caffeine consumption does not appear to be harmful. If you would like to reduce your caffeine intake, do so gradually. Stopping caffeine abruptly can lead to withdrawal headaches. Start reducing your caffeine intake by mixing increasing amounts of decaffeinated coffee in with your regular brew. Substitute juice or sparkling water with a twist of lemon or lime for caffeinated sodas.

THE BENEFITS OF EXERCISE

Along with a healthy diet, exercise is the cornerstone of good health. Physical activity produces a multitude of benefits for your overall health and well-being. Being active helps prevent heart disease and stroke by lowering cholesterol levels and making the heart pump more efficiently. It reduces the risk of dying prematurely, especially of heart disease. Physical activity helps control your weight and prevent obesity, which is a risk factor for high blood pressure and diabetes. Regular exercise also can improve your mood, reduce stress, and relieve depression, not to mention build muscular strength and tone, increase your flexibility, and enhance endurance. Just a small increase in your activity level can yield big results, especially if you lead a sedentary lifestyle.

Doctors recommend that all men engage in at least 30 minutes of moderate exercise every day. But you don't have to exercise for half an hour all at once. You can accumulate several shorter sessions throughout the day, as long as it adds up to about 30 minutes. For example, you could walk briskly to the bus for 10 minutes in the morning and home again for 10 minutes at night. Add another 10-minute period of stair climbing or yard work in the middle of the day and you've met your goal. Lack of time doesn't have to be a barrier any longer. You can reap the benefits of exercise with either shorter but more frequent periods of activity or one long, sustained session.

You don't have to aspire to be a long-distance runner or pump heavy iron to attain health benefits from exercise. Any type of physical activity—washing the car, mowing the lawn, taking the stairs, even walking—is good for you and will cut your risk of heart disease. Of course, the more exercise you engage in, the more benefits you gain. So once you begin to exercise moderately on a regular basis, try to boost your activity level by including more vigorous activities such as jogging or swimming in your exercise program (see page 59).

The good news is that even if you start exercising later in life you will still see positive results. Previously sedentary men who begin exercising in their 40s, 50s, or 60s can trim their risk of dying prematurely of heart disease by almost half, even if they already have a heart condition. All you need to do is get up and move—walk instead of drive, pull some weeds in the garden, or do light house-work several times a week. Better yet, ride a bike, swim, or jog regularly.

If you have not been very active, you need to start exercising slowly. Gradually increase the length of time you exercise. Take a walk around the block a few times each night after dinner, then walk longer distances as you feel more fit. Talk to your doctor about the types of activities that are safe. Be sure to choose activities you enjoy so you will be more likely to continue exercising. Take part in a variety of activities so you won't get bored. Walk, swim, ride a bike, climb stairs, go dancing, or play volleyball—any activity counts as long as you keep moving. Get your family involved. Family members can improve their health and spend time together on a hike, bicycle ride, or other physical activity.

Most important, make exercising a regular part of your routine. Remember to drink plenty of water before you begin exercising, and drink more afterward to prevent dehydration.

If you already exercise regularly, make sure the activity is strenuous enough that you reach your target heart rate, which is 50 to 80 percent of your maximum heart rate for your age. To find your maximum heart rate, subtract your age from 220. That number multiplied by .50 gives you 50 percent of your maximum heart rate. Multiply that same number by .80 and you get 80 percent of your maximum rate. Your target heart rate lies between these two numbers.

Immediately after you stop exercising, take your pulse for 15 seconds and multiply the number of beats by 4 to find your heart rate in beats per minute. If you are not reaching your target heart rate, exercise a bit harder the next time you work out. If your heart rate is above your target rate, work out a little less vigorously.

What Type of Exercise Is Best for You?

Choosing the best type of exercise for your lifestyle can be as easy as participating in an activity you like, whether it's biking with the family or playing a not-so-serious game of basketball. All forms of exercise are beneficial for your health. Aerobic exercises are prolonged physical activities that you can perform continuously for at least 12 minutes and that use oxygen to provide energy for your muscles. Aerobic exercises such as brisk walking, jogging, swimming, and bicycling use the large muscles in your trunk, upper body, and legs in repeated rhythmic movements that you sustain for long periods. This type of exercise strengthens your heart, making it work more efficiently during exercise and at rest.

If you are just starting an exercise program and have been inactive, ask your doctor to recommend activities that are safe, especially if you have an existing health problem such as diabetes or high blood pressure. Men who are already fit should add other types of exercises to their aerobic routine. Strength-conditioning exercises using free weights or exercise machines can also strengthen your heart and can help you build strength, improve posture, and reduce your risk of lower-back injury. Flexibility exercises such as stretching help you to maintain complete range of motion in your joints and can prevent injury and muscle soreness.

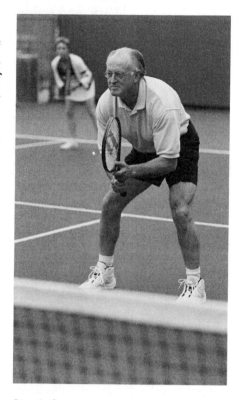

Stay Active
Regular exercise can provide health benefits at any age. In addition to keeping your heart, muscles, and bones strong, it makes you feel good. Incorporate it into your daily routine.

Before beginning any new exercise program, always consult with your doctor if you are over age 40, smoke, or have any risk factors for heart disease, including high blood pressure, a high cholesterol level, diabetes, or a family history of heart disease.

Getting Started and Staying Motivated

It may seem overwhelming to even think about exercising every day, but remember that any type of physical activity counts toward your goal. If you are over age 40 or are a smoker, you should get a thorough physical examination from your doctor before participating in any type of vigorous exercise program. After the doctor gives you the all-clear signal, try these tips to get you off to a good start and help you stick to your exercise regimen:

- Set reasonable goals. If you can only jog lightly for 5 minutes at first, don't try to do more right away.
- Listen to your body. It will tell you when to slow down or rest.
- Vary your routine. It's too easy to get bored with only one activity.
- Wear comfortable clothing and shoes that fit well and support your feet.
- Slowly increase the duration and intensity of your workouts. Start with moderate-level activities.
- Seek support from family and friends. Ask them to exercise with you.
- Keep an exercise log. Seeing your own progress is a great motivator.
- Reward yourself. Buy a special treat when you reach a milestone.

The Dangers of Anabolic Steroids

Professional and amateur athletes sometimes use supplements or drugs to improve their physical performance. Anabolic steroids are probably the most well-known performance-enhancing drugs, and the most dangerous. These synthetic drugs imitate the effects of the male hormone testosterone. The drugs have approved medical uses, but athletes use them to make their muscles bulkier and stronger.

Anabolic steroids are especially risky because they have a number of unwanted side effects. Steroids can cause acne, raise blood pressure, damage the liver, reduce sperm counts, decrease the size of the testicles, increase the size of the breasts, cause erectile dysfunction, and speed up the development of baldness. Anabolic steroids also can cause mood swings, aggression, and violent behavior. In adolescents they can prematurely stop growth and development. The drugs are either taken in pill form or injected with a hypodermic needle and, if an athlete shares the needle with a friend, he puts himself at risk of contracting a blood-borne infection such as hepatitis (see page 191) or human immunodeficiency virus (HIV), which causes acquired immunodeficiency syndrome (AIDS) (see page 186). If that is not enough to convince you not to use these drugs, you should also know that possessing or selling anabolic steroids without a prescription from a doctor is illegal.

Anabolic steroids are not worth the risks. It's much safer to increase your muscle mass and strength by performing resistance exercises regularly and eating a healthy diet.

Warming Up and Cooling Down

Always begin your exercise routine with a thorough warm-up period. Warm-up exercises heighten your flexibility and prevent muscle soreness. The purpose of warm-up exercises is to take each joint in your body through its full range of motion. Stretching exercises combined with low-intensity walking, jogging, or bicycling for about 5 minutes also prepare your body for more vigorous activity. After you finish your workout, repeat the same exercises to cool your muscles and joints down. Here are some effective warm-up and cool-down stretches you can try. Do each exercise slowly, spending 1 or 2 minutes on each stretch. If any warm-up exercise gives you pain, stop doing it. Begin by stretching your arms and spine.

Spine and Arm Stretch Stand with your feet facing forward and your knees slightly bent. Try to keep your body straight as you reach your arms over your head with your hands together, palms facing forward. Hold the stretch for 10 to 20 seconds. Slowly bring your arms down, reaching out with your hands as you go down, and bend down at the waist. Keep your knees slightly bent. Try to touch the ground, but don't stretch too far if it hurts, and avoid bouncing. Slowly rise and let your arms fall to your sides. Repeat three times.

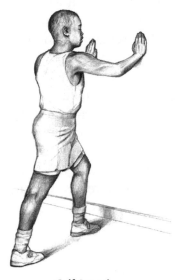

Calf Stretch Stand erect in front of a wall or a doorframe. While moving forward, bend one leg and move the other back, with both of your heels on the floor, keeping the back leg straight. Move forward as far as is comfortable until you feel a pull in the back of your outstretched leg. Relax and hold for 10 seconds. Repeat with the other leg.

Thigh Stretch Balance on your left leg. If you can't balance easily, hold on to a chair. Bend your right leg back and hold your right foot with your right hand, pressing in as far as is comfortable. Raise your left arm. Hold for 10 seconds. Repeat with your other leg.

Calf Stretch

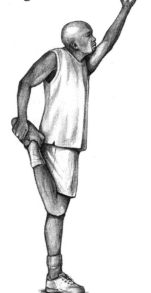

Thigh Stretch

Arm Circles Hold both of your arms out straight. Draw a one-foot circle in the air with both arms at once. Repeat five times in each direction.

Side Stretch Stand with your feet about a foot apart. Raise one arm, with the fingers pointing inward. Bend in the direction of your raised fingers. (If you can't bend at all, just hold the arm-up position for a few seconds.) You should be able to feel a stretching in your side. Repeat with your other arm raised. Stretch each side three times.

Neck Stretch Clasp your hands behind your head and slowly turn, looking over your left shoulder. Bring your head down and to the front and look to the floor as you slowly turn to the opposite shoulder. Repeat the exercise three times.

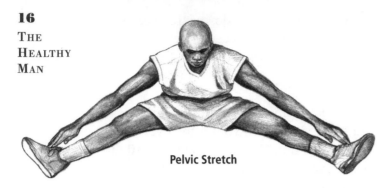

Pelvic Stretch

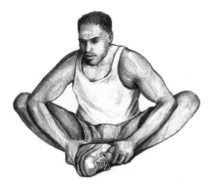

Inner-Thigh Stretch

Pelvic Stretch   This exercise will stretch your thigh muscles. Sit on the floor with your legs apart as far as they will comfortably go. Bend over and reach forward with your arms on the floor as far as you can go. Hold for 30 seconds.

Inner-Thigh Stretch   To stretch your inner-thigh muscles, sit on the floor, bring your feet together, and pull them toward your body. Push your knees down with your elbows. Keep your head up and your back straight. Stretch only as far as you can while remaining comfortable. Hold for 30 seconds.

After your exercise period, don't just stop cold and rest. As you exercise, lactic acid builds up in your muscles, causing soreness, fatigue, and possibly cramping. To reduce the amount of lactic acid in your muscles, you need to cool down by continuing to exercise at a lower intensity for 5 to 10 minutes and then do some stretching exercises. Cooling down will make you feel better as well as reduce muscle soreness.

Knowing When to Stop Exercising

Exercise- and sports-related injuries usually arise from overuse of a muscle, tendon, ligament, or joint (see page 63). If you have a condition, such as arthritis, that can be aggravated by exercise, talk to your doctor before you begin any exercise program. If you experience any pain, or if you injure yourself, stop exercising immediately. Never ignore an injury or attempt to "work through" the pain; you may make your injury worse. Instead, stop exercising for a few days and follow the RICE routine (see page 65). If you think the injury may be serious, or if you still experience pain after a few days of the RICE routine, talk to your doctor. You should also stop exercising immediately if you have any symptoms of a heart attack (see page 66).

Some athletes exercise too much, especially if they are training for an upcoming event such as a marathon. Overtraining is self-defeating. It causes physical exhaustion and adversely affects your athletic performance. If you think you may be overtraining, you need to recognize when to stop exercising and rest, before you reach exhaustion. You should always exercise at your own pace, keeping in mind your own fitness level. Don't try to work out for an hour or more every day just because a friend does. Your body will quickly tell you when it's had enough. Signs of overtraining include:

- loss of coordination
- a prolonged period of recovery after exercise
- elevated morning heart rate
- headaches
- appetite loss
- muscle soreness
- digestive system problems
- lowered ability to fight infection
- irritability and depression
- poor concentration

If you have any of these symptoms, stop exercising for a day or more to give your body time to rest. Decrease your activity level in both duration and frequency. If exercise becomes a compulsive act for you, talk to your doctor. Exercising beyond the point of exhaustion, when injured, or to the exclusion of other activities and life interests can be signs of exercise addiction. Excessive exercising produces results that are completely the opposite of those you intend to achieve. Moderation is the key to success when it comes to exercise and fitness.

A HEALTHY WEIGHT

Carrying excess weight is a known health risk. Excess weight increases the heart's workload and can raise your chances of getting a number of serious medical conditions such as heart disease, high blood pressure, adult-onset diabetes, and certain forms of cancer. It also can adversely affect your self-image and make it difficult to exercise. But how can you find out what is your ideal weight?

A healthy weight is actually a range of weight related to your height, but the number of pounds you register on your bathroom scale doesn't tell the whole story. Your body composition—the percentage of your body that is made up of lean tissue, composed mainly of muscle and bone, or fat—also is important. Your body composition is partly determined by your genetic makeup and partly by your activity level. The more fat you have in relation to lean tissue, the less healthy you are, but it is somewhat difficult to measure how much of your weight is made up of fat. The best way to judge the percentage of body fat that you carry may be by looking at how active you are. The more physically active you are, the less body fat you are likely to carry. One easy way to assess your weight and whether it puts you at risk for health problems is to consult a table that gives you your body mass index (BMI) (see page 18).

If your weight falls outside the upper end of the range for your height, you may be moderately or severely overweight. Obesity (weighing more than 20 percent over the upper ideal weight range for your height) contributes to the development of diabetes, heart disease, and gallbladder disease. Obesity also complicates the treatment of and lowers the chances of survival of people with stroke, kidney disease, and numerous other disorders. Although the idea that obesity results from a lack of willpower is outdated, doctors are still unsure exactly why some people are overweight while others are not. Losing weight and keeping it off for life can be extremely difficult, but you can control your weight if your motivation stays high.

Where on your body you carry excess weight also is important. Most men store excess fat weight around their waists and abdomens, putting them at higher risk for early heart disease, high blood pressure, and diabetes than people (mainly women) who carry excess weight predominantly in the hips, buttocks, and thighs. You can determine your waist-to-hip ratio by first measuring your waist at its narrowest point and then measuring your hips at their widest point. Divide your waist measurement by your hip measurement. If the number is 1.0, or close to it, you are a typical "apple-shaped" man. If the number is a lot less than 1.0, you are "pear-shaped" and have less risk of future health problems. Where your body stores fat is largely an inherited tendency, although strenuous exercise has been shown to reduce body fat in general and fat stored at the abdomen in particular.

Doctors no longer believe that, as you age, it's acceptable to gain up to 10 pounds over your normal weight when you were younger. Any additional weight over the accepted range for your height is now known to be a health risk, and the more you gain, the bigger your risk. So maintain your weight within the range that is normal for you and you'll be better off in the long run (see weight chart on page 69).

The Body Mass Index

The body mass index (BMI) is a helpful tool for gauging whether your body weight falls in the healthful range or puts you at risk for future health problems. You can figure out your own BMI using the following formula:

1. Convert your weight to kilograms (1 kilogram = 2.2 pounds). For example, if you weigh 198 pounds, divide 198 by 2.2 to get 90 kilograms.
2. Convert your height to meters (1 meter = 39.37 inches). If you are 6 feet tall (72 inches), divide 72 inches by 39.37 to get 1.83 meters.
3. Divide your weight by your height squared to calculate your BMI. Divide 90 kilograms by 1.83 squared ($1.83 \times 1.83 = 3.35$; $90 \div 3.35 = 26.9$) to get a BMI of 27.

Then consult the following chart to see your risk for health problems.

BMI	Weight-Related Health Status
Less than 18.5	Underweight
18.5–24.9	Healthy weight
25–29.9	Overweight
30 or more	Obese

With a BMI of 27, you are overweight. Talk to your doctor about starting a diet and exercise program to help you lose the excess weight.

It's even simpler to consult the following table to find out your BMI. Find your height in the left-hand column and move across the row to your weight. The number at the top of the column is your BMI.

Body Mass Index Table

BMI

Height (inches)	19	20	21	22	23	24	25	26	27	28	29	30	31	32	33	34	35
							Body Weight (pounds)										
58	91	96	100	105	110	115	119	124	129	134	138	143	148	153	158	162	167
59	94	99	104	109	114	119	124	128	133	138	143	148	153	158	163	168	173
60	97	102	107	112	118	123	128	133	138	143	148	153	158	163	168	174	179
61	100	106	111	116	122	127	132	137	143	148	153	158	164	169	174	180	185
62	104	109	115	120	126	131	136	142	147	153	158	164	169	175	180	186	191
63	107	113	118	124	130	135	141	146	152	158	163	169	175	180	186	191	197
64	110	116	122	128	134	140	145	151	157	163	169	174	180	186	192	197	204
65	114	120	126	132	138	144	150	156	162	168	174	180	186	192	198	204	210
66	118	124	130	136	142	148	155	161	167	173	179	186	192	198	204	210	216
67	121	127	134	140	146	153	159	166	172	178	185	191	198	204	211	217	223
68	125	131	138	144	151	158	164	171	177	184	190	197	203	210	216	223	230
69	128	135	142	149	155	162	169	176	182	189	196	203	209	216	223	230	236
70	132	139	146	153	160	167	174	181	188	195	202	209	216	222	229	236	243
71	136	143	150	157	165	172	179	186	193	200	208	215	222	229	236	243	250
72	140	147	154	162	169	177	184	191	199	206	213	221	228	235	242	250	258
73	144	151	159	166	174	182	189	197	204	212	219	227	235	242	250	257	265
74	148	155	163	171	179	186	194	202	210	218	225	233	241	249	256	264	272
75	152	160	168	176	184	192	200	208	216	224	232	240	248	256	264	272	279
76	156	164	172	180	189	197	205	213	221	230	238	246	254	263	271	279	287

Tips for Dieting

If you have a weight problem, you can find many programs to help you lose extra pounds, but the only proven method to lose weight and keep it off is to eat less and become more active. A calorie- and fat-restricted diet that follows the Food Guide Pyramid (see page 5) recommendations, combined with a regular exercise program, will help you reach your target weight range safely. You should realistically aim to shed only 1 to 2½ pounds per week by consuming about 500 calories less per day than usual. During your weight-loss regimen, periods may occur during which you may not lose any weight at all, but don't get discouraged. This is normal. The pounds will start to come off again in a week or two.

Avoid crash or fad diets because they may not provide all the nutrients you need, and extreme diets can be harmful to your health. Even worse, such diets often do not work over the long term. Here are some suggestions that can help you lose weight successfully:

- Don't skip meals, including breakfast, because you will be tempted to eat more later in the day.
- Keep a diary of your food intake before and after you begin your diet, so you can compare the difference and make sure you are getting enough nutrients.
- Start an exercise log so that, as you build stamina and endurance, you can see your progress and stay motivated.
- Don't consume fewer than 1,400 calories a day, to make sure you get all the nutrients you need.
- Cut back on fat by buying low-fat substitutes for mayonnaise and other higher-fat foods. Trim fat from meat. Drink 1 percent or fat-free milk.
- Reduce your intake of sugar by having fresh fruit or yogurt for dessert.
- Experiment with herbs and spices to add flavor to food and to make up for less sugar, salt, and fat.
- Ask your family to support your diet and exercise program by encouraging you or participating with you.

How Exercise Helps You Lose Weight

Reducing your intake of food is only half of the weight-loss equation. The other half is becoming more physically active. To lose 1 pound, you have to burn 3,500 calories. Exercise burns calories quickly, helping you shed those excess pounds even faster. Physical exercise builds muscle and lean body mass (see The Body Mass Index, page 18). Having more muscle gives you a higher metabolism (the process in your cells that produces energy), so you naturally burn more calories, even when you are at rest. Your metabolism stays especially high for several hours after you exercise, meaning that your body burns additional calories after you are physically active. Regular exercise also can suppress your appetite, so you don't feel like eating as much as usual. The following table lists various types of sustained physical activity. Each of these activities, which vary in time and level of intensity, can help you burn an additional 100 to 200 calories per day.

Comparing Types of Physical Activity

Washing and waxing car for 45 to 60 minutes   Less vigorous, more time

Washing windows or floors for 45 to 60 minutes

Playing volleyball for 45 minutes

Playing touch football for 30 to 45 minutes

Gardening for 30 to 45 minutes

Wheeling self in wheelchair for 30 to 40 minutes

Walking 1¾ miles for 35 minutes
  (20 minutes per mile)

Shooting baskets for 30 minutes

Bicycling 5 miles in 30 minutes

Dancing fast for 30 minutes

Pushing a stroller 1½ miles in 30 minutes

Raking leaves for 30 minutes

Walking 2 miles in 30 minutes (15 minutes per mile)

Doing water aerobics for 30 minutes

Swimming laps for 20 minutes

Playing wheelchair basketball for 20 minutes

Playing a game of basketball for 15 to 20 minutes

Bicycling 4 miles in 15 minutes

Jumping rope for 15 minutes

Running 1½ miles in 15 minutes
  (10 minutes per mile)

Stair climbing for 15 minutes   More vigorous, less time

Choose an activity you enjoy or one you regularly perform. Start slowly, and gradually increase the intensity of your workout. You may want to begin by walking for 30 minutes 3 days per week. Then gradually work your way up to 45 minutes of walking 5 days per week. Your goal should be to exercise for at least 30 minutes or more most (if not all) days of the week. You can do your exercise all at one time or in shorter segments throughout the day. Eventually, as you become more physically fit, you may be able to participate in more vigorous activities for longer periods of time. But don't expect miracles to happen right away. Focus on the realistic goal of losing 1 to 2½ pounds per week. Remember that you are not just trying to lose weight, you also want to keep it off. After you have reached your weight-loss target, continue to exercise regularly to keep the pounds off.

THE DANGERS OF ALCOHOL AND OTHER DRUGS

Drinking alcoholic beverages is an accepted social activity. Consumed in moderate amounts, alcohol relaxes you, stimulates your appetite, and produces mild euphoria. It also loosens inhibitions, making you feel more friendly and outgoing. While moderate drinking is not detrimental to your health, excessive drinking (defined as four drinks or more per day) or binge drinking (defined as four drinks at one sitting) can eventually lead to alcoholism and other serious health problems. There is evidence that some people have an inherited predisposition toward alcoholism. The disorders produced by alcoholism are very costly in terms of human suffering and economic hardship.

According to scientific research, the incidence of heart disease in men who consume a moderate amount of alcohol (two drinks a day or less) is lower than in men who do not drink. But there is not much difference between moderate drinking and heavy drinking. A typical drink is 5 ounces of wine, 1½ ounces of 80-proof distilled spirits, 12 ounces of wine cooler, or 12 ounces of beer (see page 24). Although moderate drinking may reduce your risk of heart disease, doctors do not recommend drinking alcohol because it carries many health risks, including cancer of the liver, mouth, throat, and esophagus. Excessive alcohol consumption also increases your chances of having an accident, makes you more prone to violence, and makes you more apt to engage in risky behaviors such as illicit drug use or unsafe sex (see page 111). Nutritional deficiencies and even malnutrition also can result from overconsumption of alcohol.

Alcohol affects every organ in your body, even in moderate amounts, but overconsumption takes its most serious toll on the liver, heart, and brain. When you drink alcohol, some of the alcohol is absorbed in your stomach, but most enters the small intestine, where it passes into the bloodstream, which carries it throughout your body. As alcohol enters your brain, it numbs nerve cells, slowing down their ability to send messages to your body. If you continue to drink, the nerve centers in the brain may lose control over speech, vision, balance, and judgment, and you may have a blackout.

Alcohol depresses the activity of your heart muscle; the heart compensates by quickening your pulse. Enzymes in the liver break down alcohol, but the alcohol interferes with the natural breakdown of fats in the liver. When you drink excessively, fats accumulate in the liver, resulting in a condition known as fatty liver, the first step—and the only reversible one—in the continuum of alcoholic liver disease. The next phase, early fibrosis, happens when fibrous scar tissue appears around the central veins in the liver and impairs liver function. Continued heavy drinking rapidly produces the final two stages of liver disease: alcoholic hepatitis and cirrhosis. Alcoholic hepatitis produces jaundice (a yellowing of the skin and eyes), appetite and weight loss, fever, an enlarged and inflamed liver, and accumulation of fluid in the abdomen. Permanent abstinence from alcohol is the only cure for alcoholic hepatitis.

The hallmark feature of cirrhosis of the liver is the presence of scar tissue that destroys the normal structure of the liver. The liver can no longer remove toxins from the blood, and the toxins accumulate in the bloodstream. Cirrhosis usually leads to liver failure or liver cancer.

Other long-term effects of excessive drinking include inflammation of the pancreas, bleeding in the stomach and intestinal tract, obstruction of blood flow to the liver, varicose veins in the esophagus (the muscular passage that leads from the mouth to the stomach), and heart failure.

Alcohol is not the only drug that is easy to abuse. Men use a number of other recreational drugs—marijuana, cocaine, amphetamines, inhalants, hallucinogens, tranquilizers, designer drugs such as ecstasy, and heroin and other opiates. All carry certain risks, some deadly. Marijuana has received much publicity for its alleged medical uses, but that fact does not mean that marijuana is risk-free. Marijuana affects short-term memory, impairs the ability to concentrate, inhibits alertness and reaction time (making driving dangerous), and reduces athletic performance. Prolonged use can irritate the upper respiratory system, making you more susceptible to respiratory infections. Marijuana smoke also contains some of the same cancer-causing chemicals found in cigarettes.

Cocaine is a dangerous stimulant that boosts the heart rate while constricting the blood vessels, increasing your chances of having a heart attack, stroke, seizure, or an abnormal heart rhythm. While usually inhaled as a powder, cocaine is sometimes injected. In another form known as crack, cocaine can be smoked. Another class of stimulants, amphetamines (also known as speed or uppers), are prescription drugs taken in pill form that may boost energy and alertness, but also produce rapid heartbeat and can raise the blood pressure so dangerously high that a stroke can occur. Habitual use of amphetamines can cause addiction. In general, stimulants can cause agitation, dilation of the pupils of the eye, visual and auditory hallucinations, seizures, and depression of the respiratory system.

Young boys may be tempted to inhale the fumes of glue, typewriter correction fluid, nail polish remover, or household cleaning products because of the availability of an easy "high." Sniffing such highly toxic fumes produces euphoria but also can damage the nerves that control breathing and can cause the heart to stop suddenly, leading to coma or death, even in first-time users.

Hallucinogens such as lysergic acid diethylamide (LSD) and mescaline create dreamlike visual hallucinations and unexplained bizarre behavior that may mimic psychosis. These drugs can foster psychological dependence. Hallucinogenic plants such as peyote have similar effects.

The most common opiates, including heroin, morphine, and codeine, are highly addictive compounds taken to acquire a feeling of profound well-being. Undesirable effects include depression of the respiratory system and swelling of the brain. When injected, these drugs increase the risk for blood clots, inflamed veins, and transmission of blood-borne infections, such as hepatitis (see page 191) and the human immunodeficiency virus (HIV). Overdoses of these drugs may lead to seizures, coma, and death from the sudden stopping of

How Much Alcohol Is in One Drink?

The type of alcohol that is found in most alcoholic drinks is ethyl alcohol, also known as ethanol or grain alcohol. The amount of alcohol in a given drink can vary considerably. Hard liquors such as whiskey, gin, vodka, and brandy are made up of about 40 to 50 percent pure alcohol (80 to 100 proof). Beer has about a 4 percent alcohol content and wine 14 percent, but beer and wine are typically served in larger portions than are distilled spirits. So, **although the proportion of alcohol varies, the actual alcohol intake is about the same.** Having some food in your stomach will delay the absorption of alcohol into your bloodstream. Also, watery drinks such as beer will be absorbed more slowly than drinks, such as hard liquor, in which the alcohol is more concentrated.

- Hard liquor: 40–50 percent
- Wine: 12–14 percent
- Wine cooler: 3–5 percent
- Beer: 3.5–9 percent

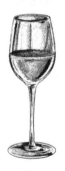 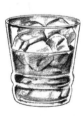 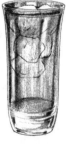 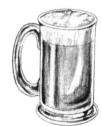

Wine	Hard Liquor	Wine Cooler	Beer
5 ounces	1½ ounces	12 ounces	12 ounces

Different Drinks: Same Amount of Alcohol
Ounce for ounce the alcohol content varies widely from one alcoholic beverage to another. A 5-ounce glass of wine contains about the same amount of alcohol as a mixed drink with 1½ ounces of 80-proof liquor or a 12-ounce wine cooler or glass of beer.

the heart or the inhalation of vomit, which can cause suffocation. Withdrawal from these substances produces serious effects such as anxiety, severe diarrhea, vomiting, cramps, and seizures.

It is also possible to become addicted to prescription drugs that you may have received for a medical purpose. Drugs that may become habit-forming include narcotic painkillers prescribed for conditions such as chronic back pain or taken after surgery, or sedatives or tranquilizers prescribed for chronic insomnia or anxiety. Ask your doctor about the potential for addiction when he or she prescribes any medication. Always take medication according to your doctor's instructions and only for the period of time specified on the prescription.

Any type of drug, including alcohol, has the potential to alter your judgment and perception and increase your chances of having a motor vehicle collision or other type of accident. Alcohol and other drug use also is linked with higher incidences of homicide and suicide in men. Moderation is the key when it comes to the use of alcohol (see previous page). Experimentation with other recreational drugs is a risky behavior that can increase your chances of continued substance abuse, accidental injury, and death.

The Warning Signs of Substance Abuse

The spectrum of behaviors that gradually lead to alcohol or drug abuse and addiction begins with experimentation, usually in adolescence. Experimentation progresses to casual use, which can easily become regular use, heavy use, abuse, and finally dependence. Once a person becomes addicted to alcohol or drugs, he often conceals his use, abandoning family and friends in favor of the social group that abuses the substance. The only way out of the cycle of drug dependence is abstinence, fortified by a formal substance abuse treatment program. Relapse is not uncommon following treatment. The warning signs of substance abuse vary, depending on the substance being used. In general, however, certain behaviors such as the following may indicate a problem with alcohol or another drug. Call your doctor, an employee assistance program, or a substance abuse hot line if you or anyone you know displays any of the following warning signs:

- absenteeism or a decline in quality of work at job or school
- uncharacteristic outbreaks of temper
- avoidance of responsibility
- deterioration of appearance and grooming
- wearing sunglasses indoors or at night, or a glazed appearance to the eyes
- wearing only long-sleeved shirts, even in hot weather
- repeatedly borrowing money
- stealing from home or employer
- secretive behavior, including frequent, unexplained trips to the rest room or basement
- acquaintance with known drug abusers

How to Treat a Hangover

A hangover manifests itself as a combination of symptoms, including headache, dry mouth, and mild dizziness. It is still unclear exactly why overindulging in alcohol produces a hangover, but several factors come into play. Alcohol causes your body to lose water by stimulating your kidneys to excrete more water than you drink, resulting in dehydration. The more alcohol you drink, the more water passes out of your body. Alcohol also widens blood vessels, and the widening of vessels around the brain may cause pain, much as it does in a migraine headache.

Once you have a hangover, there isn't very much you can do to make yourself feel better. You just may have to let it run its course. Be sure to drink plenty of liquids, such as water, fruit juice, or bland soda. Avoid drinking coffee because the caffeine it contains will make you even more dehydrated. Never fight a hangover by having another alcoholic drink in the morning because your body will take even longer to eliminate the alcohol circulating in your bloodstream. Use an over-the-counter pain medication such as aspirin, acetaminophen, or ibuprofen if you have a headache, but remember that these painkillers can irritate your stomach, and excessive doses of acetaminophen may be toxic to your liver when combined with alcohol (see warning box below).

The best way to handle a hangover is to avoid getting one by not drinking too much in the first place. Always have a couple of glasses of water with your drinks, and drink more water before going to bed to avoid becoming dehydrated.

The Effects of Alcohol on Your Sexual Performance

Social drinking lowers your inhibitions and may make you feel more ready to have sex, but too much alcohol can actually impair your sexual function. Alcohol is neither an aphrodisiac nor a stimulant. It is a central nervous system depressant that slows down your responses, making it harder to get an erection or to ejaculate. Drinking alcohol also can impair your judgment, making you less likely to practice safer sex (see page 181).

But the sexual problems that can arise after having a few drinks are mild compared with the effects of chronic alcoholism on your body. Alcoholism can obstruct the blood supply to the nerves in the penis, resulting in erectile dysfunction (see page 146). The liver damage caused by alcohol can increase the levels of the female hormone estrogen and lower the levels of the male hormone testosterone in your body, leading to breast enlargement, shrunken testicles, and a reduced sperm count.

Warning! Acetaminophen and Alcohol Can Cause Liver Damage

Taking doses of a painkiller containing acetaminophen that are in excess of those recommended on the package can cause serious liver damage if you regularly consume more than two alcoholic drinks per day. Never take more than six doses of regular-strength acetaminophen in 24 hours if you consume moderate amounts of alcohol regularly.

If you have a problem getting or maintaining an erection and you think it may be related to excessive alcohol consumption, cut back on your drinking for a few weeks to see if your ability to have an erection improves. You need to get help for your drinking problem. Ask your doctor what kind of alcohol-treatment programs are in your community, or call the local chapter of Alcoholics Anonymous.

THE HAZARDS OF TOBACCO

Tobacco use is by far the top avoidable cause of disease, disability, and death in the United States, responsible for nearly one in five deaths. Currently about 50 million adults in this country, mostly men, smoke cigarettes. Although smoking is generally declining, the number of adolescents and young adults who are beginning to smoke is on the rise. Cigarette smoke contains more than 4,000 different chemicals; about 200 of them are poisonous, and more than 40 are cancer-causing. Smoking is so dangerous that approximately 400,000 deaths are attributed to smoking-related causes in the United States each year. The health problems caused by smoking are the number one cause of death in men in this country.

If you smoke, you will notice the gradual onset of a host of long-term problems. Your senses of smell and taste will weaken, you will get more frequent colds than before, facial wrinkling will intensify, and you will develop a nagging "smoker's cough," which is actually a symptom of a serious disease called chronic bronchitis (see page 246). You also increase your chances of developing cancers of the lung and other organs, emphysema, high blood pressure, stroke, and heart disease. You also place your family at risk of the same health problems by exposing them to secondhand smoke (see page 31).

Most men first experiment with smoking in adolescence because it makes them feel more adult and rebellious. The earlier someone starts smoking, the less likely he is to quit. Experimentation quickly turns into tolerance of and then addiction to nicotine, the habit-forming drug in tobacco that keeps smokers hooked. Nicotine creates a persistent craving for more tobacco, and the amount and frequency of use usually increases, so that a smoker may feel the need to smoke two packs a day to get the same satisfaction that one daily pack once provided. Not smoking for as few as several hours produces uncomfortable nicotine withdrawal symptoms, including irritability, limited concentration, and intense cravings. These symptoms compel the person to smoke even when he knows the adverse health risks. Many social activities, such as having drinks in a bar with friends, also are conducive to smoking, making it a difficult habit to break.

Tobacco advertising has a major role in encouraging adolescents to take up smoking before they are mature enough to understand the long-term health risks.

Young people serve as the largest pool of new customers for the tobacco industry; they replace adult smokers who have quit or died. Tobacco advertising is no longer allowed on television, but the tobacco industry still spends about $5 billion each year on advertising in magazines, on billboards, and at music and sporting events to lure new smokers with the promise of sex appeal, glamour, or rugged adventure. The following pages will describe how smoking damages your body, outline the hazardous effects of secondhand smoke, and explain the risks of cigar smoking and smokeless tobacco use.

Smoking's Damaging Effects on Your Body

In addition to the addictive drug nicotine, the other principal harmful substances in cigarettes are tar and carbon monoxide. Tar is a sticky, brown residue that collects in the lungs. Primarily made up of chemicals known as hydrocarbons, tar is a powerful cancer-causing agent that has been linked to the development of lung cancer. Carbon monoxide is a poison that partially replaces the oxygen normally carried throughout the body by red blood cells, robbing the body of sufficient oxygen. Switching to a low-tar cigarette usually does not help because the person usually compensates for the change by inhaling longer or by smoking more cigarettes.

Other toxic chemicals in tobacco smoke include arsenic, formaldehyde, ammonia, lead, benzene, and vinyl chloride. The airways try to fight these poisons by producing excess mucus, which obstructs the airways, producing the telltale smoker's cough that indicates the development of chronic bronchitis.

Tobacco smoke damages not only the cells inside the lungs but also the tiny hairlike projections called cilia that line and protect the airways, hindering the respiratory system's ability to fight infection. Smoke inflames lung tissue, causing the airways to release chemicals that destroy the tiny air sacs in the lungs called alveoli, where oxygen is transferred into the bloodstream. The alveoli merge into fewer but larger air sacs, reducing the surface area in the lungs available for oxygen transfer. Because the level of oxygen in the blood is reduced, the affected person becomes breathless. This process describes the development of the disease known as emphysema (see page 247).

Cigarette smoking causes cancer of the lung, mouth, tongue, throat, pancreas, kidney, and bladder by producing cell changes that cause the cells to reproduce uncontrollably. Smoking is responsible for about 87 percent of all cases of lung cancer in the United States. Most lung cancers begin in a bronchus, one of the two main air passages that enter the lungs.

Smoking also is a major contributor to the development of heart disease (see page 204), by reducing blood levels of high-density lipoprotein (HDL), the "good" cholesterol that protects against heart disease. Additionally, smoking adversely affects the arteries that supply the heart with blood and nutrients. Men who smoke have twice the risk of having a heart attack as do nonsmoking men. Nonsmokers exposed to secondhand smoke also endure an increased risk of heart disease. Up to 30 percent of all deaths from heart disease in the nation can be attributed to cigarette smoking, and the risk increases with the number of cigarettes smoked and the number of years of smoking. Smoking cigarettes also doubles your risk of having a stroke.

In spite of the dire health prospects facing smokers, many of them continue their habit because of nicotine's addictive properties. But if you smoke, effective methods exist to help you quit and avoid starting again.

How to Quit Smoking

The most important thing you should know about quitting smoking is that the harmful effects of the habit begin to reverse almost as soon as you stop. Within 20 minutes of your last cigarette, your heart rate and blood pressure drop to normal. After 8 hours of being smoke-free, your blood levels of carbon monoxide and oxygen return to normal. Your risk of having a heart attack decreases after only 24 hours, and in 2 weeks your circulation will improve and your lung function will increase up to 30 percent. These beneficial effects continue until, after 10 years of not smoking, your chances of dying of lung cancer become about the same as for a nonsmoker.

There is no underestimating the difficulty of breaking the smoking habit because of the highly addictive properties of nicotine. You need to build a strong support system within your family and circle of friends and coworkers. You may find that some of the people you know who still smoke may feel uncomfortable or threatened by your efforts to quit. It may be best for you to stay away from them until you feel certain that you can avoid the temptation to smoke. Pick a nonsmoker or another person who is trying to quit as a "buddy" whom you can call when the going gets rough. Meet with your buddy once a week, communicate through e-mail, or talk regularly on the phone. Make a bet with him or her that you can go for 1 month, then 6 months without a cigarette, then celebrate when you have reached your goal.

Experts say that you should prepare yourself to quit in advance of smoking your last cigarette. Identify several strategies, such as relaxation exercises, that can help you cope with your cravings for tobacco. First try to establish one or two other new habits, such as regular exercise, so you will be giving up tobacco in the context of a complete lifestyle change. Exercise is important; it is the highest predictor of success when quitting tobacco use. When you are ready to quit, take the following steps to ensure success:

Step 1 Take a look at your smoking habits. Make a chart and mark down on it every cigarette you smoke in 24 hours, including the first cigarette you smoke in the morning, the one you automatically light up with a cup of coffee or a drink, and the ones you smoke while on break. Keep monitoring your cigarette use for 3 weeks.

Step 2   Write down all of the reasons why you want to stop smoking—for example, to get rid of your smoker's cough and to stop exposing your family to secondhand smoke.

Step 3   Set a date by which you intend to quit smoking. Announce the date to all of the people you know and ask them to help you in your effort so they can support you if you lose your resolve.

Step 4   Ask your doctor about using nicotine gum, a nicotine patch, a prescription nicotine inhaler, or prescription medication (see warning box, page 31) to help you quit smoking. Try sucking on hard candy or chewing gum, munching on raw vegetables, or exercising more. Stay away from places and situations, such as having drinks with friends in a bar, that you associate with smoking. Sit in the nonsmoking section of restaurants. You may want to join a stop-smoking group; ask your doctor to recommend one.

Step 5   When you quit smoking, you probably will feel like eating more often and may gain a few pounds. Don't stop yourself from eating when you feel tense during the first few weeks; it will be hard enough to stay away from cigarettes. Stock up on fresh fruits and vegetables, sugar-free candy and soda, and fat-free pretzels or crackers. Drink plenty of water. Your most intense cravings for nicotine will subside after about 8 weeks, when you can resume your usual eating pattern.

When you quit smoking, you remove an important source of pleasure and a way to reduce stress from your daily routine. You need to replace the nicotine with something else that gives you pleasure and deal with your stress in more positive ways (see page 118). Maintaining your focus on negative reasons for quitting, such as worrying about your health, will not help you succeed. Forget the "no pain, no gain" attitude. Instead, embrace your new, more healthy lifestyle positively, without guilt for your past smoking habit. Praise yourself liberally by telling yourself how much better your life is going to be from now on. And remember the following positive things about quitting each time you feel the urge to take a puff:

- Stopping smoking will free up time that you can now use to exercise, take up a hobby, or spend time with your family.
- You can use the money you used to spend on cigarettes to treat yourself or a loved one to something special.
- Your breath will smell better, your fingers will no longer be yellow, and your clothes and hair will no longer smell like smoke.
- Food will taste better because your sense of smell will improve, and the senses of smell and taste are closely linked.

- Your smoker's cough will go away in a few months, a sign that your body is healing itself.
- Being a nonsmoker makes you more attractive.
- You will no longer have to stand awkwardly outside of your workplace in the rain and the cold to smoke on breaks or at lunchtime.

Warning! Potential Health Risks of Misusing Stop-Smoking Aids

Several products containing nicotine are available today to help you stop smoking, including nicotine gum, the nicotine patch, and the nicotine inhaler. Both the patch and the gum are available over-the-counter, while the inhaler requires a doctor's prescription. All three methods put nicotine into your system to help you curb your craving for tobacco and, when used according to directions, can help you kick your nicotine habit. However, if you exceed recommended dosages, continue to smoke while using these methods, or use more than one method at a time, you can overdose on nicotine. Too much nicotine in your bloodstream can overstimulate your heart and pose life-threatening risks to your health—high blood pressure, heart attack, and stroke. If you are considering using a stop-smoking aid that contains nicotine, talk to your doctor so you can learn more about these products and how to properly use them and make an informed decision. If you are already using one of these treatments, carefully follow the directions and note the warnings on the packaging.

The Health Risks of Secondhand Smoke

Secondhand smoke is the smoke given off by a burning cigarette, cigar, or pipe mixed with the smoke exhaled by the person smoking. This smoke contains the same 200 poisonous and 40 cancer-causing chemicals contained in cigarettes. Because secondhand smoke is distributed throughout the air inhaled by everyone—smokers and nonsmokers alike—present in an enclosed space, exposure to it is called passive or involuntary smoking. The US Environmental Protection Agency (EPA) has classified secondhand smoke as a group A carcinogen (cancer-causing agent) and estimates that it causes 3,000 lung cancer deaths in nonsmokers every year.

Secondhand smoke is an especially dangerous health threat to children. A child's developing lungs are highly susceptible to irritants, producing a cough, wheezing, and excess mucus. Children exposed to secondhand smoke have an increased risk for pneumonia; bronchitis; accumulation of fluid in the ear; and irritation of the eyes, nose, and throat. Children who have asthma (see page 245) and are exposed to secondhand smoke experience more severe symptoms and have asthma attacks more often than those who live in a smoke-free home. Passive smoking is thought to cause the development of asthma in thousands of children each year.

If you smoke, don't smoke in your home, in your car with the windows closed, or around children. If the weather is too bad to smoke outside, smoke in a room with the windows open enough to provide cross-ventilation. If you are a non-smoker, don't allow anyone to smoke in your house or car, especially around children. Find out about your employer's smoking policy so you can protect yourself from secondhand smoke at work. In a restaurant, ask to sit in the non-smoking section, as far away from the smoking area as possible. If your community does not have a smoking control ordinance, become active and urge your local government officials to enact one.

Cigars Pose Health Risks, Too

Cigar sales have soared in recent years as cigar smoking has become more socially acceptable. A blitz of cigar advertising in magazines and prominent cigar placement in movies and music videos has made cigar smoking fashionable, even glamorous. Men who smoke cigars may believe that they are less harmful to their health than cigarettes, but this idea is false. Cigar smoking has been linked to the development of cancer of the mouth, larynx (voice box), esophagus (the muscular passage that connects the mouth and the stomach), and lungs. Men who smoke cigars regularly, especially those who smoke several cigars a day, raise their risk of heart disease and lung diseases such as chronic bronchitis (see page 246) and emphysema (see page 247). Drinking three or more alcoholic drinks a day combined with cigar smoking seems to raise the risk of cancers of the mouth, larynx, and throat exponentially. The harmful effects of secondhand smoke (see page 31) from a cigarette also apply to smoke given off by cigars.

While very occasional cigar smoking—for example, one cigar per month—may pose only a minimal health risk, a growing number of men smoke cigars on a far more regular basis, some even daily. Cigars are not an acceptable alternative to cigarettes when it comes to your health or the health of nonsmokers exposed to secondhand smoke from your cigar. It is best for your health to abstain from cigar smoking altogether.

How Smokeless Tobacco Damages Your Body

The use of smokeless tobacco, including snuff and chewing tobacco, increases each year, mainly among adolescent boys. Snuff consists of moist, shredded tobacco leaves that come in packages resembling tea bags. The user places the snuff between his lip and gum. Chewing tobacco is made of shredded or compressed tobacco and is placed inside the cheek and chewed. The average quantity of chewing tobacco contains the nicotine found in two cigarettes, but the nicotine in chewing tobacco is more addictive because it is more easily absorbed into the bloodstream.

Although made fashionable by professional baseball players, smokeless tobacco is not a harmless alternative to cigarettes. It wears away tooth enamel, causes the gums to recede and the teeth to loosen, and contributes to tooth decay and discoloration as well as bad breath. Most important, smokeless tobacco use has been linked to development of cancer of the mouth, throat, larynx, and esophagus. When the irritating tobacco is left in contact with the cheeks, gums, or lips for long periods, it produces sores or white patches that do not heal and can eventually become cancerous. Other early signs of oral cancer from smokeless tobacco include a prolonged sore throat and difficulty chewing or swallowing. Cancerous changes can occur after only 4 years of smokeless tobacco use. Disfiguring oral surgery may have to be performed to remove cancerous tissue.

Men who use smokeless tobacco need regular dental cleanings and checkups to look for the early signs of oral cancer, but the best approach is to stop using smokeless tobacco products. Pick a date to quit, cut back on your use before then, and stay tobacco-free for life.

SAFETY AND YOUR HEALTH

You may not often think about the effect safety has on your health, but accidental injury, motor vehicle collisions, fires, violent crime, and firearms constitute major causes of death and disability in the United States. Working in your home and community to prevent accidental and violent injury is an important but often neglected responsibility. Safety issues arise in countless places, from the dead battery in the smoke detector to the seat belt left unbuckled in the car. Drinking alcohol greatly increases your risk of injury. For example, men have a much higher risk of accidental drowning than do women, and alcohol is implicated in about 40 percent of such incidents. Drinking alcohol also heightens the risk of accidents from motor vehicle collisions, including those involving motorcycles, all-terrain vehicles, and bicycles.

You can do a lot to make your home safer. Many home safety hazards are easy to overlook but also easy to fix (see page 36). Check all areas of your home to make sure that electrical and telephone cords are unfrayed, rugs and mats have nonslip backings, smoke and carbon monoxide detectors are in working order, and space heaters and wood-burning stoves are properly installed and functioning. Have an emergency exit plan and practice it with all members of your family. Keep hallways and stairways free of clutter. Place a fire extinguisher in the kitchen. Make sure that your power tools and any flammable liquids or poisonous chemicals are properly labeled and stored in your basement, garage, and workshop.

Home security measures can go a long way toward making your home even safer. Install secure, deadbolt locks on all doors and windows and make sure your entry doors are constructed of solid materials. Outdoor lighting kept on at night discourages intruders from approaching your home. When you are away from home, ask a neighbor to pick up your newspapers and mail, and put a timer on some indoor lights to simulate a lived-in appearance. Join or organize a neighborhood watch group so you and your neighbors can look out for each other's property.

When you are out early in the morning or late at night, stay alert for potential threats. Always keep your wallet inside your coat pocket or front pants pocket, not in your back pocket. Keep your car in good running order, and never pick up hitchhikers. If someone does try to rob you, give up your wallet; it's less important than your life. Be sure to report the crime to the police.

You can easily incorporate such protective measures into your daily routine to make your life more safety-conscious. This section of the book looks at the causes of accidental injury and suggests practical safety measures you can take to prevent injury to yourself and others in your home and community.

Safe-Driving Tips

The motor-vehicle death rate has been declining in recent years, but motor vehicle collisions still cause more than 40,000 deaths in the United States each year and account for $200 billion in annual economic losses. Take responsibility for your own safety and that of your family when driving a car, sport utility vehicle, van, or motorcycle by following these safe-driving tips each and every time you drive:

- Always wear a seat belt, and position it correctly. Wear the lap belt snugly and place it low across your hips, never across your stomach or abdomen. Position the shoulder belt across your chest and collarbone. Don't wear the shoulder belt under your arm; it could break your ribs or cause internal injuries in a collision.
- Always place a child weighing fewer than 40 pounds in a properly installed child safety seat. Place the seat in the middle of the backseat. Infants under 20 pounds must ride in a safety seat that faces the rear of the car; they should also ride in the backseat.
- Keep your gas tank full and your car in good running condition. Keep the windows, lights, and mirrors clean and free of ice.
- Stay within the speed limit. Drive slower in bad weather or under unsafe road conditions.
- Drive defensively. Stay far enough behind the car in front of you to be able to stop safely, and stay even farther behind a reckless or erratic driver.
- In bad weather, find out the current road conditions and weather forecast before you leave. Leave early to allow extra time to reach your destination.

- Keep an emergency driving kit in your car. Some things to include in the kit are jumper cables, reflectors or road flares, jack, lug wrench, adjustable wrench, insulated pliers, insulated screwdrivers, all-purpose wire, duct tape, spare light fuses, spare fan belt, pocketknife, quart of oil, gallon of water, blanket, shovel, bag of sand, and first-aid kit. And make sure your spare tire is in good condition.
- Watch out for pedestrians and bicyclists, especially children and the elderly. Remember that pedestrians have the right of way at a crosswalk with no traffic control signal.
- Never drink alcohol and drive. Alcohol affects your judgment and timing. Always appoint a nondrinking designated driver if you know you will be drinking.
- In rural areas, be alert for lowered speed limits when approaching towns or curves.
- Comply with no-passing zones. Look out for slowly moving farm machinery, as well as livestock and wildlife.
- Be extra cautious at railroad crossings. Never drive around lowered gates or flashing lights. Don't drive onto a railroad crossing unless you are sure you can clear the tracks. If your vehicle stalls on a track, get everyone out of the car immediately.
- Don't stay in the blind spots of large commercial trucks and buses. Large vehicles have long blind spots on each side of and directly behind them. If you cannot see one of the vehicle's sideview mirrors, the driver cannot see you.
- Take special precautions when driving a motorcycle. Always wear a helmet and bright clothing or reflective material so you can be seen clearly.

Protecting Yourself from Violence

To protect yourself from violent crime, you need to develop a basic street sense that can guide you away from questionable or dangerous places. But dark alleys and wooded areas are not the only places where you are at risk. Violence can occur in broad daylight on the street, at the office, or while waiting for the train or subway. Intruders also can enter your home if it is not securely protected. No matter where you are, stay alert and aware of your surroundings to forestall the possibility of encountering a violent act. Here are some tips for protecting yourself from personal violence:

- Become familiar with the neighborhoods in which you live and work. Find out where the police and fire stations and hospitals are and which stores and restaurants stay open late in case you need to run in for protection.
- Stay on well-traveled streets. Avoid shortcuts through parking lots, alleys, or other deserted areas.
- Don't carry or openly flaunt large amounts of cash. Refrain from wearing expensive clothing or jewelry.

- Use automated teller machines only in the daytime. If you must use one at night, do so under well-lit conditions on a busy street.
- Make your neighborhood safer. Help to clean up vacant lots and report such problems as broken streetlights and abandoned cars.
- Keep your own property clean. Trim your bushes so intruders have nowhere to hide. Add outdoor lighting. Secure windows and doors and keep a list of your valuables, or photograph or videotape them.
- Ask for identification before admitting meter readers or other public utility workers into your home.
- Make your home look occupied when you are away. Install timers on lights and have a neighbor pick up your mail and newspapers.
- Don't carry a weapon or keep a gun in your home (see page 39). Guns cause accidental deaths in the home more often than they are used to defend family or property. If you own a gun, store it properly, unloaded, locked with a safety lock, with the ammunition kept in a separate place.

Preventing Falls in and out of Your Home

In only a fraction of a second, you could unexpectedly lose your balance and fall on a sidewalk or down a flight of stairs. Each year many Americans become injured after a fall in and around their own homes. Falls can happen to anyone, but they are the primary cause of injury in people over age 65, and the risk of falling increases as you get older. The most common injuries resulting from a fall are head injuries, wrist fractures, spinal fractures, and hip fractures. In fact, about 90 percent of all hip fractures occur as the result of a fall. Many of these injuries could have been prevented by taking simple precautions in the home, where most falls occur. It is prudent to make a room-by-room check of your own home to eliminate any potential safety hazards:

Bathroom   Keep a night-light on during the night, or replace the light switch with a "glow switch." Use rugs and bath mats with nonskid backings, and place textured strips or a nonskid mat in the tub or the shower. Leave the bathroom door unlocked when you are inside so someone else can open it if you fall. Consider installing handrails in the tub and near the toilet.

Kitchen   Don't stand on chairs, boxes, or other makeshift items to reach objects on high shelves; buy a step stool with handrails. Store as much as you can at counter level. Improve lighting by opening curtains and installing under-cabinet lighting. Clean up spills promptly. Don't wax your floors because they may become too slippery, and avoid walking on wet floors.

Bedroom   Keep clutter to a minimum. Don't throw soiled laundry on the floor; put it in a laundry basket. Remove loose throw rugs and make sure electrical and telephone cords are kept close to the wall. Don't buy an excessively high bed. Keep a night-light on during the night, or locate your bed close to a lamp or a light switch.

Living and Family Rooms   Arrange your furniture so it provides an open pathway between rooms. Keep low tables and other small pieces of furniture out of the pathway. Ensure that electrical and telephone cords stay against the wall. Purchase rugs with nonskid backing, apply double-faced adhesive carpet tape to all rugs, or put rubber padding under them.

Stairways   Use a high-wattage bulb in the stairway light fixture to see the steps clearly. Remove objects from the stairs. Install carpeting or nonskid treads on all stairways. Make sure handrails and supporting posts are sturdy and not loose.

Basement/Garage/Workshop   Make sure lighting is adequate. Store power tools when not in use so you won't trip on the electrical cords. Keep clutter to a minimum, and store all boxes against the wall.

All Areas of the House or Apartment   Avoid wearing only socks in the house, especially if you have polished wood floors you can slip on; put on shoes with nonskid soles, and tie up the laces. Keep a flashlight and extra batteries handy so you can see any tripping hazards if the electricity fails. Check all electrical and telephone cords to make sure they lie against the wall, not across the floor. Maintain good lighting. Use nonskid rugs and mats. Pick up toys, boxes, and other clutter regularly. Repair any crumbling concrete on outside stairs or sidewalks. In the winter, hire someone to shovel snow away from walkways and remove icy patches. Mark any outside steps that have unusually high or low risers with bright tape, or paint them a different color.

Regular, weight-bearing exercise, such as brisk walking and stair climbing, puts stress on the large muscles of your lower body and can help you avoid falls by increasing your strength, improving flexibility, and boosting your coordination and balance. Exercise also maintains bone strength so that, if you do fall, your chances of breaking a bone are reduced. In the event of a fall, try not to panic. Slide or crawl across the floor to the nearest chair and try to get up. If you cannot, call someone else to help you, or crawl to the telephone and dial 911 or your local emergency telephone number.

Managing Your Medications Safely

When your doctor prescribes a medication, he or she will give you instructions about how, when, and how often to take it. In addition to your doctor's orders, there are a number of other rules you should follow when taking and storing your medications to make sure you use them safely. If you are taking more than one medication, write down all of the medications your doctor has prescribed, the number of times a day you need to take them, and the times of day, such as with meals, or in the morning. Don't be afraid to ask your doctor or pharmacist about your medication, including any side effects it may cause or interactions it may have with other drugs you are taking. Be sure to tell your doctor if any prescribed drug makes you feel unusual or sick, and try to describe how it makes you feel as accurately as you can.

The following guidelines will help you manage your medications safely:

- Follow your doctor's orders. Take the exact dose at the exact time ordered. Follow the label instructions about how to take it—for example, with a meal. Don't drink alcohol if your doctor or pharmacist has told you it can interact with your medication or make it ineffective.
- Take only the prescription medicines that are prescribed for you. Never take someone else's prescription drug or give anyone else your own.
- Store medications in their original containers. Don't mix more than one drug in a container.
- Always read the label before you take any prescription drug, to minimize mistakes. If you need glasses to read, wear them when you take your medication so you can easily read the label.
- Tell your doctor about any over-the-counter drugs, vitamin and mineral supplements, or herbal medications you are taking. These medications can make your prescription drugs ineffective or cause dangerous side effects when taken with certain prescription drugs. Also tell your doctor about any allergies you might have, to help prevent an unexpected reaction to a medicine.
- Tell your doctor if you are taking medication prescribed by another healthcare provider, such as another doctor or a dentist.
- Discard expired medications or ones you no longer need to take. Flush them down the toilet so pets and children cannot get ahold of them.
- Consider that sunlight, temperature, and humidity may alter the effectiveness of your medications. The medicine cabinet or a kitchen cupboard may not be the best storage place. Store your medications in a cool, dry place.
- Keep all medications out of the reach of children. This warning also applies to over-the-counter drugs and vitamins. Iron pills are a serious poisoning hazard to children.
- If you miss your regular dose, check the patient information sheet that came with the medication to find out when to take the next dose. Don't assume you know; it is always better to ask. If the sheet does not have this information, call your doctor's office.
- Keep the phone number of your local poison-control center next to the telephone. Call the number in case you take an overdose or have questions about the effects of your medications.

- Ask the doctor if you need to modify your lifestyle. For example, is it safe to drive or operate machinery?

Fire Prevention Checklist

A few simple precautions can prevent a fire from occurring in your home. Place new batteries in your smoke detectors once a year on a memorable date, such as your child's birthday or the date that the time changes from daylight savings time to standard time. Call your gas company if you smell gas or if the pilot light on your furnace goes out. Never smoke in bed. To gauge whether your home is fire-safe, use the following checklist:

	Yes	No
Do you inspect electrical cords for signs of fraying and avoid placing cords under carpets?	☐	☐
Do you check to make sure your electrical outlets are not overloaded?	☐	☐
Do you keep any portable heater or space heater a safe distance from draperies, bedding, furniture, and other flammable items?	☐	☐
Do you have a smoke alarm on each floor of your house?	☐	☐
Do you check the batteries in your smoke alarms regularly?	☐	☐
Do you keep a fire extinguisher in your kitchen?	☐	☐
Do you have a fire emergency escape plan?	☐	☐

If you answered "yes" to all of these questions, you are well on your way to a fire safe home. If you answered "no" to any of these questions, you need to take additional steps to prevent fires in your home. Contact your local fire department for more information on fire safety.

Safety with Firearms

Fifty percent of all homes in the United States contain a gun, but having a gun in your home is dangerous. A firearm is 40 times more likely to be used to harm or kill a family member than to stop a criminal act. Having a gun in your home raises the likelihood of suicide fivefold and the likelihood of homicide threefold in your family. If you keep a gun in your home for personal protection or are thinking of getting one, explore some other ways of protecting your home and family first. You can invest in an alarm system, reinforced bars on your windows, a guard dog, and motion-detecting outdoor lighting. All of these measures are far better for your personal safety than having a firearm in your home.

If you choose to own a firearm—whether for personal safety or a sport such as hunting—you can lessen the chances of injury or death by taking certain precautions. Store the gun unloaded, trigger-locked, and in a locked gun case, then place it in a locked cabinet or drawer. Lock up your ammunition in a separate box and keep it in a different location. Check your gun and ammunition periodically to make sure they remain securely stored. Make the key available only to other trusted adults.

Learn how to use your weapon properly, and have every adult in your family take a training course in firearms safety from a certified instructor. Teach your children never to touch a gun, and tell them what to do if they find a gun anywhere: don't touch it, and tell a trusted adult right away. Also tell your children that if they are visitors in someone's home and are not sure if a gun is real or a toy, they should treat it as a real gun. Responsible gun ownership can reduce the risks inherent in having a firearm in the home and make your home a safer place to live.

PART TWO

STAYING HEALTHY

CHAPTER 1

Diet and Nutrition

Eating a balanced diet that includes plenty of whole grains, vegetables, and fruits can help you maintain or reduce your weight, be more productive at work, and perform better in sports—as we have seen in part one, "The Healthy Man." But the most important benefit of a nutritious diet is that it can dramatically reduce your risk of getting the most common chronic diseases affecting American men, including heart disease, high blood pressure, stroke, diabetes, and certain forms of cancer.

Diet has a profound role in preventive medicine and a direct effect on the development of heart disease, high blood pressure, and stroke. To lower your risk of heart disease, doctors recommend consuming a diet with less than 30 percent of its total calories from fat and less than 10 percent of total calories from saturated fat. You also need to watch your consumption of cholesterol, consuming no more than an average of 300 milligrams of cholesterol per day. On the other hand, foods containing high amounts of soluble fiber, such as oat bran and whole barley, can actually lower your blood levels of LDL cholesterol (see page 89), the "bad" cholesterol, without reducing the levels of HDL cholesterol (see page 89), the "good" cholesterol. Sodium, as found in table salt, may raise blood pressure in certain people, but the individual response to a low-salt diet varies. You should check with your doctor to see if you have this type of salt sensitivity.

Reducing your intake of fatty foods is important in preventing heart disease, but eating a wide variety of fruits and vegetables also is heart-healthy. Vegetables and fruits are rich in antioxidant vitamins (see page 9) and other nutrients that help protect your body from disease. One antioxidant in particular, vitamin E, has been singled out for its benefits to the heart. Vitamin E seems to prevent free-radical damage (see page 9) to LDL cholesterol, a process that has been implicated in the fatty buildup known as atherosclerosis on the walls of the arteries that supply blood to the heart. Be cautious when considering taking high doses of vitamin E, however, because it is a fat-soluble vitamin. This means that it can be stored in your body's cells, leading to a potentially dangerous accumulation over time. Doctors agree that the best way to get your vitamin E—and any other vitamin or mineral—is by consuming a variety of foods as part of a balanced, nutritious diet.

Being overweight is a major health problem for many American men. Maintaining your weight within a healthful range (see page 68) is an important way to lower your risk of developing diabetes, because obesity is a major contributor to this disease. If you already have diabetes, the proper diet can help you regulate your blood sugar level. For example, soluble fiber (see page 11) has been shown to slow down the digestion of starches, thus helping people with diabetes to avoid the elevation in blood sugar level that often occurs after meals. But you need to work with your doctor to plan an individualized diet that works best for you because some people with diabetes have better results on a diet that is a bit higher in fat and lower in carbohydrates than the diet recommended by the Dietary Guidelines for Americans (see page 6).

Medical research shows that eating a diet rich in vegetables and fruits, as recommended in the Food Guide Pyramid (see page 5), can actually help to prevent the development of cancers of the stomach, prostate, and lung. Cancer of the colon in particular has a strong link to dietary factors. A high consumption of fiber-rich foods, such as whole-grain breads and dried beans, combined with a limited consumption of meat (especially high-fat meats), has a strong protective effect against this form of cancer. A high-fat diet also has been implicated in the development of rectal and prostate cancer.

Moderate alcohol consumption (two drinks per day or less) has been linked to a reduction in death from heart disease, but this does not mean that doctors advise that you drink alcohol to reduce your risk of the disease. Alcohol has too many negative effects on health—the potential for addiction, liver damage and disease, an increase in the likelihood of injury or death from accidents—to be recommended as a preventive measure. The best advice is, if you don't drink alcohol, don't start drinking now. If you do choose to consume alcoholic beverages, do so only in moderation, defined in the Dietary Guidelines for Americans as two drinks a day or less for men.

Don't underestimate the health benefits of a nutritious breakfast (see page 7). The first meal of the day not only provides the nutrients and energy that your body needs to move and think but also makes you less hungry later in the day. Men who don't eat breakfast tend to eat more at lunch and dinner, resulting in an overall increase in calorie intake when compared with breakfast eaters. If you are pressed for time, breakfast need not be elaborate; a bagel and piece of fruit, a bowl of cereal, or last night's leftovers can be enough to fuel your body adequately as you begin your day.

The Basics of Nutrition

The foods that you eat come in a vast array of colors, textures, and sizes, but they are all made up primarily of three components: carbohydrates, protein, and fats. All three of these components contain calories, meaning that they produce energy in your body. In addition to carbohydrates, protein, and fats, your body needs other nutrients, including vitamins, minerals, and water. Together these categories of nutrients are known as the building blocks of nutrition.

Carbohydrates

Carbohydrates supply the main source of energy for your body, so many nutritionists recommend that they should make up the majority—50 or 60 percent—of your intake of calories. Carbohydrates consist of the starches, sugars, and fiber found in foods that come from plants. There are two types of carbohydrates: simple and complex. Simple carbohydrates, also known as simple sugars, taste sweet and are quickly absorbed and digested. Examples of simple carbohydrates are table sugar, honey, corn syrup, and the type of sugar found in fruit. Complex carbohydrates refer to the starches or fiber found in rice, pasta, bread, potatoes, beans, and some fruits (such as bananas).

Complex carbohydrates are better for you than simple carbohydrates because complex carbohydrates are absorbed by your digestive system more slowly, giving your body a more sustained source of energy and preventing steep rises and falls in blood sugar levels. They also contain many nutrients, such as vitamins and minerals, while the simple carbohydrates in foods such as candy, pastries, and other sugary desserts provide only calories. By far, most of the carbohydrates you consume should be the complex carbohydrates found in grains (preferably whole grains), vegetables, and fruits.

The problem with sugar and foods containing high amounts of sugar is that they supply "empty calories"—that is, they contain many calories but no nutrients. For example, one 12-ounce can of soda contains about 9 teaspoons of sugar. Sugary desserts taste good, but when you fill up on simple sugars, you leave no room for more nutrient-rich foods. Sweet desserts often also contain large amounts of fat; the high consumption of fat has been shown to have health risks. Overindulgence in these foods also leads to excess weight gain.

Fiber is a special type of carbohydrate that is found in foods such as whole bran and other grains, vegetables, and fruits. Fiber is the part of the plant that is not digestible and provides no nutrients, but it has many beneficial health functions. It comes in two forms: soluble and insoluble. Soluble fiber, present in oat bran and oatmeal, barley, dried beans, vegetables, and fruits, can improve your blood cholesterol levels (see page 89), especially when consumed as part of a low-fat diet. Insoluble fiber is found in whole bran cereals, whole-wheat bread, and fruit and vegetable skins. Its main function is to increase the bulk in your stools, thereby preventing constipation and protecting against certain other digestive disorders, such as colon cancer. Eating according to the Food Guide Pyramid (see page 5) will easily provide the recommended 25 grams of fiber per day.

If you want to begin increasing your intake of fiber, do it gradually, because a sudden increase can cause abdominal bloating and excess intestinal gas. Drink plenty of water to minimize these effects. Your body will eventually adapt to the higher levels of fiber. Doctors do not usually recommend fiber supplements because they lack the vital nutrients found in whole grains, vegetables, and fruits.

Protein

The primary function of protein-rich foods is to form muscle, bone, and skin and to repair body tissue. Certain proteins also carry hormones and other essential elements throughout your body by way of the bloodstream. Protein-rich foods include meat, poultry, fish, eggs, dried beans, nuts, and dairy products. Grain foods such as breads and cereals are a secondary source of protein.

Proteins are made up of combinations of 21 different chemicals called amino acids. Nine of these chemicals, called essential amino acids, cannot be manufactured by your body and must be obtained from the food you eat. Others, known as nonessential amino acids, are made from the essential type. Proteins from animal sources are called complete proteins because they are rich in essential amino acids. Because proteins in plant foods such as beans or nuts have fewer of the essential amino acids, they are referred to as incomplete proteins. In the past doctors and nutrition experts recommended combining plant proteins such as rice and beans at a given meal to ensure getting enough essential amino acids. But unless you have a protein deficiency, which is rare in the United States, or are a vegetarian, the experts now know that combining proteins is unnecessary as long as your total diet is balanced.

Many men believe that they need to consume an abundance of protein to eat healthfully, but the Recommended Dietary Allowance (RDA) for protein set by the Food and Nutrition Board of the National Research Council is actually quite low. The RDA for protein is 63 grams per day for an adult male, which is about 10 to 15 percent of your total calorie intake. Consuming this amount of protein each day is not difficult. Simply eat 6 to 8 ounces of meat, poultry, or fish and drink a couple of glasses of milk and you have met your RDA. Most Americans eat more protein than that each day—more than they need.

Fat

Fat enhances the flavor and texture of food, which helps explain why high-fat foods usually taste good. Fat has important functions in the body, including helping to make the male hormone testosterone. But most people in developed countries consume too much fat, which leads to the development of heart disease, some types of cancer, and other chronic diseases. This explains why the Dietary Guidelines for Americans (see page 6) advises deriving no more than 30 percent of your total calorie intake from fat, and no more than 10 percent of total calories from saturated fat (see below).

There are three main types of fat in the foods you eat: saturated, polyunsaturated, and monounsaturated. Cholesterol is also a type of fat found in foods of animal origin. Don't be confused by the difference between the cholesterol found in food and the cholesterol that circulates in your blood. Your liver manufactures most of the cholesterol in your blood from the saturated fat you consume; a smaller percentage comes from the cholesterol in the food you eat. Some men's blood cholesterol levels are affected more than other men's by the amount of cholesterol they eat. Having a high cholesterol level increases your risk of heart disease.

Another category of fat, known as trans fatty acids, also is present in certain foods. Trans fatty acids are synthetic fats made during food processing. The following table describes the differences in the various types of fats.

Understanding Dietary Fats

Type of Fat	Food Sources	Effects on the Body
Saturated	Red meat, cheese, butter, coconut and palm oils	Elevates total cholesterol and LDL ("bad" cholesterol)
Polyunsaturated	Vegetable oils, fish, seafood	Lowers both total cholesterol and HDL ("good" cholesterol)
Monounsaturated	Olive and canola oils, meat, fish, poultry	Lowers total cholesterol and LDL
Cholesterol	Lobster, shrimp, liver	May elevate total cholesterol
Trans fatty acids	Margarine, processed foods	Elevates total cholesterol and LDL

Water

Water is an essential nutrient, just like the nutrients in food. Your body is made up primarily of water, which accounts for 50 to 80 percent of your body weight. Your requirement for water varies, depending on such factors as the temperature and humidity or your activity level. Water loss through perspiration during physical exertion can increase your body's need for water dramatically. Having diarrhea also can cause excess water loss from your intestines, so it's important to drink plenty of fluids when you have a bout of diarrhea.

In general, thirst is the best indicator that you need water. Don't quench your thirst with caffeinated soda or alcoholic beverages because caffeine and alcohol will only dehydrate you further. Older people may find that their thirst sensation has become dulled. If you are an older man, remember to drink at least eight glasses of water and other fluids, 8 ounces each, every day, regardless of whether you are thirsty, and especially in hot weather. It's easy to become dangerously dehydrated without realizing it when the weather is hot and humid.

The federal government sets standards for the safety and purity of drinking water, and most municipalities meet these guidelines. Occasionally, however, contaminants enter public drinking water supplies. If you are told that your local water facility is having problems with high bacteria counts or other contamination, boil your tap water before you drink it or use it for cooking. The plumbing in older homes sometimes leeches lead into tap water. If you suspect that your plumbing might have lead-containing solder, run your tap water for several minutes every morning before drinking it. Always use cold water when cooking because hot water can cause lead to leech from pipes even faster.

Fluoride is an element that occurs naturally in the water found in some parts of the United States. In other regions, local municipalities add fluoride to public water supplies to help prevent tooth decay. Fluoridation of water is safe and is largely responsible for a substantial nationwide decrease in tooth decay.

Vitamins and Minerals

Vitamins are compounds that your body needs but cannot manufacture on its own (with the exception of vitamin D, which is produced by your skin when exposed to sunlight). As noted in part one, "The Healthy Man," there are two types of vitamins: fat-soluble and water-soluble. The fat-soluble vitamins—A, D, E, and K—can be stored by your body in the fat inside your cells. Taking large doses of these vitamins can be risky because they can build up in your body and cause unwanted effects. Water-soluble vitamins, composed of the eight B vitamins and vitamin C, are not stored by your body and need to be replaced every day in the food you eat.

The antioxidants (see page 9) vitamin C, beta carotene (which your body converts into vitamin A), and vitamin E have been getting a lot of publicity because of their supposed disease-preventing qualities, prompting some people to take large—in some cases massive—doses of antioxidant supplements. However, much of the scientific research that has been done on antioxidants remains conflicting, so doctors still recommend getting most of your antioxidant vitamins from the foods you eat, rather than from supplements.

Minerals are chemicals that plants absorb from soil and water. Small amounts of many of these minerals are essential for normal body function. When you eat fruits, vegetables, and grains, you receive the benefit of the minerals they contain. Two important minerals are calcium and iron. Calcium is important for building strong bones and preventing the bone-thinning disease known as osteoporosis. Too much calcium can cause health problems such as constipation and kidney stones. Men between ages 25 and 65 should take in about 1,000 milligrams of calcium per day. Men over 65 should take in about 1,500 milligrams of calcium per day. Low-fat and nonfat dairy products are excellent sources of calcium. Adequate iron intake ensures that your red blood cells have enough hemoglobin, a compound needed to transport oxygen throughout the body. However, too much iron has been linked to an increased risk of heart and liver disease in men. You need only about 10 milligrams of iron per day. Good sources of iron include red meat, raisins, nuts, and enriched breads, cereals, rice, and pasta.

Vitamin and mineral deficiencies are rare in the United States. Although many men take vitamin and mineral supplements, the best way to get your daily allowances of these nutrients is from the food you eat. This is another reason why it is so important to consume a wide variety of foods—to ensure a balanced diet.

Healthy Diet Guidelines

What is the best diet to follow to ensure good health? Doctors advise that the Dietary Guidelines for Americans (see page 6) and the Food Guide Pyramid (see page 5) are the best general guidelines for healthy people. You can adapt these guidelines to meet your individual needs by working with your doctor to find out your personal health risks. As part of a thorough physical examination, your doctor will check your cholesterol and blood sugar levels and your blood pressure. He or she also will ask you a series of questions to find out your family health history (see page 80). You can also calculate your body mass index (see page 18) and waist-to-hip ratio (see page 18) yourself to find out the distribution of fat on your body. By using this information you and your doctor can tailor your diet to lower your personal risk of disease.

For example, if you have a high cholesterol level and a family history of heart disease, your doctor probably will recommend that you lower your intake of high-fat foods. On the other hand, if you have a family history of diabetes and are overweight, your doctor probably will advise that you go on a weight-loss diet. A family history of colon cancer might prompt your doctor to advise you to reduce your consumption of red meat.

But for most men, both the Dietary Guidelines for Americans and the Food Guide Pyramid recommend consuming a diet that is low in fat and high in fiber-rich whole grains, vegetables, and fruits—at least five servings of vegetables and fruits and at least six servings of grain products per day. Eating too much fat, especially saturated fat (see page 46), elevates your blood cholesterol level and raises your risk for heart disease and stroke. Whole-grain foods that are high in fiber can help improve cholesterol levels and maintain a healthy digestive system. Grains, vegetables, and fruits contain an abundance of nutrients, such as essential vitamins and minerals, many of which have disease-preventing properties. It is important to eat a wide variety of foods to make sure that you are consuming as many of these nutrients as possible.

Eating a healthful diet does not mean that you have to eliminate your favorite high-fat foods altogether. If you occasionally indulge in a cheeseburger or a hot fudge sundae, just make sure that you make up for it by eating low-fat foods at your next few meals, a concept known as "fat budgeting." Again, you should look at your diet over several days, not meal by meal, when applying the principles recommended by the Food Guide Pyramid. Choose lower-fat foods more often—for example, broiled rather than fried chicken and reduced-fat mayonnaise or mustard on sandwiches instead of full-fat spreads.

The Dietary Guidelines for Americans and the Food Guide Pyramid both stress moderation when it comes to the consumption of sugar, sodium, and alcohol. Sugar not only causes tooth decay, but sugary foods such as soda, candy, doughnuts, and pastries contain mostly "empty calories," meaning that they have many calories but few nutrients. You can easily fill up on such foods, leaving no room for more nutritious food choices. Many foods that are high in sugar are also high in fat, which doctors recommend you keep to a minimum.

Eating a lot of salt and foods containing sodium can raise blood pressure in salt-sensitive people. Salt-sensitive means that your blood pressure goes up when you take in too much salt (sodium). Not everyone is salt-sensitive, but unless you have been tested by your doctor, it is probably wise to limit your salt intake. Many processed and commercially packaged foods—such as canned soups, hot dogs, the flavor packets in rice and noodle packages, and crackers and pretzels—contain very high amounts of sodium. Look for reduced-salt or low-sodium versions of such foods in the supermarket.

Like sugar, alcohol provides plenty of calories, but not much nutrition. Again, moderation is the key. Men should consume no more than two alco-

Ask the Doctor

Q. Are vegetarian diets healthy?

A. Yes, a vegetarian diet can provide all the nutrients you need. In fact, some research has shown that vegetarians are less likely to develop heart disease, high blood pressure, and obesity than meat-eaters. There are three types of vegetarians. Ovolactovegetarians eat eggs and dairy products along with plant foods. Lactovegetarians consume dairy products and plant foods but not eggs. A vegan diet is the strictest vegetarian diet of all. Vegans avoid all foods of animal origin, such as eggs and dairy foods, and consume only plant foods. A vegan diet can be deficient in vitamin B_{12}, iron, calcium, and vitamin D, so vegans probably should take supplements of these nutrients. Also, vegetarians who eat dairy products have to be just as careful about the amount of fat in their diet as nonvegetarians, because full-fat dairy products have as much fat, saturated fat, and cholesterol as fatty meats. If you are considering becoming a vegetarian, plan your meals carefully to make sure your diet is balanced. You may want to discuss your diet with a dietitian. Ask your doctor for a referral.

holic drinks (two cans or bottles of beer, two glasses of wine, or two mixed drinks) per day. In addition to the many health risks that overconsumption of alcohol can cause (see page 22), it also can lead to nutrient deficiencies and even malnutrition. In addition, alcohol can adversely affect how your body absorbs nutrients from the food you eat.

Changing Nutritional Needs throughout Life

Age affects our nutritional needs. Sometimes the differences are obvious. It is easy to see the difference in the amount and types of food an infant, school-age child, teenager, and adult need. Other differences are more subtle. You may not realize that, as you get older, your calorie needs decrease, especially if you become less active. Being aware of such changes can help you to plan your meals more carefully, so you eat foods that provide plenty of nutrients for their calorie count.

If you have children, there are a number of things you should know about their nutritional needs. For example, doctors now recommend that infants breast-feed for the first 12 months of their lives. Breast milk supplies better nutrition than commercial formula, promotes brain development, and provides infection-fighting antibodies to help the infant stay healthy. Provide your partner with lots of support and encouragement while she breast-feeds your infant. Note that infants should not begin to drink cow's milk until they are 1 year old because it can cause an allergic reaction and is too concentrated for an infant.

Toddlers and preschoolers sometimes become picky eaters as their newfound independence propels them into a variety of activities that seem much more interesting than eating. The best solution is to keep offering your young child a variety of foods while not forcing him or her to eat any one food in particular. A good rule of thumb to use when portioning out food is 1 tablespoon of food for every year of age, so, for example, a 3-year-old would get 3 tablespoons of each food at mealtime. Children under 2 years should not yet follow the Dietary Guidelines for Americans (see page 6) because they need fat in their diet for brain development.

As your child enters school, he or she will continue to need plenty of calories for proper growth, but be sure to encourage your child to engage in physical activity to balance his or her calorie intake. More and more American children are becoming overweight, a problem that can cause health problems such as obesity and diabetes in adulthood. Getting more exercise is generally a better solution for an overweight child than dieting. Of course, you should limit high-calorie snacks. Encourage your child to snack on cut-up fruits and vegetables such as apple slices and carrot sticks.

The rapid body changes that occur in adolescence are sustained by good nutrition. Teenage boys between ages 15 and 19 can require up to 4,000 calories per day. But many teenagers get most of their calories from fast food and junk food.

Even though your teenager may be more readily influenced by his or her friends than by you when it comes to food choices, you should do all you can to make nutritious food available in your home. Keep healthy snacks—cut-up vegetables, whole-grain crackers and pretzels, fresh fruit, cheese—in your kitchen. Resist the temptation to buy high-fat, high-calorie foods. Stress the importance of having a good breakfast (see page 7) to your teenage children.

Once you reach about 25 years of age, your nutritional needs stabilize and stay about the same until your senior years. Eating a low-fat, high-fiber diet that is rich in whole grains, vegetables, and fruits remains the most sensible dietary advice you can follow. The average man should consume about 2,500 calories per day—less if you are sedentary, and more if you are very active. Watch for weight gain as you age. Doctors no longer think that a moderate amount of weight gain is acceptable in the middle years of life (see the weight table on page 69). It is now known that any excess weight over the range recommended for your height is unhealthy and can increase your risk for common chronic health problems such as diabetes, high blood pressure, and heart disease. Regular exercise is an excellent way to help maintain a desirable weight at any age.

If you are very athletic, your calorie needs are higher than those of less active men. Athletes who compete in endurance events such as a marathon or a triathlon may require 5,000 calories per day or more. Some endurance athletes can become anemic because vigorous exercise causes a lower concentration of iron in the blood. Eating a balanced diet containing iron-rich foods such as beef, pork, the dark meat of poultry, dried beans, and enriched breads and cereals is usually enough to prevent sports anemia. Athletes do not need more protein than the average man, so protein supplements are usually unnecessary. Many runners practice "carbohydrate loading" before an event, believing that the extra carbohydrate intake will better fuel performance, but this popular practice is probably not helpful unless you are training at an extreme level.

The most important thing to remember when working out or competing in any athletic event is to drink enough fluids. Water loss from breathing and perspiration can quickly dehydrate you, especially in hot or humid weather. It is critical to drink a lot of fluids before exercising, about every 15 minutes during the workout, and for about 2 hours afterward. Water is the best thirst-quenching liquid, although sports drinks can replace the electrolytes (sodium, potassium, and other minerals) that you can lose during vigorous exercise in hot weather. However, sports drinks also contain a lot of sugar.

As you get older, your metabolism (the chemical processes that take place in your body) slows down and your calorie needs drop. But you still require the same amount of vitamins and minerals. Eating healthfully can be difficult when you are dealing with aging-related physical problems from chronic conditions such as arthritis, deteriorating eyesight, and gum disease. Emotional problems also can affect your diet. For example, depression, bereavement over the loss of a loved one, and loneliness can significantly diminish your interest in cooking or eating. Also, living on a fixed income often limits the type and the amount of food you can buy, and medications you are taking can sometimes affect your appetite. To make sure you continue to get all of the nutrients you need, take advantage of community programs for senior citizens. Ask your local senior citizens' center whether they offer inexpensive meals. Talk to your doctor or a social worker at a local hospital to find out what other kinds of programs, such as food stamps, home-delivered meals, or church-sponsored meal programs, are available in your community.

Food Allergies and Intolerances

Do you suspect that something you eat is causing those unusual symptoms you get from time to time? Food allergies are relatively rare in adults. They most commonly occur in children, who usually outgrow them over time. Foods that most often cause a true allergic reaction in children include egg whites, shellfish, nuts, and milk.

Dairy products can produce stomach cramps, bloating, gas, and diarrhea in adults, but these symptoms most often indicate lactose intolerance, an inability to digest lactose, the sugar that is found in milk and other dairy products. Lactose intolerance is much more common than you may think. Most people (except those of northern European descent) develop lactose intolerance in adulthood because their bodies gradually stop producing lactase, an intestinal enzyme that helps to digest lactose. If you think you may have lactose intolerance, switch to the many low-lactose or lactose-free dairy products that are now available. Lactase also is available over the counter in pill form.

Some people are sensitive to certain foods but are not actually allergic to them because the food does not trigger an allergic reaction. Food preservatives called sulfites and flavor enhancers such as monosodium glutamate (MSG) can produce headaches and other symptoms. Some people get migraine headaches after consuming red wine, cheese, or chocolate. Talk to your doctor about any symptoms you may be experiencing that you think may be food-related.

Buying, Preparing, and Storing Food

When you go to the grocery store, keep a few tips in mind to help you make the healthiest food choices. First, remember the Food Guide Pyramid and buy your groceries accordingly. That means filling your shopping cart with a wide variety of grain foods (such as breads, pasta, rice, and cereals), vegetables, and fruits. Choose whole-grain varieties of breads and pastas more often than those containing refined white flour. Buy only lean meats. Choose low-fat or fat-free dairy products. Limit foods containing high amounts of fats or sugar, such as doughnuts, pastries, chips, and cookies.

Second, select mostly fresh foods; processed and prepared foods can contain high amounts of fat, sodium, and added preservatives. Choose the freshest foods possible. Check the expiration date on food packages, especially on perishable foods such as milk and other dairy products, eggs, and frozen vegetables. Put perishable items in your cart last to help prevent them from spoiling by limiting the time they remain out of the refrigerator. Avoid buying food in cans with bulging tops or dents; they could cause food poisoning. When you get home, put your perishable groceries in the refrigerator or freezer right away so harmful bacteria cannot multiply.

Proper food storage can guarantee that your foods will stay fresher longer and will also minimize the chances of contamination with bacteria. The temperature inside your refrigerator should be below 40 degrees Fahrenheit at all times. Avoid opening the refrigerator door unnecessarily, and don't leave the door open for long periods. Keeping fresh fruits and vegetables in the refrigerator will prolong their shelf life (tomatoes and bananas should be stored outside of the refrigerator, however). Bread will keep longer if you store it in the freezer, but don't put it in the refrigerator or it will dry out.

You should use up milk within 1 week after opening it and keep eggs, stored in their carton, no longer than 3 weeks. Consume fresh fruit stored in the refrigerator within 3 to 7 days, depending on the fruit. Keep uncooked meat, fish, and poultry in the refrigerator no longer than 2 days. Note that if you defrost meat, fish, or poultry, you cannot refreeze it. Bread, however, can be thawed and refrozen.

Canned foods can be stored for up to 2 years in a cool, dry place. It's a good idea to keep a stock of food staples, such as canned and frozen vegetables and fruits, rice, and pasta, along with seasonings and condiments, so you can put together a quick meal in a hurry. For example, heating up a can of black beans mixed with a can of diced and seasoned tomatoes and a chopped onion, served over rice, can be an easy and nutritious meal to make after a long day at work.

Safe food handling is essential to prevent food contamination and food poisoning. Always wash your hands thoroughly before you start preparing food. It is very easy to contaminate foods in your kitchen with other foods, such as raw meat, poultry, or eggs, that can have high bacterial counts. In particular, uncooked or undercooked poultry is a leading source of bacterial contamination. Always wash any knives, cutting boards, and countertops that have come into contact with raw poultry, meat, or eggs using hot, soapy water, and wash your hands again after handling them. Never put cooked food onto a plate that had raw food on it. And be sure to cook all meat, poultry, and eggs thoroughly (to 140 degrees Fahrenheit) to kill any bacteria.

Another common cause of food poisoning is food that has been left out at room temperature when it should have been refrigerated, especially in hot weather. It is best to thaw frozen food in the refrigerator or the microwave, not on the countertop. At a picnic or backyard barbeque, make sure that you keep hot foods hot and cold foods cold. And be sure to refrigerate any leftover food promptly. As a general rule, do not keep leftovers for more than 3 days.

CHAPTER 2
Exercise and Fitness

Lack of exercise is a serious public health problem in the United States, contributing to chronic disease and premature death. Regular physical exercise is one of the most important steps you can take to protect your health and live longer. Each year, millions of Americans experience health problems that could have been prevented or relieved through regular physical activity.

The benefits of exercise are numerous and affect virtually every part of your body. One important benefit is that exercise can reduce your risk of developing certain common chronic diseases. For example, regular physical activity has been proven to reduce the risk of premature death from heart disease by preventing its development. Regular daily exercise can make your heart stronger, improve blood flow through the arteries that lead to your heart, and lower the level of cholesterol (see page 89) in your blood.

Exercise also lowers your risk of developing diabetes, high blood pressure, and colon cancer, and helps to reduce blood pressure in people who have high blood pressure. Exercise helps build and maintain healthy bones, muscles, and joints and prevents back pain by increasing your strength and flexibility and improving your posture. Physical activity also helps to decrease your percentage of body fat by preserving muscle mass. Exercise helps you lose weight and maintain your loss; this is another way exercise helps you stay healthy and live longer. It can help

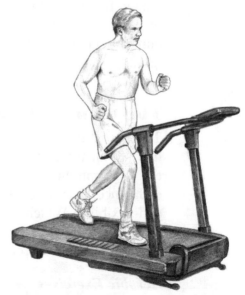

The Benefits of Exercise
Exercise—even moderate exercise such as walking briskly—can reduce your risk of major disorders such as heart disease, diabetes, and high blood pressure and can help you maintain a healthy weight. Make exercise a regular part of your life.

curb your appetite, and it burns a large number of calories. Regular exercise also helps you sleep better.

The health benefits you gain from exercise are not only physical, they are also psychological. Exercise promotes your sense of well-being by diminishing feelings of depression and anxiety. A good workout also can help you better manage the stress in your life (see page 118). When you stick to a regular exercise regimen you gain a sense of accomplishment that boosts your self-esteem. Also, because physical activity helps you control your weight and look fit, you will feel better about the way you look.

Regular exercise is extremely important for older men because it can increase the strength of muscles, bones, and joints significantly, which helps to prevent falls (see page 36), a major cause of disability in older adults. Even if you have been inactive for some time, your strength will improve with exercise, especially strength-conditioning exercises (see next page). Maintaining or improving your strength and flexibility will help you to better perform daily tasks so you can continue to live on your own and maintain a high quality of life as you get older.

While a small amount of exercise is better for you than none at all, the more you exercise, the more you will benefit. Once you start exercising regularly, your capacity for exercise will increase. That means that you will be able to exercise longer and more efficiently. If you have been inactive for some time, start with a 30-minute walk each evening before dinner and work gradually up to an hour or longer. If your doctor approves, gradually work your way up to a slow jog, and then a run. The more you work your heart muscle, the more efficiently it will pump, and the more health benefits you will gain—for both your body and your mind. Work with your doctor to find the best type of exercise regimen for your own personal health profile.

The Different Types of Exercise

There are different types of exercise, and each type has different effects on your body. Some types of exercise improve flexibility and muscle strength. Others use the large muscles in your body to build heart strength. Still others increase endurance. Exercises fall into three categories—aerobic, strength conditioning, and flexibility. Which type is best for you? Ideally, you should include all three types of exercise to achieve a complete fitness program but, if you have time for only one, aerobic exercises provide the most health benefits.

Aerobic Exercises

Aerobic exercises are any type of activity that uses oxygen to fuel your muscles. When you engage in aerobic exercises, your muscles and joints send messages to your brain, which stimulates your heart to beat faster and your breathing rate to increase so you take in more oxygen. Because aerobic exercises make your heart work harder, they improve the heart's ability to pump, even when you are at rest.

Any exercise that repetitively uses the large muscles of your arms and legs for a sustained period of time can be aerobic. Aerobic exercises are sometimes called endurance-training exercises because they make your muscles able to sustain the activity for longer and longer periods as they build muscle strength. Examples of aerobic exercises include brisk walking, running, jumping rope, bicycling or stationary cycling, swimming, stair climbing, rowing, and cross-country skiing. Sports that involve continuous running, such as basketball and soccer, also are aerobic exercises.

Regular aerobic exercises are a great way to burn calories and help control your weight. They also lower the proportion of fat on your body and increase the proportion of muscle. Men who maintain a healthy weight are less likely to develop diabetes and other chronic health problems that have been linked to obesity and being overweight.

For optimal health, doctors recommend engaging in aerobic exercises for at least 30 minutes every day. But you don't need to exercise for one 30-minute period. Three 10-minute sessions are just as effective and provide the same health benefits as 30 minutes of sustained exercise. Breaking up your exercise periods may make it easier for you to fit them into your daily activities. When you exercise, you should strive to reach a heart rate that is 50 to 80 percent of the maximum heart rate for your age. This rate is called your target heart rate (see page 12). If your heart rate does not fall within this range, adjust your activity level so it will increase or decrease your heart rate until it falls within the recommended range.

Don't forget to warm up for 5 minutes before every exercise session and to cool down afterward (see page 14). Start by stretching the muscles and joints in your spine, arms, and legs. Then begin moving your body repetitively by walking or slowly jogging or biking to elevate your heart rate slightly in preparation for your more intense activity. Warm-up and cool-down exercises can help prevent injury to muscles and joints.

Be aware that, if you don't keep doing your aerobic exercises, the hard-won health benefits you have worked for will not stay with you for very long. To remain at the healthier level you have attained, you must stick with your exercise program, whether it involves running, stair climbing, swimming, biking, or simply brisk walking.

Strength-Conditioning Exercises

Strength-conditioning exercises complement aerobic exercises by building muscular strength. Weight training, using either free weights or weight machines, is an efficient way to strengthen your muscles, but sit-ups, push-ups, and leg lifts accomplish the same goal. Strength-conditioning exercises are sometimes called resistance exercises because they force your muscles to work against, or resist, an object, such as a 5-pound weight.

You don't have to join a health club or buy an expensive weight-training machine to reap the benefits of strength conditioning. For example, simply add some push-ups and sit-ups to your exercise routine, or do some leg lifts on the floor while you are watching television. You can also purchase inexpensive hand weights in various sizes. Take a pair of 3-pound weights with you when you walk or jog to increase your level of exercise intensity. Use 5- or 10-pound weights to exercise the biceps and triceps muscles in your upper arms. Start with the heaviest weight that allows you to perform six to eight repetitions without stopping—even if it is only a 1-pound weight—and gradually work your way up to heavier weights. (Lighter weights will increase your endurance but not your strength.) Continue using the weights until you can repeat a set of six to eight lifts two or three times without stopping. Rest between sets of repetitions.

Men who are experienced weight trainers might find it helpful to seek advice from an exercise physiologist or a doctor who specializes in sports medicine when planning a new exercise routine or training for an upcoming athletic event. Remember that anabolic steroids (see page 14) are prescription drugs that may build muscle mass but also lead to serious health problems, including abnormal breast development in men, baldness, shrinking of the testicles, and a reduced sperm count, and therefore should not be used.

Even if you are older—in your 80s or 90s—weight training will increase your muscular strength. This type of exercise can help you to perform daily tasks, such as lifting grocery or trash bags, that often become more difficult as you get older. Strength conditioning can mean the difference between leading an independent life and relying on friends, family, or healthcare workers to meet everyday needs.

Flexibility Exercises

As you age, your ability to move your muscles and joints through their full range of motion diminishes. "Use it or lose it" is the principle that applies here. You may not be able to blame the stiffness you feel after sitting for long periods solely on arthritis. As it becomes more difficult to move about, you will probably want to move even less. Such immobility can threaten your ability to perform everyday tasks. Flexibility exercises such as stretching can help you to maintain the ability to move your muscles and joints easily. Stretching also protects your muscles from the normal wear and tear of both exercise and your daily routine.

Some men are more flexible than other men, and certain joints in your body may have more flexibility than other joints. But whatever your individual differences may be, you can increase your overall flexibility through stretching. Make stretching a regular part of your warm-up and your cool-down routines (see page 14). The muscle cramping or pain that can occur after vigorous exercise, especially when you are just beginning to exercise after having been inactive or have been overexercising, can often be relieved by doing stretching exercises.

The most important muscles to stretch include the hamstring (rear thigh), lower back, and shoulder muscles. When you are stretching, keep the following tips in mind. First, do not stretch to the point at which you feel discomfort or pain. Stay within a comfortable range; any discomfort is a signal that you have stretched too far. Second, stretch slowly and smoothly, and never bounce or make jerking movements. Third, sustain the stretch. Pause for 10 to 20 seconds when you have reached a full stretch, and hold the position so your muscles and joints have enough time to benefit from the stretch.

Ask the Doctor

Q. I'm disabled and confined to a wheelchair. Are there any activities I can do to get the benefits of aerobic exercise?

A. Men with a disability are less likely to engage in physical activity than men who are not physically challenged, but they have the same need for exercise. Remember that physical activity doesn't have to be strenuous to achieve health benefits. You can attain significant benefits with moderate, daily activity. First, you should consult your doctor before beginning an exercise program. Ask him or her if it would be safe for you to spend 30 to 40 minutes each day wheeling yourself in your wheelchair through a shopping mall. Wheelchair basketball is another option that would provide excellent exercise and would vary your routine. You can also lift hand weights and do stretching exercises with your arms to build upper-body strength and flexibility. Check with a local YMCA or community center to see what exercise programs may be available for people who are physically challenged.

Your Personal Exercise Program

You will be more successful if you develop a complete, personal exercise program, rather than just becoming more active in general. If you are over age 40, remember to check with your doctor before starting any exercise program, especially if you have been inactive, or if you already have a health problem. Start slowly with an easy activity that you enjoy, such as walking. Walk for as long as you feel comfortable. Gradually increase the distance you walk, and walk at a faster pace as you get used to exercising. Try to exercise for at least 30 minutes every day. Other good aerobic activities are swimming, stair climbing, jogging, biking, and cross-country skiing. The best way to make sure you will stick with your exercise program is to choose an activity you enjoy.

Varying your weekly exercise program by including two or three different aerobic activities—for example, walking or jogging 3 days a week, swimming 2 days a week, and biking 1 day a week—will help to keep your routine interesting. This concept is called cross-training, and it is a good way to prevent boredom. Cross-training also helps give your entire body a workout.

In addition to aerobic exercises, work some weight training into your routine to build muscle strength. Do push-ups and sit-ups or use hand weights to perform repetitive sets of lifting exercises. Increase your flexibility by stretching your arms, legs, and lower back before and after your aerobic workout (see page 58).

The time of day you choose to exercise can be important. There is some evidence that exercise workouts are more productive when your body temperature is highest, which is usually in the late afternoon. At this time, your muscles are more flexible and your resting heart rate and blood pressure are both low. Of course, if your schedule does not allow you to exercise late in the day, or if you already have an established exercise time and are happy with it, do not switch to an afternoon workout. Exercising at any time of the day is better than being inactive.

Making Exercise a Part of Your Daily Routine

Some men may think of exercise as something to do only when they need to lose a few pounds. But regular physical activity should be a permanent part of every man's lifestyle. The health benefits you gain (see page 55) won't last unless you exercise regularly. Here are some easy ways to incorporate physical activity into your daily routine:

• Make time for exercise every day. Get up half an hour earlier in the morning to work out. Better yet, watch television half an hour less each day and spend the time exercising.

• Work exercise into your usual routine. Stop using the elevator at work; take the stairs instead. Park a few blocks away from work or from the store and walk the extra distance. Take the dog for a nightly walk. Push the baby in a stroller or pull your children in a wagon or on a sled for half an hour every day.

• Exercise with a friend or family member. Working out with someone is a good strategy because you can motivate each other.

• Exercise while doing other things. Lift hand weights while you are talking on the phone. Do some sit-ups or leg lifts or ride a stationary bicycle while you are watching television.

• Break up your exercise time. Exercise for three 10-minute periods throughout the day instead of one long session. The exercise benefits will remain the same.

• Draw up an exercise contract. Write down weekly fitness goals and sign the contract. Then have a friend or family member witness it.

Don't forget to warm up before exercising and to cool down afterward (see page 14). And remember, you are making a change for the long term. Once exercise becomes a permanent part of your daily routine, it will cease being an effort. And you will feel better and look better—two of the best motivators you can find.

Choosing and Using Athletic Equipment

A wide variety of exercise equipment is available for home use, but how do you determine which equipment is best for your needs? Experts say to choose equipment that you are familiar with and comfortable using and to make sure that you will use it regularly before making your purchase. In other words, you have to try it before you buy it. Let's begin with the basics. The most important athletic equipment you can own is appropriate shoes.

There are many different types of shoes for various athletic activities—running shoes differ from walking shoes, which differ from basketball shoes. Cross-training shoes can be used for more than one activity, such as running and walking. First you need to decide which activity you will most often perform and then shop for an appropriate shoe. Wearing the proper shoe for a particular activity can prevent blisters or injuries such as shin splints and stress fractures (see page 63). When trying on shoes, wear the kind of socks you will be wearing when you exercise to ensure the proper fit. A stable shoe is one that prevents excessive movement of your foot inside the shoe. The insole should be cushioned, and the sole should provide traction while retaining flexibility. Athletic shoes usually have a midsole, which absorbs shock when the foot strikes the ground during walking or running.

The midsole is the layer that will wear out first on any athletic shoe. That is why fitness experts recommend replacing your athletic shoe every 350 to 500 miles of use. If you are heavy, buy new shoes closer to the 350-mile mark. If you walk 15 miles per week, you will have to replace your shoes in 6 to 8 months. Your shoes may not look worn and you may be reluctant to replace your shoes so often, but the price of a good shoe is a small investment when it comes to injury prevention.

Your athletic socks are also important. Appropriate socks can reduce the likelihood of blisters, toenail injuries, infections, and bone problems. The right socks can also enhance performance. Cotton socks effectively absorb perspiration from your feet, but if you perspire excessively or exercise in the rain, your cotton socks may reach the saturation point. If that happens, your socks will stretch and lose their shape, and your feet will begin to slide around inside your shoes, leading to friction blisters and skin irritation. Socks made of acrylic or other synthetic materials may perform better under "wet" conditions. Try wearing different types of socks when you exercise to determine which type of sock works best for each type of activity.

When considering the many different types of exercise machines you can purchase for home use, choose carefully. Remember that exercise equipment does not have to be expensive to be effective; you can use a length of rope to skip rope, and walking requires little more than sturdy shoes. If you are interested in purchasing strength-training machines or equipment that delivers an aerobic workout, here is a short equipment guide:

Treadmill

Americans buy more treadmills for home use than any other piece of fitness equipment. The motorized track of a treadmill allows you to walk, jog, or run at a pace you choose. Many treadmills have programmed inclines to simulate the intensity of jogging uphill. Others include resistance levers that give your arms and upper body a workout. If you hold the handrails, you can lower the intensity of your workout.

Stationary Bicycle

Stationary bicycles are good for exercising when the weather is bad and, unlike running, have only moderate impact on your knees. You can increase the intensity of your workout by pedaling faster or adjusting the resistance on the wheel. Some models offer movable handlebars for an upper-body workout. To avoid injuring your knees, you should adjust the seat so that your knees are still slightly bent when the pedals are at the lowest point of their cycle.

Stair-Climbing Machine

Stair climbing is one of the most intense forms of aerobic exercise you can perform. Stair-climbing machines give you a rhythmic workout that does not put a lot of stress on your knees. You can adjust the resistance for a more intense workout. Be sure to place your entire foot flat on the step to protect your Achilles tendon, which runs from the back of your calf to your heel, from injury. Do not climb using only your toes.

Cross-country Ski Machine

Because this type of equipment uses the muscles in both your upper body and lower body, it is an excellent form of exercise that burns plenty of calories. Cross-country ski machines place little stress from impact upon your joints. Some models allow you to raise the front of the machine so that you can simulate uphill skiing for a more intense workout.

Rowing Machine

Rowing machines simulate the effort exerted when rowing a boat. Rowing machines work the upper body and the legs. Some rowing machines are electric, while others are manual. You can adjust the resistance to vary the intensity of your workout. Sitting upright as you row will help prevent back strain.

Exercise Rider

This type of exercise machine combines the motions of rowing with those of leg presses to provide a total-body workout. You can adjust the resistance to alter the intensity of your workout. Exercise riders provide a more intense workout for men of average fitness than for very fit men.

It is important that before you purchase a piece of exercise equipment for your home, you try it out for 5 to 10 minutes in the store to make sure your lower back and joints feel comfortable. Do you like the "feel" of the machine? Does it seem sturdy? Is it noisy? Does it operate smoothly? Are all of the handrails and bars padded? Are the controls easy to use? Ask the salesperson how long it takes to assemble the machine and how much extra features cost. Think about your home and determine whether you have enough room to set up and store the machine. And consider honestly whether you will actually use it.

To purchase good-quality, dependable equipment, be prepared to spend at least a few hundred dollars on each piece. Once you have the equipment, be sure to follow the manufacturer's instructions carefully and use it properly to avoid injury.

Common Exercise-Related Injuries

Weight-bearing exercise such as jogging, running, or even brisk walking can place a lot of stress on joints and muscles. If you are overweight, you may be at greater risk for discomfort, pain, or injury from weight-bearing exercise early in your fitness program or when increasing your level of intensity or duration. Overuse injuries affect most men who exercise from time to time. There are a number of things you can do to prevent common exercise-related injuries such as sprains, strains, inflammation, and pain. Minor injuries usually can be treated with simple first-aid measures (see RICE routine, page 65). However, if you have a more serious injury, such as a broken bone, go directly to a hospital emergency department.

Rubbing or irritation inside your shoe can cause a blister to appear on your foot. Good-fitting athletic shoes can help prevent blisters. However, if a blister develops while you are walking or jogging, wipe the blister and a needle with alcohol to kill any bacteria that are present. Then carefully prick the blister with the needle to let the fluid out. Do not remove the overlying layer of skin; it will help protect the underlying skin. Cover the blister with a bandage. The blister will heal on its own in a few days.

Pain is your body's way of telling you that something is wrong. When pain occurs during or after exercise, it usually signals the overuse of a muscle, tendon, or joint. Most overuse injuries respond well to the RICE routine, a first-aid treatment you can perform at home.

Here are descriptions of some common preventable exercise- and sports-related injuries and tips on how to prevent them:

Tendinitis

Tendons are fibrous tissues that attach your muscles to your bones. Tendons can become inflamed from overuse, causing pain and swelling in the affected area. For example, running can cause inflammation in your Achilles tendon, which stretches from the back of the calf to the heel. This inflammation is known as Achilles tendinitis. The tendons in your forearm that attach to your elbow can become inflamed while playing tennis, causing a condition known as tennis elbow. The tendons in your forearm also can become inflamed by other activities, such as bowling or playing softball. Swimming can irritate the tendons in your shoulder, producing an overuse injury known as swimmer's shoulder. Adequate stretching (see page 58) before and after exercise helps prevent all forms of tendinitis. Exercises that strengthen your forearms, such as push-ups and lifting weights, can help prevent tennis elbow. Raising and lowering your heels and standing on your toes can strengthen your calves and prevent Achilles tendinitis. Strength-conditioning exercises (see page 57) can prevent the development of swimmer's shoulder.

Shin Splints

Pain felt along the front or the back of your shin that occurs during or after exercise such as jogging or running is called shin splints. This type of injury occurs when you exercise too much without taking enough rest periods. The best treatment for shin splints is rest. Stretching your legs before and after you exercise is the best way to prevent shin splints.

Plantar Fasciitis

This term refers to the pain and inflammation felt in the arch and heel of your foot when the plantar fascia (the band of tough connective tissue that runs along the bottom of your foot from your heel to your toes) becomes partially detached from the heel. This condition often occurs in runners. The pain is usually strongest in the morning and gradually diminishes throughout the day. After using the RICE routine (see page 65), or to prevent this type of injury, try strengthening the muscles in your feet by using your toes to pick up objects off the floor.

Strains and Sprains

Overstretching or tearing of a muscle or a tendon is known as a strain. The hamstring muscle in the back of your thigh is a common site for a type of strain called a hamstring pull. Inadequate stretching before sprinting or distance running contributes to the development of this condition. A sprain occurs when a ligament (a fibrous band of tissue that attaches one bone to another) is pulled or torn. Sprained ankles can occur when you are walking or running, especially if you step into a broken area of a sidewalk or trip over something in your path and your ankle is forced into an abnormal position. You may hear a snapping sound at the time of injury. Pain and swelling follow. Use the RICE routine (see page 65) and see your doctor. For the first 24 hours after a sprain or a strain, avoid applying heat to the affected area—for example, from a heating pad or a hot shower—because heat will increase the swelling.

Stress Fractures

Stress fractures are hairline cracks that occur in bones when the muscles, tendons, or ligaments that surround them become weakened by overuse during exercise and can no longer protect the bones. Stress fractures can occur in these bones, especially in your feet, after the repetitive impact of jogging or running. Stress fractures usually heal on their own, but if you experience severe pain, stop exercising and see your doctor as soon as possible.

In general, the best way to prevent exercise-related injury is to start exercising slowly and increase your intensity gradually. Being overly zealous in your workouts, especially in the beginning, will quickly result in an injury that will put you on the sidelines.

The RICE Routine for Athletic Injuries

The standard first-aid routine for most strains, sprains, and pulls caused by overuse during exercise is RICE, which stands for rest, ice, compression, and elevation. If you think your injury may be serious, or if it does not heal after using the RICE routine for several days, see your doctor.

Rest: Stop exercising immediately. Don't put any weight on the affected area for 24 hours.

Ice: Apply an ice pack to the affected area to reduce swelling. (Place the ice in a sealable plastic bag and wrap it in a towel.) Reapply ice for 20 minutes every hour during the first 24 to 48 hours while you're awake.

Compression: Wrap an elastic bandage around the area, being careful not to wrap it so tightly as to interfere with blood flow. Compression also helps control swelling.

Elevation: Raise the affected joint or limb higher than your heart so that gravity can help prevent blood and other body fluids from collecting at the injury site.

You can take an over-the-counter painkiller such as aspirin, acetaminophen, or ibuprofen. Aspirin and ibuprofen also help reduce inflammation. After 1 or 2 days of RICE, begin gently stretching the affected area. Don't stretch to the point at which it becomes painful, or you could damage the muscle again. Your doctor or a physical therapist can recommend simple exercises tailored to the specific injury to help you regain strength.

Heat Injury

When the weather is very hot and humid, it is a good idea to avoid exercising in order to prevent heat injury. In optimal weather conditions, sweating cools your body. But if high humidity prevents sweat from evaporating, your body cannot cool itself properly. Continuing to exercise produces more and more sweat, and dehydration can quickly occur, especially if you aren't drinking enough fluids.

Heat injury occurs in stages. In the first stage, called heat exhaustion, you experience muscle cramps, dizziness, weakness, and profuse sweating. At this stage you need to lie down in an air-conditioned room and sip cool water to recover. The next stage, called heat stroke, includes symptoms such as cool and pale or hot and red skin, no sweating, headache, nausea and vomiting, an unusually high or low blood pressure, and a temperature of 105 degrees Fahrenheit or higher. Loss of consciousness and coma can soon follow. **Warning:** Heat stroke is a medical emergency. Call 911 or your local emergency number and request an ambulance. While you wait for medical help to arrive, lie down in a cool place and have someone place cool, wet cloths on your skin or ice packs under your armpits and at the wrists and the groin area.

Remember to drink plenty of fluids whenever you exercise, but especially in hot, humid weather. Try to work out indoors when the heat or the humidity rises, or skip your exercise routine until the weather turns cooler.

When to Stop Exercising

Exercise provides many health benefits, but it is important to know when to stop exercising. If you feel any unusual symptoms, such as difficulty breathing, joint pain, dizziness, chest pain, or an irregular heartbeat, stop exercising immediately. Although regular exercise can reduce your risk of heart attack and early death from heart disease, overexercising can also bring on a heart attack, especially in sedentary men who have one or more risk factors for heart disease (see page 204). Become familiar with the warning signs of a heart attack so you recognize them if they ever occur—in yourself or in someone else. The most common warning signs of a heart attack include:

- a feeling of pressure or fullness, a squeezing sensation, or crushing pain in the center of the chest that lasts more than just a few minutes and is not relieved by rest
- chest pain that spreads to the shoulders, neck, jaw, or arms
- chest discomfort accompanied by light-headedness, fainting, sweating, nausea or vomiting, cold or clammy skin, or shortness of breath

A heart attack is a medical emergency. If you have any of these symptoms, stop exercising immediately and call 911 or your local emergency number, or go directly to the nearest hospital emergency department.

CHAPTER 3

Maintaining a Healthy Weight

Being overweight is a major health problem in the United States, and there are many good reasons to keep your weight within a healthy range. You will feel better, look better, and have more energy than men who are overweight. Having more energy makes you more likely to exercise, which can help you fall asleep faster and sleep more restfully. But the most important reason to keep your weight within a healthy range is that you will lower your risk for certain chronic diseases, including heart disease, high blood pressure, diabetes, and certain forms of cancer. Doctors no longer believe that it is acceptable to gain a few pounds as you age. Maintaining your weight at a reasonable level throughout your life is key when it comes to reducing your risk for disease.

Many overweight men have difficulty reaching their healthy body weight, and the more you weigh above your ideal weight, the harder it can be to lose the extra pounds. It is encouraging to learn, then, that losing even a relatively small amount of weight can reduce your chances of developing heart disease or stroke. For example, reducing your weight by just 10 percent can improve the efficiency of your heart, lower your blood pressure, and reduce the level of cholesterol in your blood. In fact, you can increase your overall health by losing as few as 10 to 20 pounds.

Slow and steady weight loss of no more than 2 pounds per week is the safest way to lose weight. Too rapid a weight loss can cause you to lose muscle mass rather than fat tissue and also can increase your chances of developing other health problems, such as gallstones, gout, and nutrient deficiencies. Making long-term improvements in your diet combined with exercising more is the best way to lose weight and keep it off.

When trying to lose or maintain weight, look at your eating habits and try to improve them. Follow the eating guidelines recommended in the Food Guide

Pyramid (see page 5) for the best dietary advice. Physical activity is also essential to weight control. Try to exercise for at least 30 minutes every day; start exercising slowly, and gradually increase the intensity of your workout.

If you are not currently overweight, but if weight problems appear to run in your family, you still need to watch your weight. Men who have close family members, such as grandparents, parents, and siblings, with weight-related health problems such as diabetes are more likely to develop similar health problems. If you are not sure of your risks of developing a weight-related health problem, talk to your doctor.

Although most men with a weight problem are those who struggle to lose extra pounds, a small percentage of men are actually underweight for their height. Men tend to diet for different reasons than women—to improve athletic performance, for example—and some men develop eating disorders, such as anorexia or bulimia (see page 71), from extreme dieting, although these conditions are much less common in men than in women.

Keeping your weight within a healthy range over the years requires self-control and a commitment to your health. If you are already overweight, work with your doctor to develop a safe and effective weight-loss plan that can help you keep your weight down over the long term. If you are underweight, your doctor can help you plan a diet that will allow you to gain weight sensibly.

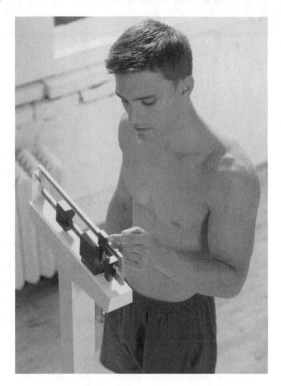

Watch Your Weight

Maintaining a healthy weight is one of the most beneficial, although most difficult, things you can do. A healthy weight not only boosts your confidence, but also minimizes your risk for major disorders such as diabetes, heart disease, high blood pressure, and some cancers.

How to Determine Your Ideal Weight

Check the following weight-for-height table to find out if your weight falls into the healthy range. Look up your height on the left side of the table, and move across the table to find your weight. If your weight is not in the healthy range for your height, you are more likely to develop weight-related health problems.

Height	Weight (in pounds)	Height	Weight (in pounds)
5'	97–128	5'10"	132–174
5'1"	101–132	5'11"	136–179
5'2"	104–137	6'	140–184
5'3"	107–141	6'1"	144–189
5'4"	111–146	6'2"	148–195
5'5"	114–150	6'3"	152–200
5'6"	118–155	6'4"	156–205
5'7"	121–160	6'5"	160–211
5'8"	125–164	6'6"	164–216
5'9"	129–169		

Weights above these ranges are less healthy for most people. The farther you are above thc healthy weight range for your height, the higher your risk of weight-related health problems. A weight slightly below the range may be healthy for some people but sometimes results from health problems, especially when weight loss is unintentional.

The Health Risks of Being Overweight or Underweight

More than half of all American men are overweight, and a third of all American men are obese (weigh more than 20 percent more than their ideal body weight). Being overweight is a major risk factor for a number of chronic diseases, including heart disease, high blood pressure, stroke, diabetes, and certain forms of cancer. Even a small reduction—as little as 10 percent—in body weight can decrease your chances of developing the most common chronic disorders as you get older. If you already have a health problem, losing weight can help you manage your condition. In some disorders, such as diabetes, weight loss can help reduce and even eliminate the need for medication.

Heart disease is the number one cause of death in American men. High blood pressure is a major risk factor for stroke, which can lead to permanent disability and death. You can reduce your risk of developing heart disease, high blood pressure, and stroke if you keep your weight within a healthy range. However, the number of pounds you weigh is not the whole story. You also need to know where your body stores fat. If you are like most men, your body stores fat around the abdomen, and a large amount of abdominal fat raises your likelihood of developing heart disease and diabetes. Regular aerobic exercise (see page 56) is the best way to get rid of abdominal fat. Also, if your waist measures more than 40 inches, you are more likely to develop heart disease, high blood pressure, or diabetes. Your body mass index (BMI; see page 18) is another important indicator of heart disease risk. Strive to maintain your BMI between 18.5 and 24.9 for optimal health.

Obesity is the top contributing factor to high blood pressure. Losing a modest amount of weight—even just 10 pounds—could return blood pressure levels to normal in many of the millions of men who have high blood pressure. Men who take blood pressure medication could substantially reduce or even eliminate their need for the drugs if they lost a modest amount of weight. Blood pressure readings go down within the first 2 or 3 weeks of such a weight loss. The percentage of your body weight made up of fat seems to affect your blood pressure more than total body weight, so exercise that builds muscle, such as strength-conditioning exercises (see page 57), also can help keep your blood pressure lower.

More than 16 million Americans have type 2 diabetes (see page 367); one third of them do not know that they have the disease because it has no symptoms in the early stages. Type 2 diabetes is characterized by increased levels of sugar in the blood because the body does not respond adequately to the effects of the hormone insulin, which regulates blood sugar levels. Diabetes can eventually produce serious complications, such as blindness, kidney disease, and poor circulation (which sometimes leads to amputation of the lower limbs). Men who have diabetes also have higher rates of heart disease, stroke, and high blood pressure than do men who do not have the disease. Uncontrolled diabetes also can cause life-threatening events such as diabetic coma.

Type 2 diabetes tends to run in families, so if you have relatives who have diabetes, your own risk of developing the disease rises. But being overweight is an even stronger risk factor than heredity. Regardless of family history, overweight men are twice as likely to develop diabetes as men who are not overweight. This means that, even if you have a family history of diabetes, you can prevent or at least delay the onset of the disorder by keeping your weight within a healthy range and by increasing your level of physical activity. If you already have diabetes, losing weight and exercising regularly can help control your blood sugar levels and could make it possible for your doctor to decrease the amount of medication you need to control your diabetes.

Colorectal cancer is the second most common cause of death from cancer in the United States, and being overweight increases your risk of developing the disease. Although some risk factors, such as family history, are beyond your control, being overweight is not one of them. If you have a family history of colorectal cancer, you should be especially careful about maintaining a reasonable weight. And be sure to limit your consumption of red meat and animal fat; a high-fat diet that includes large amounts of meat also increases your risk for this type of cancer.

Being overweight puts extra pressure on your joints, especially those in your knees, hips, and lower back. Because of this extra pressure, the cartilage (the tissue that cushions and protects the joints) gradually wears away, causing a form of arthritis known as osteoarthritis (see page 308). Over the years, the damage to the joint may be so extensive that the joint must be replaced surgically. This damage is permanent and cannot be reversed. Inflammation of the tendons, called tendinitis (see page 306), is another common problem in overweight people. Tendons can become irritated and inflamed (especially the Achilles tendon, which stretches from your calf to your heel) from simple, everyday activities such as walking. Losing weight decreases the stress on your joints and tendons and reduces wear and tear. Weight loss also may reduce the pain and inflammation of osteoarthritis.

Sleep apnea is a serious condition that is closely linked to being overweight. The condition can cause you to snore heavily and to stop breathing for short periods during sleep. Breathing can halt for 20 seconds or more, sometimes causing the skin to turn blue. Sleep apnea often causes daytime sleepiness and can be a factor in heart failure because of chronically low oxygen levels in the blood. Weight loss usually improves the condition.

Another health risk of being overweight is gallbladder disease and gallstones. The risk of gallbladder disease rises as your weight increases, although doctors do not yet fully understand the connection between the two. Ironically, weight loss itself, especially if it is too rapid, can actually increase your chances of developing gallstones. A modest weight loss of about 2 pounds a week is less likely to cause gallstones.

Although less common than in women, eating disorders such as anorexia nervosa and bulimia nervosa affect men, too. Estimating the number of men affected can be difficult because men don't often talk about such problems or seek help for them. However, the incidence seems to be increasing as a new generation of men becomes more concerned about body image. Of the people being treated for eating disorders, about 10 percent of those with anorexia and about 20 percent of those with bulimia are men. Eating disorders are most common in men who are distance runners, wrestlers, and football players.

The symptoms of anorexia (self-starvation, an irrational fear of being fat, compulsive exercise) and of bulimia (binge eating followed by self-induced vomiting or laxative abuse) are the same in both men and women. However, men often develop an eating disorder as a result of a desire to enhance sports performance or to overcome past weight problems, whereas women often develop an eating disorder as a result of an unrealistic body image. Also, body building and weight lifting have a much larger part in the excessive exercising that men with an eating disorder undertake than they do for women. Some men with an eating disorder use anabolic steroids (see page 14) to increase muscle tone and to improve strength. The affected man can become so obsessed with exercise that he begins to display exercise addiction, characterized by acute anxiety when he misses a workout and preferring exercise over time spent with family or friends.

The underlying causes of an eating disorder include a lack of self-esteem, an inability to handle stress, and sometimes sexual abuse in childhood. The man feels that controlling his intake of food gives him more control over his life in general. Most men with an eating disorder first develop it in adolescence. Although homosexual men often face pressure to be thin and attractive, placing them at a higher risk for developing an eating disorder than heterosexual men, homosexual men make up only about 20 percent of all men who have an eating disorder.

In addition to severe weight loss, anorexia can produce decreased blood levels of the hormone testosterone. The problem can become so serious that the body's major organ systems are affected. As many as 10 percent of all people with anorexia die of the disorder. The binge-purge behavior that is characteristic of bulimia can interfere with the delicate balance of chemicals in the body. Fatigue, seizures, and an irregular heartbeat can result. Stomach acid contained in vomit can damage the lining of the esophagus (the muscular passage that connects the mouth and the stomach) and corrode tooth enamel.

A relatively new type of eating disorder, called muscle dysmorphia, has emerged. This condition appears mainly in body builders who, in spite of being very muscular, fear that they look thin and out of shape. The disorder arises from the same body-image issues as those contributing to anorexia and bulimia in women.

If you think you may have an eating disorder, see your doctor right away. The doctor will conduct a thorough examination to find out how severely you are affected. He or she will assess your weight and ask you a number of questions, including whether you binge and then purge yourself of food and if you use laxatives, diuretics (drugs that cause the body to pass water), diet pills, or anabolic steroids. The doctor will perform a comprehensive physical examination, including laboratory testing to find out if any hormonal imbalances are present. If your doctor determines that you have an eating disorder, he or she will probably recommend a combination of psychotherapy, nutritional education, and counseling to treat your condition. Hospitalization may be required in severe cases.

Losing Weight Sensibly

Many overweight men have tried dieting and exercising to lose weight, with only modest success. Backsliding is easy, especially during the holidays or on special occasions. Successful weight loss depends on setting attainable goals and having reasonable expectations of meeting them. Losing 10 percent of your total body weight is an example of a sensible goal that you will be likely to reach. The sense of accomplishment that you feel will encourage you to keep the weight off and lose more if you desire. Most people should lose weight gradually; a rate of 2 pounds per week is about right. If you have a serious weight-related health problem that requires you to lose weight faster, do so only under your doctor's supervision.

How much you weigh is determined by a number of factors, including the amount and type of food you eat, whether you exercise, whether you eat in response to stress, your genetic makeup, your age, and your health. If you want to lose pounds and maintain a reasonable weight, you need to deal with all of these issues. Eating less and exercising are both critical to any weight-loss program, but if you eat out of boredom or fatigue, you will have a lot of difficulty keeping those pounds off permanently. Losing weight requires permanent changes in your lifestyle—changes that might be tough to make.

Fad diets that offer quick and easy results usually deliver only empty promises. Such diets may even be harmful to your health. Be especially wary of any diet that eliminates an entire food group, such as carbohydrates, because you could become deficient in essential nutrients. The only proven way to lose weight is to cut your intake of calories—especially high-fat foods—and to increase your physical activity to burn more calories. The healthy eating advice presented in the Food Guide Pyramid (see page 5) and the Dietary Guidelines for Americans (see page 6)—to eat a diet that is low in fat; includes plenty of whole grains, vegetables, and fruits; minimizes salt and sugar; and includes alcohol only in moderation—is even more important for men who need to lose excess weight.

The first thing you should do when thinking about starting a diet is to see your doctor. He or she can tell you whether your health status allows you to undertake a weight-loss program safely. Work with your doctor to determine the type of diet that is best for you. Your doctor may want to perform a physical examination or certain tests before you begin dieting, depending on your health.

When deciding on the type of weight-loss plan you want to begin, consider several factors. Do you want to lose the weight on your own or join a commercial weight-loss program?

Before choosing a commercial weight-loss program, ask the following questions. Does the program require periodic check-ins or meetings? Is the location easy to get to, and are meeting times convenient? Do staff members have appropriate training and credentials? If you need any medication or nutritional supplements, do they have unwanted side effects? Be sure to get a full accounting of all the costs involved with the program you are considering.

If you choose to lose weight on your own, you need to become aware of your eating habits so you can learn to control or modify them. A good way of raising awareness about your eating habits is to keep a detailed journal of the food you eat, how much you consume, and when you eat. As you take in fewer calories, charting your weight loss will build your motivation. Looking back at your food journal entries, you can sometimes see eating patterns emerge because you ate when you were feeling depressed, anxious, or angry instead of because you were hungry. You will probably be surprised at your eating habits. This new awareness will inspire you to change not only how much you eat but also the way you eat.

A strong support network is key to successful weight loss. Enlist your partner, children, siblings, coworkers, and friends to help you get through the most difficult periods. Plan low-fat, lower-calorie meals with your partner. Find a buddy who is also trying to lose weight so you can share experiences and exercise together. It's a lot easier to fall back into your old eating habits when you don't have anyone to answer to but yourself. If you do return to your old eating habits, don't be too hard on yourself. It can be especially difficult to stick to your diet at restaurants, dinner parties, and on holidays. Resolve to start fresh the next day, and consider your temporary lapse a learning experience.

Exercise is one of the most important components of any weight-loss plan because it burns excess calories, increases your energy level, and improves your mood. Make time in your day for 30 minutes of physical activity—every day. If you have been very inactive, start by taking a couple of flights of stairs rather than using the elevator or by parking farther from your destination so you can walk part of the way. Spend less of your time on activities that use little energy, such as watching television, and more time on activities that get you moving, such as yard work. Then, with your doctor's permission, gradually begin doing some type of exercise that you enjoy. It could be brisk walking, bicycling, swimming, jogging, or working out on exercise machines at a health club—whatever your doctor recommends as appropriate to your age and overall health. Remember that the activity does not have to be done all at once. You will burn the same amount of calories in three 10-minute exercise sessions as you will during 30 consecutive minutes.

Keeping a record of your exercise sessions is a good way to combat a lack of motivation. You can also write down the health-related improvements, such as easier breathing, that you have noted. Overweight men often feel discomfort or pain when beginning an exercise program. If this happens to you, try switching to non–weight-bearing activities such as bicycling or swimming.

Doctors may prescribe medications or even surgery to help some severely overweight men, or men whose weight poses a very high health risk, attain a more reasonable weight. Most drugs prescribed for weight loss work by suppressing your appetite. They are most effective if you use them as part of a weight-loss program that emphasizes consuming fewer calories and exercising more to burn excess calories and fat at the same time you are taking the drug. Weight-loss drugs work differently in different people and all have side effects, which are usually mild. You should carefully talk over your options with your doctor to determine whether weight-loss medication is right for you.

Doctors perform surgery to treat obesity only in cases in which the person's health risk from being overweight is extremely serious. This type of surgery can promote weight loss in two ways. In the most common type of surgery for obesity, commonly called stomach stapling, the surgeon closes off or removes part of the stomach to restrict the amount of food the person can eat. In the second type, the surgeon connects the stomach to a lower portion of the small intestine, bypassing the first section, known as the duodenum, so that food is less effectively digested and absorbed. This type of surgery usually causes vitamin and mineral deficiencies. Weight loss is significant after either type of surgery, but men who have surgery to correct obesity need to see their doctor regularly for the rest of their lives to monitor their condition. Because any type of surgery has health risks, you and your doctor need to weigh the risks and benefits of this type of surgery to determine if it is the best option for you.

When You Need to Gain Weight

Some men are underweight because of an eating disorder or because of treatment for a chronic disease such as cancer. They need to maintain their weight and add more pounds. For these men, taking in more calories than they burn is the answer. As simple as this may sound, underweight men often have to struggle with this concept. Some of these men experience appetite loss from chemotherapy or radiation therapy taken for cancer. Others struggle with an overwhelming fear of being fat that compels them to restrict their intake of food while burning calories by obsessively exercising. If you are underweight, there are a number of steps you can take to gain additional pounds.

Between your three meals a day, consume two or three snacks. Include high-calorie foods that are rich in nutrients, such as peanut butter and milk shakes. Space your meals and snacks so that you eat more without feeling overly full. Use the Food Guide Pyramid (see page 5) as your guide to healthy eating, consuming the highest recommended number of servings. For example, try eating 11 servings of grains and three servings of dairy products every day. Choose high-calorie fruits (bananas, dried fruit, and canned fruit in syrup) and vegetables (olives, corn, and avocados).

Add extra calories to your meals by incorporating high-calorie, nutrient-rich foods into recipes. Use milk instead of water in soups and sauces. Put a slice of cheese on your sandwich or over a baked potato. Mix wheat germ or powdered milk into casseroles. Make high-calorie shakes with whole milk, yogurt, and bananas.

Make meal and snack times as pleasant as possible to eliminate feelings of boredom, loneliness, or stress that may be affecting your appetite. Put fresh flowers on the table. Invite a friend or a neighbor over for lunch or dinner. Play music that you like during meals. These practical tips can make the difference between struggling to eat and eating well.

CHAPTER 4

Preventive Healthcare

In addition to eating a healthy diet and exercising, seeing your doctor regularly for recommended screening tests is a good way to stay healthy. Regular medical checkups are an important preventive health measure. During your periodic checkup, your doctor can detect any medical problems in the early stages so they can be treated promptly. Your doctor uses numerous medical tests and screenings to check for any health problems. Before deciding which tests to order, your doctor will perform a comprehensive physical examination (see page 86) and will take a medical history, which is a record of every factor that might affect your health. To complete the medical history, your doctor will ask you a series of questions about your personal habits, your family health history (see page 80), any medical problems you had in the past, and any symptoms you might be experiencing at present. When answering your doctor's questions, it is important to provide as much information as you can without holding back any relevant facts. Don't be afraid to ask your doctor questions if you don't understand something he or she has said.

The most common tests performed in men over 40 include the PSA (prostate-specific antigen) test for prostate cancer, the fecal occult blood test for colon cancer, and a series of tests that screen for the presence of heart disease or your risk of having it. Such tests may include measuring your blood pressure and the levels of cholesterol in your blood; an electrocardiogram, which measures the electrical activity in your heart; and a stress test, which evaluates the heart's response to physical exercise. If you have a family history of a certain disease that has a strong hereditary component, such as diabetes (see page 365), you also may undergo a screening for that disorder. For example, in the case of diabetes, the doctor would perform a test known as a glucose tolerance test (see page 367).

As you get older, you probably will need more tests during your regular checkups because common disorders such as heart disease and cancer occur more frequently in older people. Use this section of the book to learn about the various tests and screenings your doctor might order so you can become better informed.

Periodic Health Checkups for Men

Your doctor will recommend that you have a physical examination and certain screening tests periodically, depending on your age and health history. The following material indicates the most common tests ordered for men.

Eye Examination

To check for any vision problems such as near- or farsightedness or eye muscle disorders and to look for any early signs of disease.

Those at risk: Men who have diabetes, high blood pressure, or a family history of glaucoma.

Dental Examination

To check for tooth decay, gum disease, and early signs of oral cancer.

Those at risk: Men who smoke or chew tobacco; men with poor oral hygiene.

Blood Pressure Measurement

To detect high blood pressure early, before it leads to stroke, heart failure, or kidney failure.

Those at risk: Men with a family history of high blood pressure, heart disease, kidney disease, or stroke; men who are overweight or have diabetes; men who smoke or use tobacco products.

Cholesterol Test

To measure the blood levels of cholesterol, which helps evaluate the risk of heart disease.

Those at risk: Men with a family history of heart disease; men who have diabetes; men who smoke or use tobacco products.

Colon and Rectum Examination

To look for signs of cancer of the colon, rectum, and prostate. Includes rectal examination performed by hand by a doctor, fecal occult blood test that checks for blood in the stool, sigmoidoscopy (see page 284), and possibly a PSA (prostate-specific antigen) test.

Those at risk: Men with a family history of colon or rectal cancer; men who have intestinal polyps or ulcerative colitis; men over age 50. African American men have an increased risk of prostate cancer.

Comprehensive Physical Examination

To regularly assess your current health status and to maintain an ongoing relationship with your doctor. Be sure to see your doctor as often as he or she recommends.

Tests in Men Younger Than 30 Years

Test	Men at Average Risk	Men at High Risk
Eye	Every 2 years if you have vision problems	Once a year
Dental	Every 6 months	As recommended by dentist
Blood pressure	Every 2½ years beginning at age 20	Once a year
Colon and rectum	Not needed	Once a year after age 20
Physical	Twice in your 20s	Twice in your 20s

Tests in Men 30 to 50 Years Old

Test	Men at Average Risk	Men at High Risk
Eye	Every 2 years if you have vision problems; otherwise starting at age 40	Once a year
Dental	Every 6 months	As recommended by dentist
Blood pressure	Every 2½ years	Once a year
Cholesterol	Every 5 years if normal	As recommended by doctor
Colon and rectum	Once a year after age 40	Rectal examination and fecal occult blood test once a year; sigmoidoscopy every 3 to 5 years
Prostate	Not needed	Once a year beginning at age 45 if you are African American or if you are a white male with a family history of prostate cancer
Physical	Every 1 to 5 years	Every 1 to 2 years

Tests in Men Older Than 50 Years

Test	Men at Average Risk	Men at High Risk
Eye	Every year	At least once a year
Dental	Every 6 months	As recommended by dentist
Blood pressure	Once a year	As recommended by doctor
Cholesterol	Every 3 to 5 years if normal	As recommended by doctor
Colon and rectum	Rectal examination and fecal occult blood test once a year; sigmoidoscopy every 3 to 5 years	Same as for men at average risk
Prostate	Once a year	Once a year
Physical	Every 1 to 2 years to age 65; once a year after age 65	Same as for men at average risk

Your Family Health History

Many diseases run in families, and you may have inherited a genetic predisposition to a certain disease or disorder if other members of your family—your parents, grandparents, aunts, or uncles—have had them. This means that, if your parents or grandparents had heart disease or cancer, you may have inherited a susceptibility that gives you an increased risk of getting the same disorder. Many common disorders, such as heart disease, colon cancer, diabetes, and alcoholism, have a genetic component.

Just because your parents or grandparents had a certain type of cancer does not necessarily mean that you will also get it, because lifestyle factors play a role. Not smoking, eating a healthful diet, exercising regularly, and drinking alcohol only in moderation can help you control your risk of getting a disease for which you may have inherited a susceptibility. Knowing the disorders that have occurred in your family can help you and your doctor determine your risk.

Ask your relatives about medical conditions they have now and have had in the past. Ask about cancer, heart disease, diabetes, allergies, birth defects, drinking problems, and emotional problems. Try to find out from them the health problems experienced by relatives who have died. You can also contact the health department in the town in which your deceased relatives lived to request a death certificate, which will list the cause of death. Once you have interviewed all of your relatives, use the information you have gathered to construct a family health history tree like the one on the next page. Review the finished family tree carefully to identify any recurring patterns of disease. Pay special attention to disorders that occur at a relatively young age, because early onset of a disorder can signal a strong inherited influence.

During a routine physical examination, your doctor asks you a series of questions to find out your current health status, what medical problems or injuries you have had in the past, and what medical conditions your family members have had. This interview is called the personal health history, and it helps your doctor become familiar with your health status so he or she can better diagnose and treat an illness you may have. Develop your own written personal health history and keep it at home so you can monitor your medications and any changes in your health.

Use the personal health history form (see page 82) to get started. Think carefully about all the details of your medical history, including dates. Write down the names of the doctors who treated you, if they were different from your current doctor. Include your lifestyle habits, too. Have you ever smoked? Do you drink alcohol or use other drugs? How often? Safety issues are important as well. Think about whether you use a seat belt every time you drive and whether you have working smoke and carbon monoxide detectors in your home. List all

Family Health History Tree

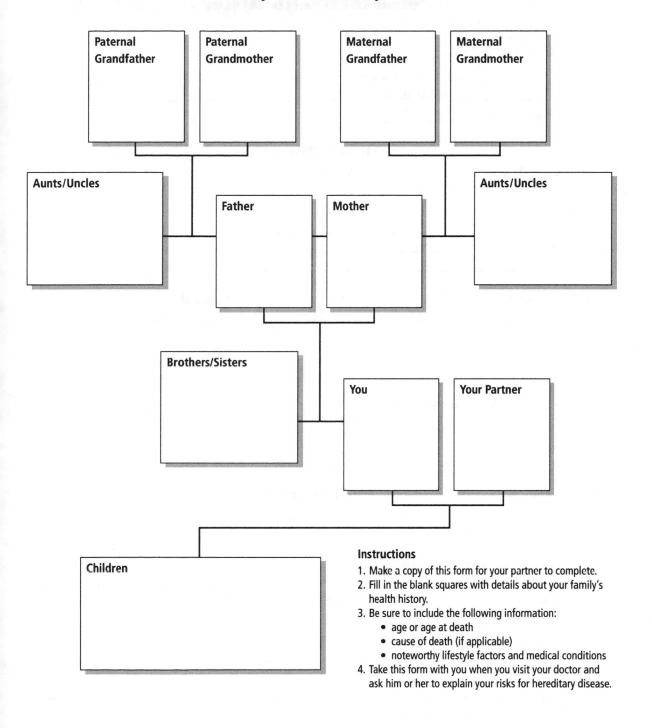

Paternal Grandfather

Paternal Grandmother

Maternal Grandfather

Maternal Grandmother

Aunts/Uncles

Father

Mother

Aunts/Uncles

Brothers/Sisters

You

Your Partner

Children

Instructions

1. Make a copy of this form for your partner to complete.
2. Fill in the blank squares with details about your family's health history.
3. Be sure to include the following information:
   - age or age at death
   - cause of death (if applicable)
   - noteworthy lifestyle factors and medical conditions
4. Take this form with you when you visit your doctor and ask him or her to explain your risks for hereditary disease.

Personal Health History

Fill out the following form.

Name: _____

Sex: _____ Birth date: _____ Age: _____

Place of birth: _____ Ethnicity: _____

Medical History

Current Conditions	Year Diagnosed
_____	_____
_____	_____
_____	_____
_____	_____
_____	_____

Previous Operations	Year	Hospital
_____	_____	_____
_____	_____	_____
_____	_____	_____
_____	_____	_____

Previous Injuries/Medical Conditions	Year
_____	_____
_____	_____
_____	_____

Mental Illnesses	Year Diagnosed
_____	_____
_____	_____

Current Prescription Medications

Medication	Dose	Length of Time You Have Taken the Medication
_____	_____	_____
_____	_____	_____
_____	_____	_____
_____	_____	_____
_____	_____	_____
_____	_____	_____
_____	_____	_____

Current Nonprescription Medications

Medication	Dose	Length of Time You Have Taken the Medication
_____	_____	_____
_____	_____	_____
_____	_____	_____
_____	_____	_____
_____	_____	_____
_____	_____	_____
_____	_____	_____
_____	_____	_____
_____	_____	_____

Drug Allergies

Medication	Reaction
_____	_____
_____	_____

Social History

Marital status: Married or single   No. of children: _____

Sexual history:

   No. of sexual partners in your lifetime: _____

   Sex of sexual partners: Male, female, or both

   Practice safer sex? Yes or No

Preventive Health History

Tobacco: Have you ever used tobacco products? Yes or No

No. of cigarettes smoked per day: _____

No. of cigars smoked per day: _____

No. of years you smoked: _____

Amount of chewing tobacco or snuff used per day: _____

No. of years you used chewing tobacco or snuff: _____

Have you ever quit? Yes or No

Alcohol: No. of drinks per week: _____
                        Have you ever quit? Yes or No
                        Have you abused alcohol? Yes or No

Illicit drugs: Have you ever used illicit drugs? Yes or No
                        Which drug(s) have you used? _____
                        When was your last use? _____

Exercise: Do you regularly exercise? Yes or No
                        If yes, what type of exercise? _____
                        How often do you exercise per week? _____
                        Length of exercise sessions: _____

Seat belt use: Yes or No

Diet: No. of meals each day: _____
                        Glasses of water per day: _____
                        No. of snacks per day: _____
                        No. of servings of fruits per day: _____
                        No. of servings of vegetables per day: _____
                        No. of servings of meat per day: _____
                        No. of servings of dairy products per day: _____
                        No. of servings of whole-grain products per day: _____

Smoke alarm in home?   Yes or No

Carbon monoxide   Yes or No
detector in home?

Gun: Do you keep a gun in the home? Yes or No
                        If yes, is it locked? Yes or No
                        If yes, is it loaded? Yes or No

Vaccinations

Vaccination	Year of Last Vaccination
Tetanus/diphtheria	_____
Pneumococcal vaccine	_____
Flu vaccine	_____
Measles, mumps, rubella	_____
Polio	_____
Varicella (chickenpox)	_____
Hepatitis A	_____
Hepatitis B	_____

Family Health History

Relative	Living (yes/no)	Age at Death	Medical Conditions and/or Cause of Death
Father	_____	_____	_____
Mother	_____	_____	_____
Partner	_____	_____	_____
Brothers	_____	_____	_____
	_____	_____	_____
Sisters	_____	_____	_____
	_____	_____	_____
Grandparents			
Paternal grandfather	_____	_____	_____
Paternal grandmother	_____	_____	_____
Maternal grandfather	_____	_____	_____
Maternal grandmother	_____	_____	_____
Uncles and aunts	_____	_____	_____
	_____	_____	_____

Doctors

Current Doctor(s)—Medical Specialty	Address	Phone No.
Primary doctor		
_____	_____	_____
_____	_____	_____
_____	_____	_____

Past Doctor(s)—Medical Specialty	Address	Phone No.
Primary doctor		
_____	_____	_____
_____	_____	_____
_____	_____	_____

Health Insurance

Health insurance company _____

Your identification no. _____

Phone no. of insurance company _____

vaccinations you have received and the dates when you last had them. Include information about sexually transmitted diseases such as genital warts.

Include information about your family health history to see if you may have inherited a predisposition to a certain disorder such as heart disease, diabetes, or cancer. Write down the name and the phone number of your health insurance company or health maintenance organization. Finally, list the names, addresses, and phone numbers of all of the doctors you now see.

Take your written personal health history with you each time you have an appointment with a new doctor or other healthcare professional. The information will help them more easily become familiar with you and your health problems.

Routine Physical Examinations

Your doctor uses the routine physical examination to assess your current physical condition and to identify any undiagnosed disorders. A routine physical examination also helps your doctor become familiar with you and your health risks or medical problems. The frequency with which you see the doctor for a routine checkup varies, depending upon your age and whether you already have a medical condition. Before beginning the examination, the doctor will take a complete medical history by asking you a series of questions about your lifestyle habits, general health, and family health history (see page 80). Taking a thorough medical history often takes as long as the physical examination itself but is just as important.

When you go to the doctor's office for a routine physical examination, a nurse or other healthcare worker will weigh you and take your temperature to find out if you have a fever, which could signal an infection. He or she also will take your blood pressure, using an inflatable cuff, pressure gauge, and stethoscope. A blood pressure reading measures how forcefully your circulating blood pushes against the walls of the blood vessels with each contraction of your heart. The reading records the pressure in the vessels both when the heart pumps blood (the systolic pressure) and when it rests (the diastolic pressure). The reading is expressed in two numbers in millimeters of mercury (mmHg)—for example, 120/80 mmHg, which is a reading within the normal range. The first number indicates the systolic pressure; the second number, the diastolic pressure. The higher the pressure in your blood vessels, the higher the reading.

You will be asked to undress and put on a cloth or paper gown. The doctor will begin by examining your skin, checking for any paleness, flushing, yellowish or bluish cast, rashes, dryness, bruising, or broken capillaries (tiny blood vessels). He or she will examine your face, which can display a number of unusual signs, such as puffy eyes, and your neck, checking for swollen glands or an enlarged thyroid (a gland just below your larynx—your voice box—that has an important role in controlling the chemical processes in your body).

Next, your doctor will look inside your mouth with a small flashlight and a tongue depressor to examine your tongue, teeth, and gums. The condition of your mouth can reveal a number of clues about your general health. For example, red, cracking areas on your lips can signal a vitamin B deficiency. The doctor also will check your throat as far back as possible. By using an illuminated instrument called an ophthalmoscope, he or she will look into your eyes to see the retina lining the back of your eyes. Another lighted instrument, known as an otoscope, helps your doctor peer into your ears, to check for any inflammation or a possible perforation of the eardrum.

Listening to your chest with a stethoscope allows your doctor to assess not only the nature of your heartbeat but also the condition of your lungs. Any abnormal heart sounds will alert your doctor to the possibility of an enlarged heart, poor blood flow through the heart, or a disorder of the heart valves. When listening to your breathing with the stethoscope, the doctor listens for wheezing, crackling, or other sounds that could signal the presence of a lung disorder such as asthma. The doctor will probably also tap your chest and place his or her hands against your chest and ask you to cough so he or she can detect any fluid in the chest. This process is called percussion. Taking your pulse is an important part of the examination because your heart rate can reveal heart or circulation problems.

The doctor will want to examine your abdomen, feeling and tapping it to detect any tenderness, abnormal masses, or fluid accumulation. He or she will continue to press on different parts of your abdomen and ask you to respond if you feel any tender areas. The doctor is also checking for the correct positioning of the spleen and the liver. As part of his or her examination of your digestive system, the doctor will probably perform a rectal examination. Your doctor will first cover his or her hands with disposable plastic gloves and lubricate the area to be examined with a cream or jelly. The doctor will gently and carefully place his or her fingers inside your rectum to feel for any tumors in the rectum or prostate. Many prostate tumors are first detected in this way.

If the doctor notices any signs that indicate that you may have a disorder of the nervous system, he or she will assess your motor ability, or ability to move, by observing the way you walk. He or she may also ask you to move your arms and legs in various ways to see whether there is a difference in movement between the two sides of your body. Testing the reflexes at your wrists, knees, ankles, and soles of your feet will also tell your doctor important information about the proper functioning of your nervous system.

To complete the physical examination, the doctor may order blood, urine, stool, or other tests (see next page) to help detect any abnormal conditions. Typical blood tests include the complete blood cell count, cholesterol testing, and a blood glucose test. The collected body fluids are sent to a laboratory for analysis. The doctor may also order X rays or other scans, depending on your condition.

After your doctor examines you, he or she will write down his or her findings, along with the information obtained during the medical history, in your medical record. The doctor will also write down his or her orders to other healthcare workers in the office about your medications, diet, tests, and recommended treatments. Your medical record serves as a means of communication for all of the doctors, specialists, nurses, therapists, and other healthcare workers who care for you. It is a confidential and legal document maintained by professional records management workers. If you would like to have a copy of your medical record, contact the medical records department of your doctor's office or hospital.

Common Screening Tests

Sometimes a physical examination of your body is not enough to tell your doctor the full condition of your health. In such cases the doctor may order a number of common screening tests. Blood tests and urinalysis help the doctor find out if all of the components of your blood or urine are at normal levels. Scanning techniques such as X rays, magnetic resonance imaging (MRI), ultrasound scanning, and computed tomography (CT) scanning produce pictures of the inside of your body without surgery to give your doctor important information about your overall health. If your doctor has ordered one of these tests for you and you don't understand what exactly is going to happen, ask questions so you can feel more comfortable about having the procedure. Diagnostic techniques are changing rapidly, and newer techniques will undoubtedly be available in the near future.

Blood Test

A sample of your blood can provide many clues about the quantity and quality of the individual blood cells and whether your blood can clot normally. To obtain a sample of your blood, a medical technician will draw blood with a needle and syringe from your forearm and send it to a laboratory. At the laboratory, your blood will be analyzed in several ways. Tests will be done to check the number of your red blood cells and the concentration of hemoglobin inside them. Hemoglobin is the substance in red blood cells that carries oxygen throughout the body. A low red blood cell count or too little hemoglobin indicates anemia. Blood tests also will be conducted to detect the number of white blood cells, which have a major part in defending the body against infection. If an infection is present, the number of white blood cells in your blood will rise. The appearance of your blood cells is also important. Abnormally shaped red or white blood cells can signal the presence of diverse conditions such as sickle-cell disease, leukemia, or mononucleosis. Finally, your blood will be checked to see how well it clots by examining the number of blood cells called platelets, which help stop bleeding.

Cholesterol Levels   Elevated levels of the fats known as cholesterol in your blood increase your risk for heart disease. When the excess fats build up inside the walls of your arteries, they narrow the arteries, obstructing blood flow to your heart. When the heart receives less blood, it gets less oxygen, which is transported by red blood cells. Your heart sends out warning signals in the form of pain and discomfort known as angina. When the blockage in the arteries supplying blood to your heart causes severe obstruction, resulting in a heart attack (see page 207), the heart muscle can become permanently damaged.

Cholesterol comes in two forms: low-density lipoprotein (LDL), the "bad" cholesterol, and high-density lipoprotein (HDL), the "good" cholesterol. Somewhat like a delivery truck, LDL cholesterol carries most of the fat in your blood and deposits the excess inside your artery walls. Like a garbage truck, HDL cholesterol removes fat from your blood, preventing it from building up in your arteries. When testing your cholesterol levels, your doctor measures your total blood cholesterol as well as your LDL and HDL levels by taking a sample of your blood and having it analyzed in a laboratory.

A desirable total blood cholesterol level falls under 200 milligrams per deciliter of blood. Doctors consider cholesterol levels above 200 to be high. One in five Americans has a total cholesterol level of 240 or greater, placing that person at risk of a heart attack. Your LDL cholesterol levels should be under 100, and HDL levels should be 40 or higher. The higher your HDL level, the lower your risk for heart disease.

All men over 20 years of age should have their total cholesterol levels checked at least once every 5 years. Your level of LDL cholesterol also should be tested if your HDL is less than 40 or if your total cholesterol is 240 or higher—200 if you have two or more risk factors for heart disease. Talk to your doctor about your personal risk factors for heart disease. Don't hesitate to ask him or her anything you do not understand about cholesterol testing.

Urinalysis

Your urine provides crucial information about the presence of any disorders of the kidneys or bladder. If your doctor orders a urinalysis, you will be asked to pass some urine and collect a midstream sample (urinate for several seconds before collecting the sample of urine) in a small container, either at home or in the doctor's office. If you are uncircumcised, you should pull back your foreskin and wash the tip of your penis with soap and water before urinating to ensure that your urine remains sterile. Your urine may be tested in a laboratory or in the doctor's office, using special strips that the doctor can dip into the urine to test for any abnormalities. The presence of particular substances such as blood or sugar in the urine can indicate certain diseases. For example, the presence of protein in the urine can signal some types of kidney disease.

X ray

The most common scanning test is the X ray, in which electromagnetic radiation passes through a body part to produce a picture of internal structures on film. X rays are a good way of showing dense areas of the body, such as bones or a tumor, that allow only a few rays to pass through. These dense areas show up as white areas on the film. Doctors use X rays to examine the chest, skull, and spine and to view a bone that may have been fractured. Even organs filled with fluid, gas, or air—such as the arteries, colon, or bladder—can be viewed with X rays if the organs are first enhanced with a special liquid dye called a contrast medium. The contrast medium is injected, swallowed, or inserted through the anus; then the doctor or technician takes a series of X rays as the contrast medium moves through the organ to facilitate viewing. Getting an X ray is safe because today's X-ray equipment minimizes your exposure to radiation.

MRI

Magnetic resonance imaging (MRI) uses a magnetic field and radio waves to produce a picture of the inside of the body. When you undergo an MRI, you lie on a table that slides into a rounded scanner containing a doughnut-shaped magnet that creates a magnetic field. Radio waves are sent to the part of your body to be viewed. The atoms in your body respond by emitting energy, and a magnetic field detector measures this energy and sends it to a computer, which translates the signal and creates a picture that your doctor can read. The procedure can take from 30 to 90 minutes and is painless, but the magnetic field can interfere with a pacemaker, hearing aid, or metal implants, so your doctor needs to know if you have any of these devices in your body. MRI scanning poses no known health risks.

Ultrasound

Ultrasound scanning uses sound waves to produce pictures of internal body structures. Doctors often use an ultrasound scan to diagnose disorders of the heart, kidneys, bladder, gallbladder, and pancreas. If your doctor orders an ultrasound scan, you will be asked to lie on a table, and the ultrasound technician will spread a gel on your skin over the area to be scanned. The technician will then move a handheld instrument called a transducer over the area, sending sound waves into your body. The sound waves bounce off of your internal organs, and the transducer transforms the waves into an image on a screen or on paper. Ultrasound is risk-free and is not painful.

CT Scan

Computed tomography (CT) scans take hundreds of X-ray images of the body from different directions that a computer then converts into cross-sectional pictures on a screen. CT scans can pick up details of abnormalities that a conventional X ray cannot detect. Doctors often order a CT scan to check for tumors or other abnormalities in the brain, liver, spleen, lungs, kidneys, pelvis, or lymph nodes (a part of the body's immune system). During a CT scan, you lie on a table that moves into a circular machine. A tube revolves around the machine, taking multiple, low-dose X-ray images from many angles. The procedure takes about 20 minutes. Although a CT scan takes a vast number of images, the amount of radiation generated in a CT scan can be the same as or even less than that from a traditional X ray.

Self-Examinations

In addition to the tests and screenings that your doctor performs during routine checkups, there are two important self-examinations that you should do regularly to detect any early signs of cancer. The testicle self-examination can help you identify any early signs of cancer of the testicle, and the skin self-examination will aid you in spotting early signs of skin cancer.

Testicle Self-Examination

Examining your testicles once a month will help you to become familiar with their normal appearance so you can tell if something unusual turns up. A small, hard, painless lump on or enlargement of a testicle could be a sign of cancer. This type of cancer usually affects young men between the ages of 15 and 35. If another man in your family had cancer of the testicle, your risk is higher than normal. Early detection and treatment of cancer of the testicle is crucial because the cure rate is very high (about 90 percent) when the disorder is found and treated early.

The best time to examine your testicles is after a shower or a bath, when the muscles in your scrotum are relaxed. To examine your testicles, follow these steps:

- While standing in front of a mirror, look for any swelling on the surface of the scrotum.
- Using both hands, examine each testicle by placing your index and middle fingers underneath the testicle with the thumbs placed on top. Gently roll the testicle between the thumbs and fingers. One testicle may seem slightly larger than the other, but that is usually normal.
- Feel for abnormal lumps, about the size of a pea, on the sides or front of each testicle. Abnormal lumps are usually painless. Do not confuse the epididymis (the soft, tubelike structure on top of and behind the testicle) with a lump.

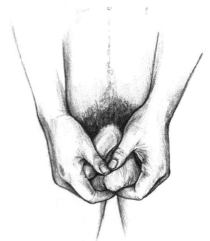

Testicle Self-Examination

If you find a lump, call your doctor right away. The lump may be an infection that requires treatment, or it may be cancer. You should also contact your doctor if one of your testicles has not descended from the abdomen, if you have pain or swelling in your scrotum, or if you feel a collection of veins above one of your testicles. These signs do not indicate the presence of cancer of the testicle but may point to another disorder of the testicles. Only a physician can make an accurate diagnosis. Be sure to see your physician regularly in addition to performing routine self-examinations. Your doctor should examine your testicles during a checkup. He or she also can check the way you perform a testicle self-examination.

Skin Self-Examination

Examining your own skin is the best way to find skin cancer in the early stages, when it is most treatable. This is especially true of malignant melanoma, the most virulent and sometimes deadly form of skin cancer. A skin self-examination should be a regular part of your health routine. To identify abnormal-looking moles, look for the following signs of skin cancer:

ABCD of Moles

 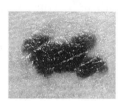 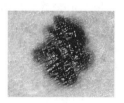 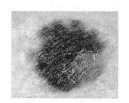

Asymmetry
One half of the mole is a different size or shape than the other half.

Border
The edges of the mole are irregular, notched, or blurred.

Color
The color may be uneven, containing shades of brown, black, white, blue, pink, or red.

Diameter
The mole is typically larger than a pencil eraser (half an inch).

Malignant melanoma may also cause a mole to change in a number of ways, becoming scaly or crusted; oozing; or becoming harder or softer. The mole might change in size, or the skin around the mole could redden, swell, bleed, or itch. A red, scaly patch or a red or flesh-colored nodule could also develop next to the mole. A change in any mole is an important warning sign.

Carefully examine your skin from head to toe every month, including your scalp, the soles of your feet, and between your toes. Use a mirror to check your back, or ask someone else to check it for you. If you see anything unusual, contact your doctor, even if you think it is nothing. Remember that skin cancer is most easily cured when detected early.

Immunizations

Immunizations are not just for children. They continue to be important in adult-hood to protect you from several dangerous infectious diseases, although the number of immunizations you need drops dramatically after age 16. The three most important immunizations are those for tetanus, influenza (flu), and pneu-mococcal disease (a type of pneumonia).

Tetanus is a bacterial infection that affects the central nervous system and can be life-threatening. The bacteria that cause tetanus are found in soil, dust, and animal feces and usually enter the body through an open cut. The bacteria pro-duce a toxin, or poison, in the body that attacks the nervous system, stiffening the muscles. Tetanus is commonly called lockjaw because the muscles in the jaw and neck are affected first. You should get a booster shot of the tetanus vaccine every 10 years throughout adulthood.

Influenza, commonly called the flu, is an infection caused by a virus that affects the respiratory system. Symptoms include fever, chills, headache, muscle aches, and a sore throat. Influenza is spread from person to person through direct contact, such as shaking hands, or by inhaling droplets containing the virus in the air after an infected person coughs or sneezes. New strains of influenza virus appear every year, so you must get a shot of the influenza vaccine yearly, in the fall, just before the flu season starts. Doctors recommend the influenza vaccine for all men over age 65 and for younger men who have medical problems such as heart disease, lung disease, or diabetes or who have close contact with high-risk people.

Pneumococcal disease is caused by a bacterium. It can lead to pneumonia and a number of other serious complications. The most common symptoms are fever, chills, chest pain, a bluish cast to the lips and under the nails, and a cough. You should have a "pneumonia shot" if you are age 65 or over or if you have a long-term health problem such as heart or lung disease, diabetes, or kidney dis-orders. The vaccine is taken once and provides long-term immunity; it can be taken at any time of the year. A person should be revaccinated if he received pneumococcal vaccine in childhood and has a chronic condition such as sickle-cell disease.

Some men may need additional immunizations, depending on several factors. Hepatitis is a potentially serious inflammation of the liver caused by different viruses. The hepatitis A virus is transmitted through food touched by an infected person or in water that has become contaminated with raw sewage. The vaccine for hepatitis A is administered in two doses. Men traveling to countries in which the disease is common should get the first dose at least 4 weeks before departure, but preferably much earlier because the second dose is given 6 to 12 months after the first. The hepatitis B virus is spread through contact with an infected person's blood or other body fluids. Healthcare workers who may be exposed to a patient's body fluids, dialysis patients, people with HIV, and men who live with people infected with hepatitis B are at risk of getting the disease and should be immunized. The hepatitis B vaccine is given in three doses. The second dose is administered 1 month after the first, and the third dose is given 5 months after the second.

A chickenpox (varicella) vaccine is now available for children and for adults who never contracted the disease in childhood. Chickenpox is a very contagious disease that causes only fever and an itchy rash in children. Although rare in adults, chickenpox can be much more serious when contracted in adulthood, causing sterility in men. Ask your doctor if he or she recommends that you get immunized for chickenpox. The vaccine is given in two doses, the second dose 1 to 2 months after the first.

Developing a Good Relationship with Your Doctor

In the past, many people saw the same doctor for years—sometimes for most of their lives. Today, people are much more mobile, making a long-standing patient-doctor relationship more difficult. People move to new locations, accept new jobs, and change healthcare coverage. Any of these situations may require a change of doctors. Some health plans restrict your choice of doctors to those who participate in their plans. Seeing a specialist may entail getting a referral from your primary care doctor. Choosing a new doctor takes more than just a word-of-mouth recommendation from a friend. You need to think carefully about what you are looking for when changing doctors.

The area of medicine in which a doctor specializes is an important consideration. If you have a particular medical problem, such as heart disease, you will probably want to see a cardiologist (a doctor who specializes in diseases of the heart). If you are generally healthy, an internist (a doctor who specializes in the care of adults) or a family physician is probably the best choice. You may also prefer a male doctor over a female doctor. Some people choose a doctor based on the hospital to which he or she admits patients. The location of the doctor's office also is a factor. It should be easy to reach from your home or workplace, especially if you rely on public transportation.

Once you have narrowed your choices, find out more about the doctors you are considering. Important information includes where they trained, how long they have been practicing, and their specialty area and whether they have been certified by the board in that specialty.

To become board-certified, a doctor must have had at least 7 years of medical training and must pass a comprehensive examination in his or her specialty (such as plastic surgery or otolaryngology). To find out if a physician is board-certified, call the American Board of Medical Specialties (ABMS) at 800-776-2378, or, if you have access to the Internet, visit the ABMS Web site (www.abms.org). Also, the American Medical Association's online Doctor Finder (www.ama-assn.org)

provides helpful information such as medical training, specialty, and board certification for more than 650,000 physicians in the United States. The least reliable source of information about doctors is probably paid advertising.

After you have compiled a list of doctors, you will need to check their credentials. There are several good sources of information about doctors. Three reference books—*Directory of Medical Specialists, Compendium of Certified Medical Specialists,* and *The Official ABMS Directory of Board Certified Medical Specialists*—that list board-certified physicians by location are available at your local public library. You also can call your local hospital or the offices of the doctors you are considering to find out the following information:

- *Training.* Where did the doctor attend medical school? Has he or she completed a residency? If so, where?
- *Board certification.* Make sure that your physician has been certified by an appropriate certifying board, such as the American Board of Internal Medicine, the American Board of Surgery, or the American Board of Dermatology.
- *Hospital privileges.* To treat patients at a given hospital, a doctor must gain official approval of his or her peers at that hospital. At which hospital in your community does the physician have staff privileges? Contact the hospital to verify this information.
- *Experience.* For example, if the doctor is a surgeon, how many times has he or she performed the type of surgery you are planning to have? When was the most recent time? The surgeon you select should be up to date on the surgery you are considering.
- *Professional society membership.* Perhaps the most important organization to which a physician can belong is his or her specialty society—the group that represents the medical specialty practiced by the doctor. Specialty societies certify their members and require that they participate in continuing medical education and adhere to a strict code of ethics.

Once you have made your choice, your next step is to develop a good working relationship with your doctor. A good relationship depends on effective communication between you and your doctor. Before you see your doctor for a scheduled visit, think about what you are going to say. Write down important questions you have or symptoms you want to tell the doctor about so you won't forget them. When describing your symptoms, be specific; explain when they started and what you experience when the symptoms occur. Write down the names of all the medications you are taking, including over-the-counter drugs and vitamin or mineral supplements. Remember to bring your notes with you.

Don't hold back any information when the doctor asks you questions about your diet, alcohol or other drug use, smoking, or sexual activity. These factors can affect your health, and the doctor needs to know about them to get a full understanding of your condition and treat your problems appropriately. If you feel embarrassed about talking over sensitive subjects, it's all right to tell your doctor about your discomfort. Rest assured that all of your conversations with your doctor will remain confidential.

Your doctor needs to communicate well with you by fully answering all of your questions and explaining medical terms and procedures in language you can understand. He or she also needs to treat you with respect and keep waiting times to a minimum. If you feel that you are not getting all the information you need to follow your doctor's instructions or that your appointment times are too rushed to address all of your medical concerns, try to talk to your doctor about the problem before switching to another doctor. Keeping an established relationship is much easier and more valuable than starting all over again.

CHAPTER 5
Avoiding Risky Behavior

A wide variety of behaviors are considered risky, which means that they have a high probability of causing or leading to personal harm and, in some cases, death. People usually choose to engage in risky behavior because of the immediate enjoyment it offers and because they are able to convince themselves that the risks are small, or that the risks can be prevented, avoided, or controlled. They may not consider the possible long-term consequences of their behavior. Risk-taking is also sometimes encouraged by others. For example, peer pressure is strong during adolescence because that period is seen as a time of becoming independent and testing limits.

There are risks associated with nearly every activity in which the consequences are unknown or uncertain. Risky behavior can include everything from adventurous activities such as skydiving or mountain climbing to routine activities such as driving to work. Some behaviors, such as gambling or gang activity, carry an identifiable risk of loss or harm that occurs each time they are performed. For other activities, such as cigarette smoking, the resulting harm often occurs in the longer term. Because of this delayed impact, people often ignore or deny the risk involved.

Many of the health risks for today's children and adolescents are related to behavior and lifestyle. For example, risky behaviors (such as drug use and smoking) and failure to follow the basics of a healthy lifestyle (such as exercising regularly and eating a healthy diet) can contribute to poor health in both children and adolescents. A variety of personality traits have been identified in young children that can be used to predict risky behavior later in life. These traits include tolerance for deviance, rebelliousness, nontraditional values, emphasis on autonomy, inability to delay gratification, deemphasis on achievement, self-centeredness, and low self-esteem.

Environmental influences on behavior during childhood include parental and peer attitudes and behavior and the impact of the wider environment (such as the media). Even in younger children, multiple influences can affect the use of (or intention to use) alcohol and other drugs. In many cases, a child's intentions to use alcohol can be predicted by whether his peers drink (or whether he thinks they do), whether family members drink, the child's involvement in family drinking, and the child's tendency toward risk-taking.

Risky Behavior of Teenagers

The greatest number of deaths among teenagers are attributable to accidents, unintentional injuries, homicides, and suicides. This means that most deaths among teenagers are related to their behavior, rather than to disease or other natural causes. Other examples of national trends in risky behavior among teenagers include the following:

- Across all races, teenage boys die more frequently than teenage girls because of accidents, injuries, homicides, or suicides.
- Adolescents are starting risky behavior at an earlier age.
- Cigarette smoking among teenagers is on the increase, even as smoking is declining for all other age groups.
- After a decline in illicit drug use among teenagers, it is again on the increase.
- More than two thirds of students have had sexual intercourse by their senior year of high school (although the incidence of teenage pregnancy is decreasing).

The greatest danger to male teenagers seems to be that a significant percentage of them multiply their risks by engaging in more than one risky behavior. Teens who become involved in one risky behavior at an early age are more likely to take other risks. For example, boys or young men who use drugs or have school problems or past criminal involvement are more likely to be sexually active.

The higher incidence of problem behaviors among teenage males suggests that the origin of these behaviors rests in genetic differences between boys and girls and in differences in social expectations about behavior. Levels of the male hormone testosterone may influence the development of problem behavior in 13-year-old boys. But the association between hormone levels and problem behavior does not persist as boys get older. During this later period, problem behavior seems to be self-perpetuating, independent of testosterone levels at that time, and more influenced by social and psychological factors. Also, there is evidence that risky behavior is also on the rise among adolescent females in urban areas across the United States, a trend that cannot be explained by testosterone levels.

Boys and young men who strongly endorse a traditional view of masculinity appear to be more likely to engage in risky behaviors, such as getting suspended from school, drinking, using drugs, having multiple sexual partners, forcing someone to have sex, or not using condoms consistently. Mistaken beliefs about being tough and getting respect, which are traditionally part of the popular concept of manhood in the United States, may lead young men to engage in behaviors that endanger their health.

Preventive health programs around the United States have typically focused on single behaviors or problems, but new approaches to prevention are emerging. For example, new prevention efforts are more broadly based and deal more with the interrelationships among various types of risky behaviors within the context of the family, neighborhood, and peer group in which these risky behaviors arise.

Alcohol and Other Drugs

Dependence on alcohol and other drugs, also called addiction, poses a triple threat to the dependent person and to society as a whole. It increases the probability that a person will do something potentially harmful, such as acting in a violent or careless manner. It leads to impaired judgment that affects certain everyday activities, such as driving a car, thereby increasing the risk of injury or death. And it creates chemical imbalances in the brain and the body that increase the risk of illness and death. Nicotine, the drug found in cigarettes and other tobacco products, is extremely addictive.

Drug Dependence

A person who uses a drug for other than a recommended or prescribed purpose is said to be abusing that drug. Drug dependence (or addiction) is an uncontrollable craving for a particular substance, which can, in some cases, take over a person's life. A person who is psychologically dependent on a drug experiences emotional distress when the drug is withdrawn. Physical dependence means that the body has adapted to the presence of the drug, causing symptoms of withdrawal when deprived of it.

Drugs that can cause addiction fall into three general categories: those that depress the central nervous system, those that stimulate the central nervous system, and those that produce hallucinations and also affect the central nervous system.

Drugs That Depress the Central Nervous System   A person who is addicted to a drug that depresses the central nervous system is both psychologically and physically dependent.

• Examples are opiates such as codeine, heroin, and morphine; barbiturates; alcohol; and antianxiety drugs.

- Short-term effects include euphoria, relief from pain, and prevention of withdrawal symptoms.
- Long-term effects include depression, malnutrition, constipation, and, when injected from a contaminated needle, an increased risk of infection with HIV or hepatitis B.
- Withdrawal symptoms for opiates include weakness, sweating, and chills, progressing to vomiting, diarrhea, and sometimes cardiac collapse, which can be fatal. Withdrawal symptoms for barbiturates and antianxiety drugs include tremor, anxiety, restlessness, and weakness, sometimes progressing to hallucinations and seizures. Withdrawal symptoms for alcohol include trembling hands, sweating, nausea, and, in some cases, cramps and vomiting. Other severe withdrawal symptoms for alcohol may include confusion, hallucinations, and seizures.

Drugs That Stimulate the Central Nervous System   Tolerance builds up quickly with drugs that stimulate the central nervous system, which means that a person must take increasingly large doses to achieve the same effects.

- Examples are cocaine and amphetamines.
- Short-term effects include excitation, sleeplessness, hyperactivity, and euphoria.
- Long-term effects include hallucinations, delusions, and depression.
- Withdrawal symptoms include severe depression, sleeplessness, mood swings, headaches, muscle pain, apathy, and drug cravings that may last up to a year.

Drugs That Produce Hallucinations   Hallucinogens do not produce physical dependence, so there are no withdrawal symptoms, but they may produce psychological dependence and genetic damage.

- Examples are LSD and mescaline.
- Short-term effects include exhilaration, sensory distortion, illusions, paranoia, and panic.
- Long-term effects include flashbacks.

Some people are more susceptible than others to drug dependence for reasons that may include both genetic and environmental factors. Heavy use of any addictive drug may encourage the use of other drugs; adolescents who use alcohol, tobacco, or marijuana are more likely than their peers who don't use these drugs to use cocaine or heroin eventually. In general, the younger people are when they start and the more types of drugs they use, the greater their risk of addiction.

People start taking a drug for a variety of reasons. They may be having problems coping with a difficult situation, such as divorce or unemployment. They may be bored or curious or under pressure to conform to the behavior patterns of their peers. Most do not realize that they are risking becoming dependent on the drug. Dependence not only causes physical problems such as lung and heart disease from tobacco smoking and liver disease from drinking excessive amounts of alcohol, but it also contributes substantially to the breakdown of families, to unemployment, and—in some cases—to crime.

Effective treatment for drug dependence consists of both physical detoxification and mental and social rehabilitation. Detoxification, or withdrawal of the drug gradually over a period of a week to 10 days, is usually done in a controlled setting such as a hospital, where the person's physical symptoms can be treated. Sometimes a less harmful drug with similar effects is substituted, such as methadone for heroin. Formal rehabilitation programs, which may include therapeutic communities and may use self-help groups such as Narcotics Anonymous or Alcoholics Anonymous, have been shown to greatly increase a person's chances of staying off drugs permanently.

Alcohol

Alcohol is the most commonly used drug in the United States. Nearly 14 million Americans are dependent on it or have other problems associated with drinking. These problems cost the nation more than $100 billion annually in medical care and lost productivity. Alcohol accounts for one of every 20 deaths and one of every four hospital stays. Nearly 60 percent of all violent acts—including murders, child abuse, family abuse, and other felonies—are associated with the consumption of alcohol. Alcohol dependence is a chronic disease characterized by a tendency to drink more than was intended, unsuccessful attempts to stop drinking, and continued drinking in the face of adverse consequences.

Moderate drinking—two drinks a day for men—has been found to have health benefits. Statistically, moderate drinkers live longer than both nondrinkers and heavy drinkers, reflecting alcohol's ability to reduce some of the risks associated with heart attack, stroke, and diabetes. For example, alcohol lowers low-density lipoprotein (LDL), the "bad" cholesterol, and elevates high-density lipoprotein (HDL), the "good" cholesterol that protects against clogged arteries. Alcohol also helps prevent the formation of blood clots and increases estrogen production in postmenopausal women. Many people, however, find it impossible to drink in moderation. If you have questions about the benefits versus the risks of having one or two drinks a day, talk to your physician.

Alcohol's Effects on the Brain   Alcohol exerts its effects by altering the function of different chemical messengers (neurotransmitters) in the brain. The initial effects of alcohol are to mildly sedate the brain: the drinker becomes a little less inhibited and anxious. The second and third drinks affect the brain's pleasure center, located in the lower midbrain, producing an emotional high.

The pleasure center evolved in all animals to ensure survival. Although the mechanism is not fully understood, sex, eating, and other behaviors that enhance evolutionary adaptation and survival produce pleasurable feelings that make people want to repeat those behaviors again and again. Sensory inputs and thoughts are sorted out by the pleasure center in the brain and tagged as being good (pleasurable) or bad (hurtful or unimportant). Good things are remembered, unimportant things forgotten, and bad things feared. This is one of the ways we learn, but it is also the process that underlies addiction to alcohol and, very likely, other drugs. Once rewarded for something, such as alcohol intake, with an emotional high, we want to do it again.

Alcohol does not affect all people in the same way. Genetic differences may account for variations in the way the pleasure center responds to alcohol. There is, however, no single "alcoholism gene." Most likely, many genes are involved in a person's response to alcohol, and these genes interact in different combinations with environmental influences, such as peer pressure and the availability of alcohol. As the genetic contribution to alcohol becomes better understood, it may be possible to test for genetic susceptibility to alcoholism.

Men are four times more likely than women to become dependent on alcohol. As with other addictions, those who cannot stop drinking eventually have difficulty maintaining personal relationships and taking care of themselves. People who are dependent on alcohol often fail to eat properly or get adequate rest, which can lead to serious health problems.

Codependence   Family members and friends who act in ways that allow a person to continue to misuse alcohol or other drugs are considered to be codependents or enablers. These people often make excuses for the addicted person's behavior, such as calling in sick to work for him or her, to hide the problem from others. A person who is codependent may plead with a loved one to stop using alcohol or other drugs but rarely does anything else to help the person change the harmful behavior.

The best thing family and friends can do is to encourage the person who is addicted not only to stop taking drugs but also to enter a treatment program. Threats to withdraw regular contact or support, combined with professional intervention or counseling, may be the only way to persuade him or her to seek help.

Prevention and Treatment   The following steps can help prevent the development of alcohol dependence:

- Limit your drinking to no more than two drinks a day.
- Drink slowly; do not have more than one drink per hour.
- Never drink to relieve anxiety, tension, or depression, or on an empty stomach.
- Do not feel embarrassed for refusing an alcoholic drink at a social occasion.

No single form of treatment works for everyone who is dependent on alcohol. Several different approaches may be used, often in combination:

- Psychological treatment usually involves psychotherapy on a one-on-one or family basis, or is carried out in groups using a variety of talk therapies.
- Social treatments often address problems at work and include family members in the treatment process.
- Physical treatment, needed by some people who are dependent on alcohol, may use a deterrent drug such as disulfiram to sensitize the person to alcohol. The drug causes extremely unpleasant symptoms when a person drinks, so that he or she eventually becomes reluctant to do so.
- Self-help organizations such as Alcoholics Anonymous (AA) are a particularly helpful form of support for people who are trying to quit drinking.

Some people require medical help in getting through physical withdrawal when they stop drinking. This process of detoxification, which takes 4 to 7 days, is usually followed by long-term treatment.

Do You Have a Drinking Problem?

If you have any doubt about your level of alcohol consumption or your ability to control it, consider these questions:

- Has a friend or a family member ever expressed concern about your drinking?
- Has such concern annoyed you?
- Do you frequently drink alone?
- Do you try to conceal your drinking?
- Do you drink to relax, relieve stress, overcome shyness, or go to sleep?
- Have you ever felt the need to cut down on your drinking?
- Have you ever felt guilty for drinking?
- Do you ever have a drink first thing in the morning?
- Have you ever missed or been late for work because of a hangover?
- Have you gotten into arguments when you have been drinking?
- Have you ever had an automobile accident or even a close call when you have been drinking?
- Have you sprained an ankle or had other injuries while drinking?
- After drinking, have you had sex with someone you would not have had sex with if you were sober?
- Have you hit your children or your partner while drinking?
- Have you gotten sick when drinking?

If you answered yes to any of these questions, you may be addicted to alcohol. If you think that you—or someone you love—has a drinking problem, seek help immediately. Stopping now will significantly improve your life and your health, no matter how long you have been drinking. Here is how you can get help:

- Ask your doctor for the name of a healthcare professional who specializes in treatment for alcohol dependency.
- Call the employee assistance program where you work.
- Call nearby hospitals or a local mental health center to ask if they provide a program for alcohol addiction.
- Call the local chapter of AA, a support group of alcoholics who meet regularly to help each other stop drinking and stay sober.
- If you are concerned about the drinking of a family member or a friend, call the local chapter of Al-Anon, a support group for relatives and friends of alcoholics.

Tobacco

Smoking, directly and indirectly, causes more death and illness in the United States than any other single activity. Each year, more than 300,000 Americans die of smoking-related illnesses, including lung cancer, emphysema, and heart disease. Although the incidence of smoking among men has declined to about 32 percent from its peak of 54 percent in the mid-1950s, smoking remains one of the most difficult habits to kick. Much of what is known today about the harmful effects of tobacco was learned from medical studies of the effects of cigarette smoking on the lungs. The effects of smoke from cigars and pipes are also dangerous, although in somewhat different ways.

Harmful Effects of Smoking   The risk of developing lung cancer is 10 times greater for cigarette smokers than for nonsmokers. Decades of study in many countries have shown a direct link between smoking and lung cancer. Since cigar and pipe smokers do not inhale as much tobacco smoke, they have a slightly lower risk of lung cancer, but the risk is still significantly higher than it is for nonsmokers. Tar and nicotine, as well as smoke, play a role in the development of lung cancer. The risks for lung cancer increase proportionately with the number of cigarettes smoked, the length of time the person has smoked, the age at which the person started smoking, and the amount of smoke inhaled.

Other types of cancer caused by cigarette smoking include cancers of the throat, esophagus, bladder, kidney, pancreas, and mouth. Pipe and cigar smokers also have an increased risk for cancers of the lip and mouth. Since some of the tars in tobacco are swallowed, there is also an increased risk of stomach cancer.

Respiratory diseases associated with smoking include chronic bronchitis, sinusitis, and emphysema. Each year in the United States, these diseases account for tens of thousands of deaths from respiratory failure. Cigarette smoking slows down the action of the cilia, tiny hairlike projections that line the airways and help clean the lungs. When the cilia are immobilized, dust and dirt particles are able to invade the lungs and cause inflammation. As a result, cigarette smokers also have more chronic coughs, phlegm production, wheezing, and other respiratory symptoms. People with allergies and asthma are particularly vulnerable to the negative effects of cigarette smoke.

For men, the most significant health hazard of smoking is coronary artery disease—the most common cause of death in men in the United States. A young man who smokes 20 cigarettes a day is three times more likely than a nonsmoker to develop coronary artery disease. The risk increases proportionately with the number of cigarettes smoked. Smokers have been shown to have severe and extensive narrowing of their coronary arteries, the vessels that deliver blood to the heart muscle. They also have higher blood levels of LDL (low-density lipoprotein), the "bad" cholesterol, and are more likely to have high blood pressure.

Smoking lowers the threshold for the onset of angina, chest pain associated with heart disease, and is a major risk factor for peripheral vascular disease, which affects the arteries of the legs, causing painful neuropathy (degeneration of the nerve endings). Smoking also affects the arteries leading to the brain, thereby increasing the risk for stroke.

Physiological Effects of Smoking   Scientists now understand the details of how and why smoking is able to exert so many different negative effects on many parts of the body. The smoke from a lighted cigarette contains a mixture of more than 3,000 different substances that are dangerous to living tissue. In addition, tobacco products contain hundreds of chemical additives used as flavors and fillers. No federal agency currently has the authority to require the tobacco industry to reveal the names of these additives, or to remove them from tobacco products if they are found to be harmful. These substances in cigarettes include tars, nicotine, and gases such as carbon monoxide, nitrogen oxide, and hydrogen cyanide. Together, these substances interact to create a huge number of different chemical compounds that have harmful effects on the body. Tobacco tar is made up of hundreds of chemicals that have been shown to cause cancer.

Nicotine is the addictive substance in tobacco. The signs of addiction include tolerance (the need to take larger doses to produce the same effects), physical dependence, continued use despite known harmful effects, euphoric effects, relapses following drug abstinence, and recurrent drug cravings. Nicotine is inhaled, along with tars and carbon monoxide, in tobacco smoke. Nicotine in smokeless tobacco is absorbed through the mucous membranes in the mouth (chewing tobacco) or the nose (snuff). Nicotine acts primarily on the nervous system, often causing an increased heart rate and elevated blood pressure.

Nearly 90 percent of the nicotine found in cigarettes is inhaled and absorbed into the bloodstream. In addition to its effects on the respiratory system and the gastrointestinal system, nicotine also affects the brain, the spinal cord, and the peripheral nervous system. Nicotine can stimulate, then depress, the production of saliva, constrict the air passages in the lungs, and increase cholesterol levels in the bloodstream.

Carbon monoxide is a deadly gas that is a by-product of burning tobacco. It is the same pollutant that is found in automobile exhaust. Carbon monoxide is deadly because it displaces the oxygen molecules in red blood cells, making oxygen less available to your muscles, brain, heart, and other organs. It also damages the lining of arteries, causing atherosclerosis (the buildup of fatty deposits called plaque in the inner lining of the arteries that supply blood to the heart). As a result, the heart must pump harder to deliver an adequate supply of oxygen to the cells.

Smokeless Tobacco   Smokeless (chewing) tobacco has been making a gradual resurgence in the United States for the past 20 years. Advertisers have presented smokeless tobacco as a healthier alternative to smoking, using the macho image of tobacco-chewing cowboys and athletes to promote their products. Apparently these advertisements have been effective, as indicated by an increase of 52 percent in sales of smokeless tobacco since 1978. It is estimated that 7 million to 11 million Americans, mostly males, use smokeless tobacco.

Smokeless tobacco comes in three forms: loose leaf, plugs, and snuff. Chewing tobacco may be packaged as loose-leaf tobacco, which is sold in a pouch. The user places the tobacco between the cheek and the gum, and when a certain amount of tobacco juice and saliva are accumulated in the mouth, it is spit out. Chewing tobacco also can be found as plug tobacco, which is a solid brick form of tobacco. The user cuts off a piece with a knife and chews it, and again, spits it out. Snuff is a finely ground tobacco, sold in cans, that is put on the back of the hand and sniffed through the nose. It also can be placed between the cheek and the gum.

Despite its macho appeal to men, few women find tobacco chewing attractive. Users of smokeless tobacco may not experience the effects of carbon monoxide, but the substance has plenty of other harmful effects, including:

- damage to the soft and hard tissues in the mouth
- excessive abrasion of tooth surfaces
- presence of nitrosonornicotine, a cancer-causing agent
- increase in heart rate and blood pressure
- development of leukoplakia, a disease that results in thick, white patches on the cheek, tongue, and other parts of the mouth
- cancer of the inner lining of the cheek
- suppressed immune response
- increase in the number of dental cavities
- inflammation of the gums
- cancers of the pharynx, esophagus, bladder, and pancreas
- darkened teeth and bad breath

Secondhand Smoke   Breathing in smoke from someone else's tobacco presents a significant risk to a nonsmoker's health. Exposure to so-called secondhand smoke (sometimes referred to as passive smoking) is a significant cause of heart disease, stroke, lung cancer, and respiratory problems such as bronchitis.

Two different types of smoke enter the air when a person smokes: exhaled smoke and the smoke that comes directly from the burning tobacco. This second, more dangerous type of smoke is what hovers in the air in smoke-filled rooms.

Secondhand smoke is especially harmful to infants and young children. Smoking by parents is known to worsen asthma in children and even to trigger asthma attacks. Children without asthma whose parents smoke have far more respiratory illnesses—coughs, colds, middle ear infections, pneumonia, and bronchitis—than children of nonsmokers.

How to Quit   If you are a smoker, kicking the habit could be the single most important thing you do for your health and your family's health. It's not easy, but millions of people have quit smoking on their own. Many programs are now available to help. The American Cancer Society (800-227-2345) and the American Lung Association (800-LUNG-USA) offer excellent support resources and information for those who want to quit on their own. You can also check your Yellow Pages for listings of other smoking treatment programs and support groups.

Most successful stop-smoking programs suggest that you tackle the job in three stages: preparation, quitting, and reinforcement. The following tips will help you prepare to quit smoking:

- Choose a target date to quit, such as a birthday or an anniversary, and stick to it.
- Make a list of reasons for quitting, and review it carefully.
- Note your smoking habits and routines; plan activities that would disrupt them.
- Condition yourself physically: start a modest exercise program, drink more fluids, and get plenty of rest.
- Think of alternative activities to do when the urge to smoke is strong.
- Go public with your intentions to quit, and gain the support of friends and family.
- If possible, get someone to quit with you.

The following tips will help you quit smoking:

- Don't be discouraged by the thought of never smoking again; think one day at a time.
- Clean your clothes to rid them of the cigarette smell.
- Get rid of all cigarettes, ashtrays, and lighters at home, in your car, and in your office at work.

- On the day you quit, keep busy: go to a movie, exercise, take long walks, buy yourself a treat, or do something special to celebrate.
- Visit the dentist and have your teeth cleaned.
- The first few weeks, spend as much free time as possible in places where smoking is not allowed.
- Avoid alcohol, coffee, and other beverages associated with smoking, but drink large quantities of water and fruit juice.

Once you have successfully quit smoking, here are some tips for helping you stay away from cigarettes:

- Keep healthy substitutes handy, such as carrots, sunflower seeds, raisins, or sugarless gum.
- Learn how to relax quickly and deeply: make yourself limp; visualize a soothing, pleasing situation; and get away from it all for a moment.
- Participate in activities that make it hard to smoke such as jogging or swimming.
- Do things that keep your hands busy such as crossword puzzles or gardening; while watching television, play with a paper clip, a pencil, or a rubber ball.
- Stretch a lot.
- Pay attention to your appearance.
- Never allow yourself to think that "one cigarette won't hurt."
- Get up from the dinner table as soon as you're finished eating and brush your teeth.
- If you are concerned about gaining weight, join an exercise group, plan menus carefully, and weigh yourself weekly; don't try to lose weight, just try to maintain your prequitting weight. Keep in mind that the benefits of giving up cigarettes far outweigh the drawbacks of gaining a few pounds.

Most smokers successfully quit only after several attempts. You may be lucky enough to quit on your first try, but if not, don't give up. Try again.

A number of products are now available to help break the smoking habit. These include nicotine patches, nicotine gum, nicotine inhalers, and drugs such as bupropion hydrochloride. The patches and gum provide a low dose of nicotine that can be used to wean your body off the drug. Bupropion hydrochloride is a nicotine-free pill that can help reduce your urge to smoke. Other approaches to quitting smoking include hypnosis, acupuncture, behavior modification, and meditation. Your physician can give you more information on smoking-cessation programs and products.

Illegal Drugs

In addition to the physical and social problems caused by dependence on drugs such as alcohol, people who become dependent on an illegal substance risk penalties for violating drug control laws and their personal safety when procuring drugs. Those who use unsterilized needles also risk exposure to HIV, hepatitis, and other sexually transmitted diseases that are transmitted through contaminated blood. More than other addictive substances, illegal drugs are a powerful force behind criminal activity that destroys families and neighborhoods, and overwhelms prisons.

If you feel you are unable to stop using illegal drugs on your own, you will need professional help to quit. Although quitting is something only you can do, it is not likely that you can quit by yourself. Talk to your doctor, or call your local hospital or clinic to ask about their drug treatment programs.

Cocaine Whether sniffed as a powder, injected as a liquid, or smoked (freebasing), cocaine acts as both a stimulant and a local anesthetic, producing a rush of euphoria and energy. Its effects wear off quickly, often leading users to take another dose in a short time. Cocaine is derived from the leaves of the South American coca bush. Crack cocaine, the purest form of the substance, is especially lethal because its effects are more intense and can lead to cardiac arrest.

The euphoria caused by cocaine use is intense but short-lived and usually followed by depression as the drug wears off. The drug causes the coronary arteries to constrict, boosting blood pressure and, with it, the risk of heart attack, stroke, and seizures. Regular use of cocaine often causes nervousness, insomnia, inability to concentrate, fatigue, depression, or anxiety; some people become aggressive, violent, or paranoid. Side effects include nausea and vomiting, bleeding of mucous membranes, and cold sweats. Cocaine also can cause hallucinations, abnormal heart rhythm, coma, and death.

A very ill person who is dependent on cocaine may need to be hospitalized. All people who are addicted to cocaine should seek counseling and rehabilitation to overcome their addiction.

Club Drugs So-called club drugs such as ecstasy, rohypnol, GHB, and ketamine are synthetic drugs made in illegal production facilities. These drugs are being used increasingly by teens and young adults as part of a nightlife scene at nightclubs, bars, and "raves." Many young people experiment with a variety of these drugs together. Combining any of these drugs with alcohol can lead to severe reactions and death.

Ecstasy comes in pill form and also can be inhaled or injected. The effects of ecstasy are similar to those of amphetamines and cocaine. Psychological effects include confusion, depression, sleep problems, severe anxiety, and paranoia. Physical effects include muscle tension, involuntary teeth clenching, nausea, blurred vision, faintness, and chills or sweating. Use of the drug is associated with increases in heart rate and blood pressure. Ecstasy also has been linked to long-term damage to those parts of the brain that are critical to thought, memory, and pleasure.

Rohypnol, GHB, and ketamine depress the central nervous system, inducing a state of dazed relaxation. They have been implicated in cases of date rape; because they are often colorless, tasteless, and odorless, they can be slipped easily into an unsuspecting victim's drink. Rohypnol can be fatal when mixed with alcohol or other depressants. Abuse of GHB can produce withdrawal effects such as insomnia, anxiety, tremors, and sweating, and can cause coma and seizures, especially when combined with ecstasy. Sometimes ketamine is used as an alternative to cocaine and usually is snorted.

Heroin   Heroin is an opiate, which means it comes from the opium poppy. Like other opiates, it can be eaten, inhaled, smoked, or injected. Because the body quickly builds up a tolerance to heroin, users can become addicted rapidly. The euphoric and tranquilizing effects of heroin come at a high price: regular use can lead to kidney dysfunction, pneumonia, lung abscesses, and brain disorders, depending on how the drug is taken. Those who inject the drug also risk skin abscesses, phlebitis (inflammation of a vein, often accompanied by formation of a blood clot), scarring, hepatitis, and HIV infection.

The drug methadone, itself addictive but much less so than heroin, is often used to treat heroin addiction; the person may need to take it for the rest of his or her life. Methadone treatment is usually given on an outpatient basis under a physician's supervision.

Marijuana   The most widely used illegal drug is marijuana, made from the leaves of the hemp plant. The drug is typically smoked in joints (cigarettes). People use marijuana to feel good and to relax. The drug can cause a distorted sense of time and a reduced ability to think and communicate clearly. Other side effects can include problems with depth perception and short-term memory, impaired motor abilities, bloodshot eyes, dry mouth, and—with chronic use—paranoia, panic, and hallucinations.

Like cigarette smoke, marijuana smoke impairs the lung's defenses against infection and can lead to bronchitis and emphysema. Smoking marijuana may pose even more of a cancer danger than cigarettes because marijuana smoke contains more of a potent cancer-causing substance than tobacco smoke and because people who smoke marijuana inhale the smoke more deeply into their lungs.

Heavy, long-term use of marijuana can cause a psychological addiction that can lead to loss of energy, ambition, and drive. People who are psychologically addicted to marijuana tend to have difficulty dealing with normal, everyday stress.

LSD   Lysergic acid diethylamide (LSD) is a powerful hallucinogen that induces a wide range of psychological effects, which can be enjoyable, terrifying, or both. "Bad trips" can cause paranoia and panic, but even ordinary episodes of LSD use can involve:

- depressed appetite
- loss of sexual desire
- distorted perceptions
- difficulty communicating
- feelings of paralysis
- hyperactivity
- dilated pupils
- increased heart rate and blood pressure
- sleeplessness
- tremors

In whatever form it is taken (blotter paper, sugar cubes, gelatin squares, or small tablets) the effects of LSD are unpredictable, in part because it is impossible to know the exact dose you are getting and in part because the effects are influenced by the user's personality and mood. A single dose of LSD can last for 12 to 18 hours, and many users experience flashbacks—recurring memories of some aspects of their experiences using the drug—for up to a year.

LSD is not considered to be addictive but, like addictive drugs, LSD can produce tolerance, which causes people who use the drug regularly to take increasingly higher doses to get the same effects. In susceptible people, LSD use may contribute to the development of mental disorders such as schizophrenia and severe depression.

Unsafe Sex

Unsafe sexual practices are the primary means for spreading sexually transmitted diseases (STDs; see page 180). Practicing safer sex not only protects your health but also the health of your partner (or future partners), as well as the health of any children you may have in the future (some STDs can be passed from a woman to a fetus and cause birth defects).

Condom use by American teenagers appears to be decreasing. For many adolescent males, as their sexual activity increases with age, their condom use decreases. This decrease in condom use may reflect one or both of the partners' primary concern with avoiding pregnancy rather than preventing the spread of STDs. As these males age, they tend to switch from reliance on condoms to use of female contraceptive methods, especially oral contraceptives (the pill). And because their level of sexual activity increases at the same time, they run a much greater risk of contracting HIV and other STDs. The young man may have one steady girlfriend who takes the pill, but he also may have sex with other partners. Unmarried males of all ages are much more likely than females to have multiple sexual partners and therefore are more likely to be exposed to STDs.

Safer sex requires taking precautions. The only guarantee against STDs is to refrain from sexual contact. If you are planning to have sexual intercourse, discuss safer sex practices with your partner—well in advance, if possible. Although you may feel uncomfortable talking about such issues with a potential sexual partner, don't let embarrassment stand in the way of your health and safety. For more information about safer sex practices, see page 181.

Safer Oral Sex

Many teenagers avoid having sexual intercourse as a way to "abstain" from having sex. Instead, they are increasingly engaging in non-intercourse sexual activities such as oral sex, which they think are safe and risk-free. They don't realize that they can contract many STDs—including chlamydia, gonorrhea, herpes, genital warts, and HIV—through oral sex. Safer oral sex is just as important as safer vaginal or anal sex. Always use a non-lubricated latex condom for oral sex. For oral sex on a woman, cover the vagina with a non-lubricated latex condom that has been cut open, a piece of plastic wrap, or a dental dam (a small sheet of latex that you can buy in drugstores).

Unsafe Driving Habits

Risky behavior is involved in the traffic accidents that kill more than 40,000 Americans each year. Driving while drunk accounts for the majority of serious traffic accidents, and more than half of all road-related fatalities are automobile passengers who might have lived had they used seat belts.

Never drive under the influence of alcohol. It slows your reaction times, distorts your vision, and impairs your judgment. And never use other psychoactive drugs (those that alter your mind or behavior, such as marijuana or methamphetamine) while driving. Be sure to read the labels on all prescription and over-the-counter medications for warnings about how they could affect your ability to drive.

Safety with Seat Belts

Every motor vehicle crash has two collisions. The first is a collision of the car with another object. But the second is more important in terms of life and death. That's when the driver or passenger collides with the vehicle's interior or is thrown out of the vehicle to collide with the ground, another car, or an object such as a wall.

Ejection from a vehicle occurs 10 times more often to occupants who are not wearing seat belts. The best protection for people in a collision is to use lap belts and shoulder restraints. In a head-on collision, these safety restraints can dramatically reduce the chance of injury to the head or the face and cut in half the risk of serious or fatal injury. Every person in the car must wear a seat belt. It's the law, and it can save your life.

If you transport small children (age 6 and under), be sure your car is equipped with a child safety seat for each child. Be sure the child safety seat is installed and secured to the vehicle's backseat the way the manufacturer recommends. Children always must ride in the backseat. Children who are too large for a child safety seat must wear a seat belt. Children who are not protected by safety restraints face increased risk of serious injury. (Traffic injuries are a leading cause of death for children.) During a crash, an unrestrained child becomes an uncontrolled missile that can crash through a windshield or careen into any object or person in the vehicle.

Do not consider air bags a substitute for safety belts. Air bags are designed to inflate only during head-on collisions and are useful only as supplements for seat belts. Also, air bags offer no protection during multiple crashes, rollovers, or side collisions. Air bags have been the cause of a number of serious injuries to children and several deaths. They are one of many reasons that children always should ride in back.

Road Rage

Another type of risky behavior that has emerged in recent years is known as "road rage." It is estimated that as many as 1,500 people are killed or injured on American highways each year as a result of aggressive driving. No single profile fits all aggressive drivers, but they are three times more likely to be male than female, generally between ages 18 and 26, and usually have no record of crime, violence, or illegal drug use.

Although the risks of becoming a victim of road rage are small, if you encounter a threatening driver, the most important thing you can do is defuse the situation by not reacting. Staying safe on the road is a two-part process. Avoid behaviors that could be interpreted as confrontational, such as:

- sudden acceleration
- blocking the passing lane
- tailgating
- braking or swerving, which could cause you to lose control of your car
- cutting off another driver or failing to signal when changing lanes
- making obscene gestures
- failing to dim high beams for oncoming traffic
- taking up multiple parking spaces or damaging another vehicle while parking

All drivers need to control their stress to avoid situations in which they become angry with discourteous or aggressive drivers. A few simple changes in the way you approach driving can significantly reduce stress, including:

- altering your schedule to avoid congestion
- improving the comfort of your vehicle
- concentrating on being relaxed (but not to the point of being distracted)
- not driving when you are angry, upset, or overtired

As a driver, you cannot control traffic, only your reaction to it. Give the other driver the benefit of the doubt. Assume that other drivers' mistakes are not intentional or aimed at you personally.

Addictive Gambling

Compulsive gambling is an addiction, like alcohol dependence or other drug addiction. Because no physical substance is ingested, gambling has been called the purest form of addiction. Although it is strictly psychological, the uncontrollable impulse to gamble can become overwhelming and eventually cause major disruption in a person's life—including loss of job, financial ruin, a broken home, criminal activity, and loss of self-respect and the respect of others. Many people have the potential to become addicted to gambling.

The term "problem gambling" includes but is not limited to the condition known as compulsive gambling. Gambling, like other addictions, is a progressive illness that cannot be cured, only kept under control. The growth and popularity of state lotteries, as well as gambling casinos on America's rivers and lakes (and land-based casinos in some states), has made gambling easily available. Horse racing, dog racing, and private illegal gambling operations attract many additional gamblers.

You may be addicted to gambling if five (or more) of the following factors apply to you:

- being preoccupied with gambling (such as reliving past gambling experiences, planning the next gambling venture, thinking of ways to get money for gambling, or fantasizing about how to spend the money once you win)
- wanting to gamble with increasing amounts of money to achieve the desired level of excitement
- trying repeatedly, but unsuccessfully, to control, cut back on, or stop gambling
- being restless or irritable when attempting to cut down on or stop gambling
- using gambling as a way of escaping problems or of relieving feelings of helplessness, guilt, anxiety, or depression
- returning another day to get even after losing money gambling
- lying to family members, a therapist, or others to conceal the extent of your involvement with gambling
- committing illegal acts such as forgery, fraud, theft, or embezzlement to finance your gambling
- losing a significant relationship, job, or educational or career opportunity because of gambling

- relying on others to provide money to relieve a desperate financial situation caused by gambling

Many addicted gamblers have the following personality traits:

- *An inability or an unwillingness to accept reality.* This attitude can lead them to escape into the world of gambling.
- *Emotional insecurity.* A compulsive gambler finds that he or she is most emotionally comfortable when gambling.
- *Immaturity.* Many gamblers seem to have a hard time accepting responsibility. They want to have all the good things in life without any great effort on their part.

If you think you may have a problem with gambling, talk to your doctor. He or she may be able to refer you to a mental health professional who can help you overcome your addiction. For more information, contact the National Council on Problem Gambling, Inc. (800-522-4700) or Gamblers Anonymous (213-386-8789) or consult your local telephone directory.

CHAPTER 6

Emotional Health and Well-being

As a boy, you were probably taught not to cry, but to act tough and "be a man." Although attitudes are changing in our society, many males are still brought up not to express their emotions, learning that any display of feeling (other than anger) is a sign of weakness. While living up to the traditional, aggressive masculine identity may give a man certain advantages in a competitive society, it also can explain why the rates of substance abuse, domestic violence, homicide, suicide, sexual abuse, automobile accidents, and stress-related chronic illness are higher in men than in women. If a man has not learned to properly deal with and express his emotions, then stressful situations may lead to inappropriate responses such as anger or violence.

If you have a son, it's important to teach him not to shut down his feelings, because such an emotional disconnection can lead to a lack of empathy, sympathy, and the ability to express himself productively. This stereotypical male image, combined with exposure to violent television programs, movies, and video games, may promote violent and remorseless behavior in boys. It also can lead to an emotional disorder such as depression. Remember that your son needs your time and understanding. Spend as much time with him as you can and encourage him to be caring rather than tough. Don't force him to suppress his emotions. Instead, tell him it's okay to cry and teach him by example to feel empathy for other people.

Fortunately, there are many hopeful signs for men with an emotional disorder, including new ways of diagnosing emotional problems and more effective methods of treating them. The social stigma once linked to emotional problems has lessened considerably as medical science has come to understand the biological basis of these disorders.

Of course, not all emotional problems can be classified as a disorder. We all feel stress to varying degrees in a variety of situations. In terms of major stresses, men are just as likely as women to undergo an emotional upheaval during a time of divorce or from the loss of a job. The death of a spouse or parent will trigger a natural and extended period of bereavement as a man comes to grips with the loss of his life partner or family member. The best way to ensure your own emotional health is to find practical ways to handle stress and restrain your feelings of anger. This section will give you important information about stress management and the control of anger. In the final analysis, your emotional health is more under your own control than you think. The key is learning effective ways to exercise this control.

Physical and Emotional Health: How They Interact

Doctors are not sure exactly how physical and mental health influence each other, but growing scientific evidence suggests that the mind/body connection is real. For example, the so-called fight or flight response, in which the nervous system and the adrenal glands flood the body with the hormone adrenaline when you are frightened, increases both heart rate and blood flow to the muscles. This response prepares the body to deal with apparent danger. In this case, the survival response is helpful.

However, when a person is under constant stress, the body steadily releases a hormone called cortisol, which can cause long-term damage to the brain and other organs. The harmful effects of this hormone include an increased tendency for blood to clot, a surge in the pressure on coronary arteries, increased blood pressure, and other demands on the heart and blood vessels.

There has been a recent surge of interest in the mind/body connection by physicians to see if positive health effects can be obtained from relaxation techniques such as meditation. The increasing complexity and pace of life and the awareness that long-term stress has a negative physiological effect on the body have triggered the exploration of relaxation techniques. By combining knowledge of meditative techniques from Eastern cultures with Western scientific techniques, doctors have developed a form of meditation that may have positive effects on blood pressure and heart disease. Meditation appears to lower metabolism—decreasing breathing rate, heart rate, and blood pressure.

An understanding of the connection between the mind and the body becomes clearer as new techniques are found to examine and to measure the nervous system's subtle control over changes in the circulatory system. The positive response of the circulatory system to a variety of relaxation techniques, such as meditation and biofeedback, can now be explained partly in physiological terms. In addition to high blood pressure, meditation has been shown to benefit people who have chronic pain, tension headaches, asthma, insomnia, and other stress-related problems.

Interest in the mind/body connection has now expanded into studying the possibility of using mental techniques to strengthen the immune system. The immune system fights germs such as viruses and eliminates cells that are damaged, are turning cancerous, or have become cancerous. Researchers are trying to determine whether stress that accompanies major, life-changing events such as divorce or moving into a nursing home can lead to changes in the immune system that make people more vulnerable to infection, heart disease, or other illnesses. Factors that can contribute to a negative response of the immune system include whether a person feels in control of a given situation and whether a person feels lonely.

One technique being tested to teach the immune system to work better is biofeedback, in which special instruments that measure the body's vital signs amplify the signs that represent relaxation, in order to train the person to recognize and replicate them. Biofeedback is being used in studies of people with diabetes who are under stress; the aim is to substitute relaxation exercises for additional insulin injections needed to deal with the stress. Other research is focused on relieving chronic lower back pain and muscle pain. Guided imagery is a system that uses symbols to imagine the desired physical changes occurring in the body during the treatment of asthma and cancer. Some people who repeatedly imagine a healing process may be able to boost their immune system. For example, a person might imagine his or her healthy white blood cells as white knights on horses subduing a source of infection. Or a patient with cancer might see his or her white blood cells as a computer game, gobbling up the cancer cells. Some people with AIDS (acquired immunodeficiency syndrome) or with cancer use complementary therapies such as meditation and massage to supplement their medical and surgical treatments.

Keep in mind, however, that few alternative and complementary therapies have been proven safe and effective through rigorous scientific testing, and some can be very expensive. If you are thinking about trying an alternative treatment, talk to your doctor. Some therapies can be harmful, especially if you forgo conventional medical treatment for a serious illness. Never stop taking a prescription medication unless your doctor tells you to.

Stress Management

Doctors don't know all of the ways that stress and illness are connected, but they do know that the central nervous system (the brain and the spinal cord) and the immune system can influence one another during stress. Short-term positive stress can be invigorating, stimulating us to respond positively to meaningful challenges and opportunities. Short-term negative stress can be life-saving, causing us to flee dangerous situations. The brain releases hormones into the bloodstream, causing the heart to beat faster, the face to flush, and the arm and leg muscles to tighten, allowing the person to run away or escape. Once the danger is over, the body repairs damaged areas and returns to its prestressed state.

In long-term stress, the hormones continue to be released but the body does not have time to make repairs or to rest and recuperate. This is the type of stress that creates health problems. Under constant stress, a person becomes so conditioned to expect potential problems that his or her body tightens and remains in that state until the stress stops. Under this long-term stress state, the body can develop stress-related problems.

Many connections between stress and chronic conditions are known. Stress increases blood levels of adrenaline and cortisol, two so-called stress hormones. Cortisol can suppress the immune system, making people more susceptible to infectious diseases such as colds and flu. The effects of stress on the circulatory system (a quicker pulse, narrowed blood vessels, and thickened blood) can make people more susceptible to heart rhythm irregularities, angina (chest pain), high blood pressure, and stroke.

Muscles tighten as stress starts, often causing intense headaches, backaches, and gastrointestinal problems. Stress also can cause testosterone levels to decrease and blood vessels in the penis to constrict, often resulting in erection problems. The rush of hormones caused by a stressful situation can bring on an asthma attack in a person with a history of asthma. Stress also draws the blood supply away from the abdominal area and encourages overproduction of acids in the digestive system, often leading to indigestion and other gastrointestinal problems. Other problems related to stress include insomnia and irritability.

The number of hours worked does not seem to cause as much stress as do two other occupational factors: lack of control and inadequate social support. Men who have little control over the demands of their jobs feel more stress than those who have more control. Men who also experience a low level of social support from coworkers have even more problems.

What is stressful to one person may be relaxing to another. Some people, for example, like to keep busy all the time, while others need to take frequent breaks. Some people can keep track of multiple tasks, while others prefer to do tasks in sequence. If you are under stress, it is important to recognize it and deal with it in a positive way. Here are some tips to help you relieve stress:

- *Exercise regularly.* You can decrease stress and release tension through regular exercise or other physical activity. Running, walking, swimming, dancing, playing tennis, or working in your garden are some activities you may want to try.
- *Talk about your stress.* For example, talk to a friend, family member, teacher, or boss about what is bothering you. If that does not help to resolve the problem, consider seeking help from a professional therapist or counselor. Ask your doctor for a referral, or contact the employee assistance program at work.

- *Know your limits.* If a stressful situation gets beyond control, walk away. Return to deal with the situation when you have calmed down.
- *Take care of yourself.* Get plenty of rest and eat a healthy diet. If you feel irritable and tense from lack of sleep or if you are not eating properly, you will be less able to deal with stressful situations.
- *Take time for yourself.* Take a break from regular work and do something you enjoy. Just relax.
- *Be a participant in life.* Help yourself by helping others. Share your abilities with other members of your community by volunteering.
- *Prioritize your tasks.* To keep your schedule from overwhelming you, make a list of your tasks and check them off as you complete them.
- *Be cooperative.* If things do not go your way, try compromise rather than confrontation. A little give and take on both sides can help you meet your goals and make everyone feel better.
- *Cry if you need to.* Crying can be a healthy way to bring relief to your tension or anxiety.

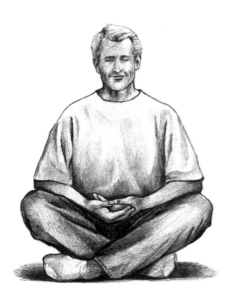

Reducing Stress by Relaxing

Learn to make yourself relax. A state of relaxation can counteract the potentially harmful effects of being under stress. When you are relaxed, your breathing and heart rate slow, your need for oxygen decreases, and the electrical activity of your brain goes into a resting pattern. Try to find at least 10 to 20 minutes in each day to relax.

- *Create a quiet scene in your mind.* You can't always get away, but you can try closing your eyes and letting your mind wander. A quiet country scene painted mentally can temporarily take you out of the turmoil of a stressful situation and help you to relax. Listening to beautiful music or reading a good book may help you achieve the same results.
- *Avoid self-medication.* When you need them, you can use prescription or over-the-counter medications to relieve stress temporarily, but realize that they don't remove the conditions that caused the stress in the first place. Becoming overly reliant on drugs or alcohol can only complicate matters in the long run. They may be habit forming, or they may interfere with your body's ability to function normally.
- *Learn to relax by using a specific relaxation strategy, such as meditation or deep-breathing exercises.* Participate in activities you can enjoy without competing. Cycle, swim, or walk the dog. Forget about always winning.

Relaxation can stimulate the release of endorphins—brain chemicals that promote feelings of well-being. Relaxation strategies work by blocking conscious thoughts, resulting in decreased tension, lower heart and breathing rates, and slower metabolism. Several relaxation techniques, such as meditation, guided imagery, muscle relaxation, and deep breathing, can be used to relieve stress and bring on the relaxation response.

   If you feel that you are under severe or long-term stress, seek help immediately. Talk about your problems with your doctor. He or she can treat any stress-related disorders you may have developed and will refer you to the appropriate mental health professional.

Getting a Grip on Your Anger

Anger is a normal human emotion. Sometimes when you become very angry, you may feel as if the emotion has taken over and can't be controlled. When your anger is getting out of control, you may run into personal problems at work or at home. But you can learn ways to handle your anger so you can gain some control over this seemingly uncontrollable feeling.

   Anger is an emotion, but it also affects you physically. When you get angry, your heart rate increases, your blood pressure rises, and the stress-response hormones adrenaline and noradrenaline surge throughout your body, preparing you for action. Back in our remote past, anger helped us respond to threats by fighting and defending ourselves when we were attacked. But in today's world you no longer need to respond so strongly to a perceived threat, which is more likely to be someone cutting you off in traffic or competing with you for a promotion than someone trying to steal your food.

   Some people have a low tolerance for frustration and seem to become angry more easily than others. Doctors are not sure why this is so, but possible causes include an inherited tendency, early childhood learning, or living in a family in which members failed to learn how to properly communicate their emotions.

   The popular notion that venting your anger is healthy has turned out to be false. Doctors now know that freely expressing your anger in the heat of the moment actually escalates the emotion and does little to help anger subside. Instead, the best solution seems to be finding out what triggers your anger so you can find ways to deal with those issues.

   Of course, if your anger is so out of control that it's affecting your relationship or your job, or if you feel the urge to hit someone, seek help. Talk to your doctor about your anger and ask him or her to refer you to a counselor. Experts say that some people with extreme anger may be able to moderate their emotions in about 10 weeks or less with counseling.

How to Get a Good Night's Sleep

Sleep is a basic requirement for good health. The mind and the body need sleep to perform maintenance and repair. Even one night of disrupted or missed sleep can drastically alter a person's chemical balance and cause daytime sleepiness and fatigue. The results of such sleep deprivation can reduce productivity as well as increase the chances of accidents at home or at work. Most adults need 7 to 8 hours of sleep each night, although sleep requirements may differ from one person to the next. For example, some people may feel rested after 5 or 6 hours of sleep, whereas others may still feel sleepy after 9 or more hours of sleep.

In general, people tend to sleep less soundly as they age. They may wake up more frequently and have a harder time getting back to sleep. Many older men may find that they simply don't need as much sleep as they did when they were younger. Overweight men may have problems getting a good night's sleep. Snoring also may contribute to a loss of sleep. Sleep apnea (a condition characterized by brief episodes of interrupted breathing during sleep) is another common reason for losing sleep. Many people who have sleep apnea find it difficult to stay awake during the day. However, the most common reason for an occasional night of lost sleep is worry or anxiety.

Here are some helpful tips for getting a good night's sleep:

- Stick to a regular schedule for going to bed and getting up. Going to bed and getting up at the same time help set your biological clock.
- Do not sleep late on weekends, and avoid napping during the day.
- Make your bedroom exclusively a place for sleep and sex. This means no TV, work, or serious discussions while in bed. Keep your bedroom comfortable, dark, quiet, and not too warm (about 60 to 65 degrees Fahrenheit).
- Exercise during the day so your metabolism has slowed by bedtime and you are ready for sleep.
- Avoid stimulants such as caffeine, nicotine, and alcohol, and rich, heavy meals before bedtime.
- If you are not lactose intolerant, drink a warm glass of milk just before bedtime. But don't drink so much that a full bladder disturbs your sleep.
- Have sex before bedtime; it may have a relaxing effect.
- Take a warm bath just before bedtime to help you relax.
- Set aside some quiet time about an hour or so before bedtime.
- If you still can't fall asleep, get up and read or do a simple chore until you become tired.

Relationships

People have a strong need to connect with others, and the central task of adulthood involves the ability to master relationships. Both men and women have a similar need to be close. But the way in which many boys are raised and socialized in our society sometimes makes it difficult for them to recognize and acknowledge this. Boys want to be like their fathers and loved by them. Similarly, boys have normal and natural wishes to be close to and to feel loved by their mothers.

Many men grow up wanting to be closer to their mother and father, yet some may feel they have to hold back to feel manly. Unfulfilled attachment needs can create a great deal of inner sadness or anger, which can continue into adulthood. For many males, a struggle with competence, independence, stoicism, and public performance can evolve, obscuring their ability to be responsive to those they love. They may have a strong drive to prove their competence. But even as they achieve competence, the urge to connect does not disappear.

The Changing Male Image

Attempts to describe behavior associated with male expectations often result in a series of negatives, such as men don't cry, men don't show their feelings, or men are never scared. Positive ways of describing masculine behavior have traditionally focused on characteristics such as physical strength, aggressiveness, and independence. Cultural or ethnic expectations, socioeconomic success, individual achievement, and education level heavily influence the perception of male characteristics.

Men who are married tend to live longer than men who are single. Does this mean that marriage is the healthiest form of relationship for men? Not necessarily. But it does mean that a stable, long-term relationship includes features that positively affect many men's emotional and physical health.

Role expectations for men in Western societies traditionally have emphasized protection and provision. In colonial times, physical strength was essential to survival. Along with these expectations was the premise that a man should hold a leadership position in the family and should be in charge of both household and community affairs. Many of these male role expectations remain today; many men see themselves as the primary provider for their families. This view is often reinforced by their partners.

However, cultural role expectations for men are changing. This has become a potential source of anxiety for both men and women. Some men may learn that providing financial support is not enough to satisfy their partner, although their ability to provide may still be used as a measure of both their worth and their suitability as a partner.

Most women also expect to have emotional support, mutual respect, stability, and a satisfying sexual life as part of their relationship. Working women expect greater participation by their partner in household chores and child rearing. Tension in marriage is often the result of different role expectations and unfulfilled needs. The role behaviors and values you learned during childhood may not work in your relationship today.

Men who remain well adjusted and healthy throughout life seem to have mastered the following values:

- intimacy—achieving an interdependent, mutually responsible, committed relationship
- satisfying work—engaging in work that is valued and rewarding
- parenting—accepting responsibility for the physical and emotional health and well-being of children

- leadership—taking responsibility for being a positive role model and inspiration to others
- integrity—following a code of moral values

Being a Father

In the past, fathers were expected to play a limited role in their childrens' lives. Once a child was conceived, the father's role was often defined primarily in terms of supporting the mother, both financially and emotionally. Often he was the major disciplinarian. Childcare was considered women's work. The father's responsibility was to be a role model for his sons, to impart sexual knowledge to them at the appropriate time, and to be a good provider. He often represented the disciplined, serious side of life.

Today, a new awareness of the importance of fathers is having a beneficial effect on the lives of children. Fathers are crucial to the emotional and intellectual growth of their children. Fathers contribute to the welfare of their families in many different ways—providing financial support or assistance; providing emotional support for their partner; performing household and childcare tasks; nurturing a caring, committed relationship with their partner; and having frequent and positive personal contact with their children.

Bonding with Your Child   In the past, many fathers of newborns sometimes found it difficult to bond with their infants and to express their feelings. Today, however, most fathers are bonding with their children and playing a nurturing role in their lives. Most fathers want to be involved, even occasionally volunteering to stay home from work to spend more time with their baby.

When fathers become involved during the pregnancy, delivery, and postpartum period, their involvement with and attachment to their infants are strong. The period immediately after delivery is especially conducive to the development of psychological ties between parents and their newborns. Fathers experience the same feelings of warmth, devotion, protectiveness, and pleasure at physical contact with their children that mothers do.

Divorce   If your marriage fails, it does not mean that you are a failure or that your role as a father is diminished. Try not to let your contact with your children drop off after your divorce. Children are at risk when they grow up without their father. They are more likely than children who have regular contact with their fathers to have psychological problems, abuse drugs and alcohol, live in poverty, and fail in school. Almost half of all divorced fathers have not seen their children in the past year. Keep in mind that your child needs and wants your continued love and emotional support even if you are no longer living together as a family.

Blended Families   A blended family, or stepfamily, includes a couple with one or more children from a previous relationship. Half of all people in the United States will experience a stepfamily relationship at some time in their lives—as a stepparent, remarried parent, or stepchild.

Children in blended families have strong emotional connections to a parent who lives in another household or to a parent who has died. In many cases, a child moves back and forth between two households that often have very different rules and expectations. This adjustment period can be even more stressful than a divorce or living in a single-parent home. Children may feel angry, anxious, or depressed and worry that they won't be able to have as much contact with either parent.

Blended families in which both adults have children from previous relationships have the biggest problems to overcome. Children in these families may worry that their own parent will have less time to spend with them, that they will have to share their bedroom or possessions with a stepsibling they hardly know, or that their place in the family hierarchy will change. Rules and family routines may be different.

All these new experiences can put stress on a child. He or she may display his or her feelings through disruptive behavior, or perform poorly in school. Give your child time to adjust to the situation, to become familiar with the new family members, and to get used to the working structure of the household. Stepfamilies who work together to solve problems eventually find a living arrangement they can all be happy with. Once you make it through the difficult early years, you will probably find that being part of a stepfamily is an enriching, fulfilling experience.

Here are some tips for helping to make living in a stepfamily rewarding for everyone involved:

- Put a priority on the couple relationship; a secure relationship between the two adults is essential for a successful blended family. In many stepfamilies, couples spend so much time dealing with child issues that they don't nurture their own relationship.
- Agree with your partner on a few important rules and spell them out to the children. Always support each other in front of the children.
- Be patient in establishing a relationship with a stepchild—it takes time. And be cautious when taking on a parenting role, especially with a teenager, who may never accept you as a parent. Your stepchildren are more likely to treat you with respect and courtesy if you treat them the same way.
- Supervision of children is especially important in a blended family, especially when their ages vary. It can be tempting for an older child to stretch the rules with a younger or smaller stepsibling when the two are left alone.
- Have regular family meetings to discuss the week's activities or any problems

that might come up. Open communication helps establish healthy relationships among all family members.

- Take most of the responsibility for disciplining your own child. Give the stepparent time to establish a trusting relationship with your child before beginning to set rules for him or her. Discipline all children in the household equally and fairly.

- Resolve any personal differences between a stepparent and a stepchild or between stepsiblings promptly and directly; unresolved problems tend to get worse over time.

- Set aside time for one-on-one activities between family members. Stepchildren need to spend time alone with their parent; stepparents should do things alone with stepchildren; and the two adults should spend time alone with each other.

- Participate in a support group for stepfamilies. You'll see that you are not alone and can learn a lot from the experiences of other stepfamilies.

- If your children are part of their other parent's stepfamily, support that family and cooperate with both of the adults involved. Competition and tension between two households can cause the children to suffer emotionally.

Family Violence

Family or domestic violence is emotional, physical, or sexual abuse committed by a spouse, former spouse, partner, parent, roommate, or other person living in the home. Domestic violence also includes emotional, physical, or sexual abuse of children, abuse of parents or grandparents, violence toward a partner of the same sex, and even date violence and date rape. Family violence is a rapidly growing public health problem that affects more than 2.5 million Americans—mainly women and children—each year.

Many theories exist that attempt to explain why men use violence against their partner, including deficient communication skills, provocation by the partner, stress, and financial hardship. While these factors may provoke an isolated incident of violence, they do not adequately explain the man's motivation. The main reason why men commit violent acts within the family is because they see violence as the best way to gain and keep control over other people without experiencing negative consequences. Many violent men have firm and inflexible ideas about traditional male and female roles and hold a distorted concept of manhood.

Violent men typically have grown up in a violent family, in which they learned that violence is a "normal" response to solving problems. They may have been victims of violence as children or watched one parent beat the other. Violent men often have a quick temper and overreact to frustration. There is a strong link between violence and alcohol or other drug abuse. Poverty and lacking at least a high school education are contributing factors, although domestic violence appears in every social and economic group.

The effects of family violence extend far beyond the physical scars produced by the abuse. People who have been physically or sexually abused at home often experience long-lasting depression (see page 345), panic attacks, sleep or eating disorders, or sexual problems. They may begin abusing alcohol or other drugs, become aggressive or neglectful, or attempt suicide (see page 346). Children who witness or experience family violence are deeply affected and often grow up to become violent or aggressive themselves. Many people are afraid to leave their abuser because they fear what the abuser will do if they try to leave or think they may lose custody of their children. Others may have nowhere else to go or no money of their own.

Domestic Violence

Domestic violence—also known as battering, spouse abuse, or partner abuse—is a pattern of psychological, economic, or sexual force used by one person in a relationship against the other. It is characterized by recurrent verbal and physical assaults that tend to escalate over time and is the most common cause of injury to women who need emergency medical treatment. It is estimated that an act of domestic violence occurs every 15 seconds somewhere in the United States. This translates to more than 2.5 million victims of domestic violence each year. Domestic violence occurs in all ethnic, racial, educational, and socio-economic groups.

The targets of domestic violence are usually women and their children. More than 90 percent of family violence cases in the United States involve women being abused by men. Six in every 10 women who are victims of homicide were murdered by someone they knew. About half of these women were murdered by a spouse or someone with whom they had been intimate. Men who commit domestic violence may be a spouse, a former spouse, a fiancé, or a boyfriend.

Children are involved in about 60 percent of domestic violence incidents. During assaults on their mothers, the children of battered women are at risk for injury themselves, either deliberate or incidental. One in 10 calls made to alert police to domestic abuse is placed by a child in the home. More than 53 percent of male abusers also beat their children. The self-perpetuating aspect of domestic violence can be seen in the fact that one of every three abused children becomes an adult abuser or victim.

Domestic violence has long-term effects on the lives of the victims as well as any children who live in the home. It may take years for the woman to become disentangled from the abusive relationship, during which time the level of abuse can increase. Attempts to escape often escalate the violence.

Domestic violence can take many forms. It usually falls into one or more of the following categories:

- *Physical battering.* The abuser's physical attacks or aggressive behavior can include grabbing, pinching, slapping, punching, hair-pulling, kicking, biting, restraining, or choking; destroying furniture or personal possessions; injuring pets; and murder.
- *Psychological battering.* This type of violence can include cursing, shouting or verbal abuse, implicit or direct threats of bodily harm, uninvited visits, stalking, malicious telephone calls or letters, throwing things, blocking a doorway passage, cornering the victim during an argument, possessiveness, embarrassing the victim in public, restricting telephone use and isolating the victim from friends and family, forbidding use of the family car, withholding money or health insurance, refusing to pay bills, and sabotaging the victim's attempts to work or to go to school.
- *Sexual abuse.* Physical attacks by the abuser are often accompanied by, or culminate in, sexual violence in which the victim is forced to take part in a sexual activity.

Battering is viewed as a set of learned controlling behaviors and the feeling of being trapped in a relationship. The batterer may find that violence is an effective method for gaining and keeping control over another person, and he often does not experience adverse consequences as a result of his behavior. Historically, violence against women has often not been treated as a "real" crime. There is no distinct personality or socioeconomic profile for men who commit domestic violence. Many batterers have no history of a mental health condition or a criminal record. Batterers come from all groups and backgrounds and have different personality profiles.

Help Stop the Violence   You can play an important role in helping to stop domestic violence in your community. Domestic violence is not an issue just for women. Family violence is everyone's concern. It's essential for men to get involved. Men are vital to violence-prevention efforts because men are more likely to open up to other men if they have a problem, and they are more likely to listen to advice from men. In addition, fathers have enormous influence over their children's developing attitudes and behavior.

There are many different ways, including the following, in which you can contribute to making your community a safe place to live:

- *Speak out against domestic violence.* Take a leadership role in community organizations such as sports clubs, churches, and neighborhood associations, and take a stand against domestic violence.
- *Be a role model for other men.* Reach out to men who are violent at home, and let them know that their behavior is not acceptable and that you want to help them break the pattern of abuse.

- *Be a role model for your son.* Show kindness and respect to your partner and you will give your son an example of a healthy, nurturing relationship.
- *Be a role model for a child who lacks a positive male figure in his life.* A male mentor and friend can provide consistent, positive support to help ensure that a child does not grow up to be a batterer.
- *Reach out to a family that is involved in violence.* Talk to family members about what is happening, and offer to help them. Follow through on your offer.

Could You Be a Batterer?

Early signs of domestic abuse can be subtle, progressing gradually from overly controlling behavior to threats, and, ultimately, to violence. If you think you may have a problem with violence, consider the following:

- Do you imagine that another person is interested in your partner or that your partner is interested in another person?
- Do you abuse your partner verbally? Do you ridicule your partner or use disparaging terms such as "stupid," "fat," "lazy," or "ugly"?
- Are you unusually concerned with your partner's whereabouts, activities, and contacts with friends and family?
- Do you threaten to do something violent if your partner does something you don't like?
- When you are angry, do you throw things, damage your partner's possessions, or threaten to hurt your partner or your partner's pets or children?
- Do you use force such as pushing, shoving, or restraining during an argument?
- Do you blame your partner for your anger or violence?
- After a violent episode, do you promise your partner that it won't happen again, say you love your partner, or buy your partner gifts, but repeat the behavior another day?

If you answered "yes" to one or more of the above questions, you are a potential batterer. Denying that you have a problem or rationalizing your behavior puts you and your loved ones at risk of escalating violence that may lead to injury or even death. It's not enough to say you are sorry and you will never do it again; that is part of the cycle of violence. It is crucial for you to recognize your abusive behavior and take responsibility for it. Before you react, think about the safety, health, and emotional well-being of your partner and children.

Call your doctor or a domestic violence hot line and find out what programs are available in your community. Your doctor may refer you to a mental health professional who can help you understand the reasons for your behavior and help you develop strategies to change it and break the pattern of abuse. Joining a support group of other men who have a similar experience also can be helpful.

Child Abuse

Child abuse includes neglect, physical abuse, emotional abuse, and sexual abuse. Girls are more likely to be sexually abused than boys. Child abuse occurs in all racial, ethnic, educational, and socioeconomic groups. The abuser is usually someone who provides care for the child—such as a biological parent, adoptive parent, foster parent, grandparent, sibling, other relative, or a friend or neighbor.

Child abuse can have serious, long-term consequences for a child. Children who are abused or who live in violent homes are more likely to see violence as an effective solution to problems. The majority of child abusers were abused or neglected when they were children.

Signs of possible child abuse include the following:

- repeated injuries with unconvincing explanations of the cause
- injuries that leave scars that resemble cigarette burns or marks from an electrical cord, especially in areas of the body that are very sensitive, such as the genitals, nipples, and face
- behavior problems—behavior that is either passive and withdrawn, or hyperactive and aggressive
- reluctance to respond or fear when asked about life at home
- self-destructive, delinquent, or reckless behaviors such as substance abuse, crime, or running away from home
- low self-esteem
- learning problems and lack of motivation in school
- neglected appearance
- no desire to make friends or invite other children home
- depression
- suicide attempts

If you think that a child you know may be a victim of abuse, do not directly confront the suspected abuser. Contact a local service agency such as a child protective service agency, welfare department or social service agency, public health department, or the police—they can assist the child and the family.

If you are abusing your child or think you may be at risk for doing so, talk to your doctor or a clergy member, or join a support group of people with similar concerns. Many communities have intervention and prevention programs to help you learn positive coping and parenting skills.

Signs of possible sexual abuse include the following:

- bruising, redness, swelling, discharge, or other signs of injury in the rectal or genital area
- regressive behavior such as bed-wetting, thumb-sucking, or excessive clinging

- frequent nightmares or fearfulness
- an increase in hostile or aggressive behavior
- withdrawal from friends, family, or school activities
- provocative, promiscuous, or sexually precocious behavior

Teach your children the difference between good touching and bad touching. A friendly hug or a pat on the back are examples of good touching. Feeling private parts (areas covered by a bathing suit) and touching (including rubbing or kissing) anywhere on their body that makes them feel uncomfortable are examples of bad touching. Make sure that your children know that their body is private and that no one may touch them without their permission.

If you suspect that your child may have been sexually abused, get help immediately. Call your pediatrician or contact the police, a social worker, or a school guidance counselor. Do not hesitate to contact local authorities. Most sex offenders have abused more than one child. Stopping a sex offender will prevent the sexual abuse of other children.

Elder Abuse

Abuse and neglect of older people can involve physical abuse, verbal intimidation, exploitation (such as mishandling of financial resources), medical neglect (such as withholding medications or treatment or devices such as dentures, eyeglasses, hearing aids, or walkers), or physical neglect or abandonment. Most abused older people are women, but men also are abused. Victims of elder abuse usually live with their abuser.

Watch for the following signs of possible abuse in older friends and family members:

Physical or emotional abuse:
- unexplained burns, bruises, cuts, or scars
- frequent falls
- noticeable fear of caregiver
- withdrawal; isolation
- lack of responsiveness
- agitation; anxiety
- confusion; disorientation
- depression
- anger
- poor hygiene
- bedsores
- unexplained weight loss
- lethargy
- changes in personality

Signs of financial exploitation:
- mismanagement of the person's assets
- diversion of the person's income
- withdrawal of funds without the person's permission
- withdrawal of funds against the person's will

If you suspect that an older friend, relative, or neighbor is being abused or exploited, try to help him or her. Stay in touch with the person. If you have not seen him or her recently and cannot reach him or her by phone, stop by unexpectedly. If you are not allowed to see the person, ask about his or her health and stop by again within a day or two. Keep trying. If your persistent attempts to see the person fail or if, when you see the person, you suspect that there is a problem, consider reporting the situation to the local protective services agency. A local senior center or senior citizens' agency can tell you where to call for help. Be prepared to provide the person's name and address, the nature of the suspected problem, the names of other people who may know about the situation, and how best to contact the person. Your identity will be kept confidential.

Dealing with End-of-Life Decisions

Over the course of a lifetime, men face a variety of inevitable stresses that create emotional responses. Dealing with death and dying presents some of life's greatest emotional stress. There are two ways in which a man finds himself confronting the issues surrounding death and dying: as someone caring for a dying person, most often a parent, and as someone who is facing his own death. In both roles he must find ways to deal with his grief. Grief affects each person differently but typically involves four stages—shock, denial, depression and withdrawal, and acceptance. If you are grieving, it is important for your emotional health to talk about your feelings—to a family member or a close friend, to others in a support group, or to a counselor. "Bottled up" emotions can lead to depression, withdrawal from friends and society, sudden irrational outbursts, feelings of anger and resentment, insomnia, and even physical illness. Here are some positive steps you can take to deal with grief:

- Rest, eat a healthy diet (see page 43), and keep warm (emotional stress will make your body temperature drop). Avoid caffeine and alcohol because they can add to your stress.
- Use relaxation techniques. Try deep breathing. People who are under stress tend to hold their breath or to breathe shallowly, which can cause fatigue and anxiety.
- Express your feelings. Talk to family, friends, members of a support group, or clergy.

- Accept help. Let others care for you. Let your friends and family make a meal for you, do some housework, or just listen to you. Such support can be healing for them as well as for you.
- Take as much time as you need. Grieving has no time frame.
- Think about how your life has changed and what that means for the future.

Family Caregiving

A large part of the stress related to the dying of family members has to do with the challenges of providing care. People who have a terminal illness usually have important and wide-ranging needs for assistance in addition to the medical care they receive from physicians and other healthcare workers. A majority of people who are dying require home nursing care, help with transportation, homemaking services, and personal care. In many cases their families must take on the substantial burden of caring for them. In some cases, home healthcare programs may help. Traditionally, women have provided most of the home care, even when the family member is the man's parent or grandparent. But today, with most women working outside the home, men and members of religious or civic organizations have an opportunity to be more actively engaged in caring for the dying. People are relying increasingly on paid workers to provide the nonmedical care needed by family members who are dying.

Hospice Care

Hospice care is a life-affirming approach to caring for people who are in the final phase of a terminal illness. Hospice regards death as a natural part of life, and emphasizes the comfort and quality of life of a dying person. The focus is on relieving pain and controlling other symptoms. With hospice care, a dying person is allowed to live his or her last days with dignity, pain-free and alert, surrounded by loved ones at home or in a homelike setting.

In general, a person becomes eligible to enter a hospice program when a doctor has determined that he or she has 6 months or less to live and refers him or her to a hospice program. Family members, friends, clergy, or healthcare professionals also can make referrals.

Under the supervision of a doctor, an interdisciplinary team—doctors, nurses, therapists, counselors, social workers, clergy, healthcare aides, and volunteers—works closely with the dying person to provide medical care and support. The team deals with the person's medical, emotional, and spiritual needs. And because the entire family is regarded as the "unit of care," the hospice team also provides support and assistance to the person's loved ones. Members of the hospice team are available to assist the person and his or her loved ones 24 hours a day, 7 days a week. After the person has died, the hospice program also provides grief counseling to the survivors.

Advance Directives

When a person becomes seriously ill and is no longer able to make decisions about his or her healthcare, those decisions are usually made by a close family member or by the person's doctor. Advance directives are legal documents designed to help ensure that healthcare decisions made on a person's behalf are consistent with his or her preferences. Advance directives may provide either general guidelines or specific instructions.

Although advance directives do not go into effect until the person is unable to make his or her own healthcare decisions, the forms should be prepared and signed long before they are needed. When the person is in a hospital or a nursing home, emotional factors may make it challenging to talk about the forms (and the issues involved). These documents should be reviewed and updated regularly. The person can revise or withdraw his or her advance directives at any time.

Advance directive forms are available through hospital social service departments and from state or local medical societies and bar associations, or you can consult a lawyer to produce your own living will and durable power of attorney for healthcare. Because requirements for advance directives vary from state to state, you should consider talking to a lawyer when preparing or filling out these documents.

Be sure to tell the doctor and the person you have chosen to make your healthcare decisions about your advance directives. Give each of them a copy, and keep a copy for yourself.

The most common types of advance directives are living wills, durable powers of attorney, do-not-resuscitate orders, and organ and tissue donor cards:

- A *living will* is a document that indicates a person's wishes regarding life-sustaining medical treatments. It is prepared by a competent person and goes into effect only when the person is unable to speak for himself or herself. A living will guides medical professionals and family members so they can make healthcare decisions that are consistent with the person's beliefs. A living will can be revised or withdrawn by the person at any time. You should consult a lawyer when preparing a living will because legal requirements vary from state to state.

- A *durable power of attorney for healthcare* is a document in which a competent person gives another person (called a healthcare proxy) the power to make healthcare decisions for him or her. It goes into effect only in the event that the person is unable to make such decisions. The durable power of attorney can be withdrawn by the person who initiated it at any time.

- A *do-not-resuscitate (DNR) order* states that no one should perform heroic measures, including CPR and the use of mechanical life support equipment, to restart a person's heart should it stop. The document must be signed by the person if he or she is competent (or by his or her healthcare proxy if he or she is not competent) and by his or her doctor. In some cases, doctors recommend that people wear a special bracelet or necklace that communicates their DNR status to emergency responders. The person should keep a copy of the document in his or her home in a prominent place where it will be noticed by emergency medical personnel called to the home; the doctor should keep a copy in the person's medical records at all times to make sure that the person's wishes are respected. DNR orders can be withdrawn at any time by the patient, as long as he or she is competent.

- An *organ and tissue donor card* informs medical personnel that your organs and tissues may be used for transplant in the event of your death. Many states provide an opportunity to register as an organ and tissue donor when you apply for a driver's license or state identification card. Your donor status is then indicated on the license or identification card. Be sure to tell your loved ones that you are a registered donor.

PART THREE

THE REPRODUCTIVE SYSTEM

CHAPTER 7

Sexuality

Sexuality is a normal part of being human. It refers to the capacity, as we mature, to develop behavior patterns, emotions, and sensations related to reproduction and sexual expression. It also can be defined as a person's attitudes, values, goals, and behaviors based on the person's perception of his or her gender. A person's concept of sexuality influences many aspects of his or her life, including priorities, aspirations, preferences, social contacts, interpersonal relationships, self-evaluation, expression of emotions, and career. In short, sexuality touches nearly every aspect of our lives.

Male Sexuality and Sexual Behavior

Gender and sexuality evolve together and become inextricably intertwined. Parents often interact with their children in different ways depending on the children's sex. Girls may be caressed and patted while boys are tickled and rough-housed.

Sexual values and feelings usually are established and reinforced during childhood. Children between ages 5 and 10 often tell stories that have sexual or romantic themes. Girls are more likely than boys to tell romantic stories and less likely than boys to tell sexually explicit stories. This fundamental difference may explain some of the difficulties in understanding and communication that sometimes occur between men and women.

During adolescence, changes in development cause boys and girls to diverge even more dramatically. Both sexes are going through a major biological event—for girls, menstruation; for boys, the ability to ejaculate. A boy's sexuality is primarily located in his genitals during puberty. Within 2 years of puberty, all but a relatively few boys have experienced orgasm, usually brought on by masturbation. Girls this age tend to focus more on developing relationships than on their sexuality.

Masturbation

For males, masturbation is touching or massaging their penis for sexual pleasure or to achieve an erection and ejaculation. Male sexual impulses, initially acted out through masturbation, are linked to physiological changes, brought on by increased production of the male hormone testosterone during puberty. At this age, boys are easily aroused. Male adolescents have frequent erections, often without apparent stimulation of any kind.

Masturbation was once considered abnormal. Today it is viewed as a normal, healthy sexual activity that starts in puberty and can continue throughout life. There is no evidence that masturbation causes any physical injury or psychological harm. For many adolescent boys masturbation is their major sexual activity, and many engage in it frequently. For many men, also, masturbation remains a satisfying, if less important, component of their sexuality.

Long-term Relationships

Most people in our society ultimately marry or make a long-term commitment to another person. Sexual commitment inside marriage or an established relationship makes up the larger part of adult sexual experience. Many couples find new and different kinds of satisfaction in long-term sexual relations with the same person: coming to know and understand each other better, learning to make each other happy through sex, and relaxing with and not having to impress the other person. For many men, not having to worry about sexual conquest any longer is a great relief; finally, love and sex can grow closer together.

In a long-term relationship, most couples find that they have sex less frequently than they did when their relationship was new. After childbirth, sleep loss and the demands of parenthood often interfere with sexual intimacy. Anger, depression, drinking too much alcohol, certain medications, and fatigue also can take their toll on your sexual drive. You should not feel pressured by the need to conform to a sexual norm you have heard about regarding the frequency with which you have intercourse. However, if you or your partner want to revitalize your relationship, you can do something to

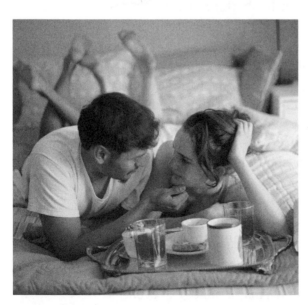

Maintain the Romance

Keeping a relationship strong requires the effort of both partners. Make your relationship a priority. Have fun together. Enjoy at least part of your leisure time together and create time to be alone with each other.

put some of that old spark back into your sexual relationship. Go out on a date, just the way you did when you first met. Or set aside some time each week to be together alone. But remember that the number of times per week you and your partner have sex is not as important as the quality of your lovemaking. If you feel that you or your partner may have a more serious sexual problem, talk to your doctor, who can refer you to a sexual therapist.

Homosexuality and Bisexuality

Men who are sexually attracted to other men are called homosexual. Women who are sexually attracted to other women are called lesbians. The term "gay" is often used to describe homosexual men and women. Bisexuality is sexual attraction to both men and women.

No one is sure what causes homosexuality, or what causes heterosexuality, for that matter. No particular hormonal, biological, or psychological influences have been identified with certainty as substantially contributing to a person's sexual orientation. Most scientists believe that a person's sexual orientation is established in childhood, through genetic or environmental influences or a combination of both. It is not a choice. Therefore, the term "sexual preference" is inaccurate.

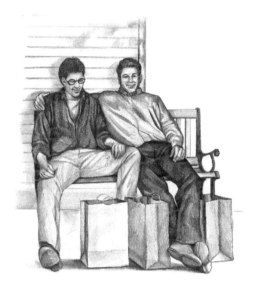

Relationships
You can benefit from forming and maintaining a close, stable, long-term relationship. Nurturing your relationship with your partner can make you happy—and it also can keep you healthy.

Scientific research indicates that parents have very little influence on their children's sexual orientation. Evidence also shows that children who are raised by homosexual parents are no more likely to grow up to be homosexual than are children raised by heterosexuals. Like heterosexuals, most gay people realize their sexual orientation during adolescence. Some, however, realize it much later, even after leading a married life.

An estimated 3 to 10 percent of American men have been involved exclusively in homosexual relationships throughout their lives. A much higher percentage of people have reported experimenting in same-sex activities during adolescence, although they identify themselves as adult heterosexuals. Although a significant number of people have bisexual feelings, a small percentage actually act on those feelings. Most homosexuals adjust well to their sexual identity, even though they often must overcome disapproval and prejudice. This adjustment can be stressful and may lead to emotional and physical health problems. Homosexual teenagers in particular may feel confused and isolated from friends and family, and they may fear rejection.

For some homosexuals and heterosexuals, frequent sexual activity with different partners is a common practice throughout life. People with multiple sex partners run the risk of developing a variety of sexually transmitted diseases (STDs; see page 180).

Health Concerns of Gay and Bisexual Men   The biggest health concern among sexually active gay men is contracting STDs including the human immunodeficiency virus (HIV), which causes acquired immunodeficiency syndrome (AIDS). Men who have sex with men make up the largest category of people infected with HIV in the United States. The risk of HIV transmission is greater for a person who is receiving anal sex because the lining of the rectum is delicate and can be easily torn, allowing easy entrance of the virus into the bloodstream. Condoms are essential to reduce the risk of transmitting HIV.

Sexually active gay men are also at increased risk for infection with hepatitis B (see page 191). This bloodborne virus can be transmitted through unprotected sex. Although condoms provide some protection, the best way to avoid hepatitis B is to be immunized. The vaccine is given in a series of three injections. Immunization against hepatitis B is recommended for all sexually active gay and bisexual men.

Anal cancer is more likely to occur in gay men than in heterosexuals. The increased risk is thought to be related to a higher risk of infection with the human papillomavirus (HPV; see page 184), a sexually transmitted virus that can cause precancerous skin changes. Men at risk for anal cancer should have regular examinations by their physician to detect the early signs of this form of cancer. Men who participate in anal sex are also at risk for urinary tract and gastrointestinal infections; when bacteria in the rectum enter the urethra, the infection can spread up the urethra into the urinary tract and into the intestines.

Drug and alcohol abuse affect a large percentage of gay men. Nearly one third of homosexual men and women abuse drugs or alcohol, while only 10 to 12 percent of the heterosexual population abuses drugs or alcohol. Drinking alcohol and abusing other drugs, such as cocaine and marijuana, not only endanger a person's health by increasing the risk for disease but also increase the chances that a person will engage in other risky behaviors, such as unprotected sex.

Societal discrimination, issues surrounding AIDS, and the lack of emotional support from family or friends can create psychological problems that weigh heavily on gay and bisexual men. Even though openly gay people are more accepted than ever before in the United States, some state laws still ban homosexual activity. Physical or verbal abuse and harrassment are relatively common experiences for gay men and women.

Without some level of acceptance and support from family members and friends, teenagers who are struggling with their sexual orientation may become depressed, turn to drugs, or run away from home, usually to large cities, where their problems are intensified. Suicides among homosexual teenagers are two to three times more likely than among heterosexual teenagers of similar age. Many homosexual and bisexual teenagers use drugs such as alcohol, marijuana, and cocaine and crack. Drug abuse not only harms teenagers directly but also increases their risk of engaging in unsafe sex and developing STDs, including HIV.

Many homosexual men may also face the stress of living in an unaccepting society, hiding their sexual orientation from those around them, and dealing with loneliness and isolation. Gay men may have difficulties finding partners and establishing meaningful relationships. The threat of AIDS also takes its toll on the emotional health of gay men in the United States. Many gay men have to deal with the deaths of partners and friends who die of AIDS, as well as pressure from some people who may blame the homosexual community for the disease. All of these issues contribute to high levels of depression, suicide, and drug abuse among gay men.

Some homosexuals may hesitate to seek medical care because they fear rejection by physicians. If you are gay or bisexual, look for a doctor you are comfortable with and who understands your healthcare needs. In many large metropolitan areas, special clinics are dedicated to meeting the healthcare needs of the local gay community.

Sexual Desire and Aging

Several factors play a role in determining whether an older person is sexually active, including the biological processes associated with normal aging, the desire to engage in some form of sexual activity, and availability of a suitable partner and privacy for sexual expression.

Biological Changes with Age

Among men, some sexual problems may increase with age, but not necessarily because of aging. The incidence of erectile dysfunction increases for men over 40 and escalates with each decade. The intensity of sexual sensation among men over 40 may be reduced, as may be the speed of erection and the force of ejaculation. Compared with younger men, middle-aged men (45 to 50 years old) are more likely to experience orgasm in one stage, involving a shorter orgasmic period and a rapid shrinking of the erection after ejaculation. The amount of time before another erection can be achieved usually increases, as does the amount of time an erection can be maintained.

Among women, biological changes leading to menopause may extend over a 20-year period, with onset generally in the mid 30s and occasionally extending beyond the mid 50s. After menopause, the intensity of sexual response may be reduced, and for some postmenopausal women intercourse may be painful due to vaginal dryness. For many women, estrogen replacement therapy can relieve vaginal dryness and other symptoms of menopause and may help restore sexual desire.

Hormone levels play a role in men's sexual expression, and changes in hormone levels may account for some of the age-related changes in sexuality. Testosterone is the key hormone that regulates sexual response in men and has some effect in women. Testosterone is produced by the adrenal glands, testicles, and ovaries. Women produce less than a tenth of the amount produced by men. Testosterone levels in men are highest in the morning right after waking and decrease throughout the day, so blood tests for testosterone are taken before 9:00 AM for accuracy. After a rise during adolescence, testosterone production declines throughout life in men. Much less is known about age-related production of testosterone in women.

Changes in Sexual Desire with Age

Although aging brings biological changes that may dampen sexual interest in some people, the demands of daily life also shape older people's sexual desires or drives. Engaging in sex at any age requires an investment of time, emotion, and energy. As for people in other age groups, older people's sexual drives may decline under the pressures of mental or physical fatigue, preoccupation with business, overindulgence in food or drink, physical illness, or fear of sexual failure. For some people, boredom within the relationship also may be a factor in a loss of sexual interest. Life events and major transitions often affect a person's interest in sex.

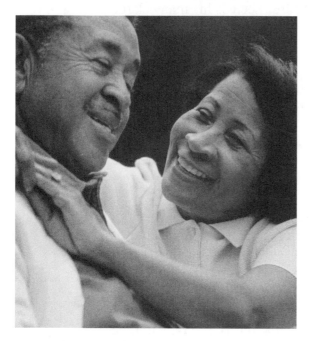

Sex and the Older Couple

Many older adults who have an active sex life say that sex feels as good or better than when they were younger. The changes that come with age, such as a man's taking longer to achieve orgasm, can provide an opportunity for couples to become more sexually compatible. Also, without the distraction and demands of children, or worries about contraception, older couples may find themselves at a stage of life that is more conducive to sexual intimacy. Retirement allows more time to enjoy each other.

Many healthy older men maintain their production of testosterone at levels equal to those of younger men. Men feel some level of sexual desire throughout life. A positive self-image is probably the single greatest contributor to sexual desire. Men and women who feel good about their bodies and who perceive themselves as physically desirable are more likely to have a satisfying sexual relationship than those who do not. Women, however, are more likely to base their self-image primarily on judgments about their appearance; men also consider appearance but give greater weight to their sexual performance. Men and women with positive attitudes toward sex are more likely to remain sexually active throughout their lives.

While the desire for sexual activity can remain strong in later years, interest often outlives opportunity. Having a suitable partner is a major factor in whether and how often older people engage in sexual activity. Although individual characteristics are important for attracting a potential partner, events that influence social relationships are even more important. For example, marriage, remarriage, separation, divorce, or death of a spouse can influence opportunities for developing relationships and having sex. Other factors, such as gender, sexual orientation, and the influence of family and other social networks also affect the chances of finding a suitable partner.

Older married people are more likely than single people of the same age to report engaging in sexual intercourse. But marriage does not guarantee a partner for life. Health problems that develop over the course of a marriage can interfere with one partner's or both partners' ability to engage in sex. Because men have a shorter life expectancy and women tend to marry older men, women are more likely to be widowed. Nearly 34 percent of women and 7 percent of men are widowed at ages 55 to 59; 60 percent of women and only 18 percent of men are widowed at age 85 or older.

Sexual activity can also include a range of behaviors that do not require a partner. Erotic dreams and fantasies represent mental sources of arousal and pleasure that can occur when one is alone. Sexual fantasies and dreams allow for an acceptable expression of sexual feelings and can provide an avenue for sexual expression when other forms of sex are unavailable. Older adults seem to enjoy both forms of sexuality. Masturbation is a healthy and readily available form of sexual activity that can be practiced alone and can provide sexual release for both men and women.

Sexual Dysfunction

The mind and the body must work together for normal sexual function. Thoughts and emotions interact with the nervous, circulatory, and endocrine (hormone) systems of the body to produce a sexual response. The sexual response has four stages:

1. *Desire* (the wish to engage in sexual activity) is triggered by thought or verbal and visual cues.
2. *Arousal* (the state of sexual excitement) occurs as blood enters the genital area, leading to an erection in the male.
3. *Orgasm* (the climax of sexual excitement) occurs at ejaculation (the emission of semen from the penis); muscle tension increases throughout the body.
4. *Resolution* (a sense of well-being and complete muscle relaxation) follows orgasm.

Erectile Dysfunction

Psychological problems, neurological problems, abnormalities in blood flow, damage to the genital organs, hormonal imbalance, and the use of drugs or medications—all can interfere with any of the four stages of normal sexual function. Erectile dysfunction occurs when one or more of these factors persistently interfere with the ability to achieve and maintain an erection sufficient to complete sexual intercourse.

Erectile dysfunction is often called impotence. Some experts object to the term "impotence" because of its negative implications and lack of precise meaning. The term "erectile dysfunction" is now used. Erectile dysfunction is defined as the inability to achieve or maintain an erection as part of the overall multifaceted process of sexual function. This definition deemphasizes intercourse as the essential or only aspect of sexual life and gives equal importance to other aspects of male sexual behavior.

At some time in their life, all men experience erectile problems. But for 30 million men in the United States, erectile dysfunction is a chronic, persistent problem. This number includes about 10 percent of the entire male population and 35 percent of men over 60. Fewer than 5 percent of men with erectile dysfunction seek treatment for this condition.

There are different levels of erectile dysfunction:

- a total inability to achieve erection
- the occasional ability to achieve erection
- an inability to maintain erections
- the ability to achieve erection, but inability to control ejaculation

Most cases of erectile dysfunction are treatable and are not the result or inevitable consequence of aging. The response in the penis that results in a normal erection depends on healthy nerves, blood vessels, muscles, and fibrous tissues, as well as on adequate blood levels of certain hormones, such as testosterone. Damage, injury, or malfunction in any of these areas can lead to erectile dysfunction. A number of phys-

The ABCs of Erection

An erection occurs when blood is pumped into the penis. The more blood that fills the penis, the harder the erection. Failure to achieve erection occurs when the penis does not fill or remain filled appropriately.

The penis has three chambers: two chambers called the corpora cavernosa, and one called the corpus spongiosum. The corpora cavernosa run the length of the penis and are filled with spongy tissue that contains smooth muscle, fibrous tissue, open spaces, veins, and arteries. A strong membrane, the tunica albuginea, surrounds the corpora cavernosa. The corpus spongiosum, which contains the urethra, runs along the underside of the corpora cavernosa.

Erection begins when a man receives an erotic sensory or mental stimulus. The brain sends impulses to the nerves around the penis, which cause the many tiny muscles of the spongy corpora cavernosa to relax, allowing blood to flow in and fill the open spaces inside the corpora cavernosa. This blood creates pressure in the corpora cavernosa, which makes the penis expand and compress the veins that normally allow the blood to drain. By helping to trap the blood in the corpora cavernosa, the tunica albuginea sustains the erection. Erection is reversed when the muscles in the penis contract, preventing blood from flowing in and opening the channels that allow blood to flow out.

ical factors such as disease or surgery, as well as psychological factors, can also cause erectile dysfunction. In the past, it was believed that erectile dysfunction was largely caused by psychological problems. Today most experts agree that, in 85 percent of cases, erectile dysfunction is the result of physical factors, most of which can be treated.

The following conditions can cause erectile dysfunction:

- *Diabetes.* High levels of blood sugar associated with diabetes can damage small blood vessels and nerves throughout the body, including those in and around the penis. Diabetes can interfere with the nerve impulses and the blood flow necessary to produce an erection. About 60 percent of men with diabetes experience erectile dysfunction.
- *Heart disease.* Atherosclerosis, which causes hardening and narrowing of the arteries, increases with age. Over time it can reduce blood flow to the penis and lead to erectile dysfunction. It accounts for most cases in men over 60 years of age.
- *Leaking veins.* When veins in the penis are not compressed during an erection, a vein can leak, leading to erectile dysfunction. A leak can be the result of injury, disease, or damage to the veins in the penis.
- *Neurological injuries or disorders.* Spinal cord and brain injuries, including paraplegia and stroke, can cause erectile dysfunction when they interrupt the transfer of nerve impulses from the brain to the penis. Other nerve disorders, such as multiple sclerosis, Parkinson's disease, and Alzheimer's disease, may also result in erectile dysfunction.
- *Drugs.* More than 200 prescription medications may directly cause or contribute to erectile dysfunction. Among these are drugs for high blood pressure, antidepressants, tranquilizers, sedatives, and a number of over-the-counter medications. Long-term, excessive consumption of alcohol and use of illegal drugs such as heroin and cocaine also can cause erectile dysfunction.
- *Hormonal imbalances.* Hormonal disorders account for fewer than 5 percent of cases of erectile dysfunction. Testosterone deficiency, which is rare, can result in the loss of libido (sexual desire). An excess of the hormone prolactin, produced by tumors in the pituitary gland, reduces levels of testosterone. Kidney and liver disease also may lead to hormonal imbalances that contribute to erectile dysfunction.
- *Peyronie's disease.* This is a relatively rare inflammatory condition that causes scarring of the erectile tissue in the penis. The scarring produces a curvature in the penis that can interfere with sexual function. In addition, it may cause erections to be painful.
- *Pelvic surgery.* With surgery of the colon, prostate, or bladder, the nerves that control the flow of blood into and out of the penis may be cut or removed. These nerves can be permanently damaged in men who have undergone radiation therapy for prostate or bladder cancer. Although these nerves do not

control sensation in the penis and, therefore, are not responsible for orgasms, they influence the firmness of the penis during erection.

Some surgeons may try to spare nerve function during these procedures, with the hope that any sexual function problem will be temporary. Usually it takes 6 to 18 months for erections to return. Partial erections may return sooner. If they do, it could be a sign that complete erectile function will eventually return.

- *Pelvic injury.* A minor injury to the pelvic area, including a fall or blow to the hip while playing sports, or a very long bike ride, can sometimes numb the nerves around the penis and block their normal functioning. A day of rest is usually enough time for the nerves to recuperate.

- *Psychological causes.* Even though most cases of erectile dysfunction are the result of physical factors, psychological factors should not be overlooked. The most common psychological cause of erectile dysfunction is performance anxiety, a man's fear that he will not be able to perform sexually. Anxiety may lead to an initial failure, which increases the anxiety, resulting in a cycle that leads to future failures to achieve an erection.

Stress, tension, depression, worry, guilt, and anger can also inhibit sexual performance. These psychological factors may occur secondary to and possibly as a result of the physical causes. They may magnify the impact of erectile dysfunction resulting from physical causes.

Problems Associated with Erectile Dysfunction

Many cases of sexual dissatisfaction are related to problems in the control of ejaculation or in the loss of sexual desire unrelated to achieving or maintaining an erection.

Premature ejaculation is ejaculation that occurs too early, usually before, upon, or shortly after penetration. This condition, also called rapid ejaculation, is the most common sexual dysfunction. As many as 30 to 40 percent of men may have this problem. Even when rapid ejaculation is not defined by a man as a problem, it limits the sexual satisfaction of his partner.

Premature ejaculation is common among adolescent boys who fear being caught having intercourse or making their partner pregnant, or who have anxiety about their sexual performance. Some boys may find the excitement of seeing a nude body or touching a female to be so overwhelming and so stimulating that they may ejaculate even before they get their pants unzipped. In most men, ejaculatory control increases with sexual experience.

When premature ejaculation persists into adulthood, it often signals a problem in the relationship. One consequence of premature ejaculation is that the man begins to feel inadequate in meeting his partner's sexual needs since he may not maintain an erection long enough for his partner to achieve orgasm. He often tries to distract himself mentally during the sexual experience or reduce his thrusting in an effort to slow ejaculation. Some men may concentrate so heavily on not ejaculating that they lose all sense of pleasure in sexual intercourse.

There is no agreed-upon amount of time that has to pass before an ejaculation is no longer considered premature. Some experts have used the number of thrusts and the partner's achievement of orgasm as criteria. But there is no standard for how long the sex act should last. Some men may feel they are accomplished lovers if they can pull off a "quickie"; others may feel they demonstrate their masculinity by prolonging intercourse to satisfy their partner.

No one is sure what causes premature ejaculation. Some question whether premature ejaculation is abnormal and point out that in the animal kingdom rapid ejaculation is an evolutionary adaptation to ensure procreation of the species. For men, however, most experts think of it as a psychological or learned problem. Although the condition rarely has a physical cause, in some cases inflammation of the prostate gland or a nervous system disorder may be involved.

Three different approaches are used to treat premature ejaculation. Counseling by a psychologist, psychiatrist, or sex therapist may be recommended based on the assumption that the problem is psychological in origin. Success rates of counseling are difficult to evaluate, since therapists use a variety of methods to measure success.

The second approach to treating premature ejaculation is behavior modification. A popular technique is the "stop-start" exercise. The male works with his partner to stop sexual stimulation just short of reaching ejaculation. The erection is allowed to subside. Then stimulation is started over and the procedure is repeated. This gives the man confidence when the deliberately subsided erection returns. The aim is to improve the man's ability to maintain higher levels of sexual excitement without ejaculating.

The third and most recently introduced treatment method is medication. One of two drugs, clomipramine or sertraline, can be used to produce a rapid and dramatic delay in the ejaculation response, which persists only as long as the drug is continued. These drugs have few side effects. While the potential benefits of these medications are significant, there are some concerns that treatment may be offered without first evaluating the man's health history, current health status, and actual need for the medication.

Retarded ejaculation is the opposite of premature ejaculation—the inability to have an orgasm even with prolonged erection. This condition is rare. But as men get older, it normally takes longer to reach orgasm. Often, however, this condition is caused by blood pressure medications, tranquilizers, and antidepressants, as well as by diabetes. Psychological causes include fear of vaginal penetration and fear of ejaculating in the partner's presence. Treatment usually involves undergoing behavioral therapy to reduce anxiety and learning techniques for timing ejaculation.

Retrograde ejaculation is a condition in which semen travels up the urethra toward the bladder instead of through the penis. This condition is seen with some spinal cord injuries, after removal of the prostate gland, or after bladder surgery. It does not have any negative effects on the man's health.

Loss of libido (sexual desire) is a decrease in sex drive that occurs in both men and women. Nearly half of those seeking sex therapy have low libido. Most often, this common condition develops after years of normal sexual desire and activity. It may be caused by boredom, stress, depression, conflict with a partner, or changes in hormone levels. Often it is related to the increased use of medications, particularly in middle age.

A loss of libido may occur as a consequence of erectile dysfunction or it may precede erectile dysfunction. There is no "normal" amount of sexual drive or desire. Having less sexual desire than your partner does not indicate that you have a problem, only that there is a difference in how much sex each of you wants. If loss of libido has become a problem in your relationship, it is important to seek a physician's help to rule out medical causes. If psychological factors are involved, sex education, counseling, or behavioral therapy may help you and your partner communicate better and achieve a more intimate sexual relationship.

Decreased orgasmic intensity is another symptom of men who have problems with sexual function. It is not quite the same as loss of libido because the man still has the same level of sexual desire, but he experiences the loss of or diminished sensation of pleasure usually associated with ejaculation. Those who lose the sensation may lose interest in sex altogether. Others may become anxious, which often leads to erectile dysfunction.

The intensity of orgasm depends on many factors, including the setting in which sexual activity occurs, feelings toward the partner, the amount of fantasy and foreplay, the partner's physical response to stimulation, and the amount of time that has passed since the previous orgasm. Men with diabetes or with a neurological condition such as multiple sclerosis often experience decreased orgasmic intensity. With age, some loss of orgasmic intensity is normal.

Effects of Erectile Dysfunction

Erectile dysfunction, regardless of cause, leads both sexual partners to experience a range of feelings and intense emotions, including a sense of hopelessness and low self-esteem. These feelings can reinforce a man's performance anxiety and create a cycle of repeated failures and increasingly negative feelings. To overcome these feelings, both partners have to acknowledge the problem and communicate openly and honestly with each other. Because sexual performance is linked so strongly to a man's self-esteem, erectile dysfunction can be devastating not only to his sex life but also to his sense of self. Men with erectile dysfunction often develop feelings of inadequacy, embarrassment, or guilt, and may consider themselves unattractive to their partner. These feelings might cause a man to avoid intimate situations, isolate himself from the relationship, or withdraw from his partner, which can increase tension in the relationship.

The psychological effects of erectile dysfunction can invade other areas of a man's life as well, such as social interactions and job performance. It is important for a man with erectile dysfunction to overcome the reluctance to talk with his partner and physician to determine effective treatment strategies.

Diagnosing Erectile Dysfunction

Since erectile dysfunction has a number of causes, the underlying problem must be found through diagnostic procedures before treatments can be suggested. A physical examination always includes a medical and sexual history. The doctor asks questions regarding the use of prescription medications, other drugs, and alcohol. He or she also will ask about possible problems at work or at home and about other diseases that may contribute to the dysfunction. In particular, the doctor will ask about your ability to have erections and how frequently you have erection problems. From this information the doctor can determine the severity of the problem.

The doctor will perform a physical examination that includes many of the procedures that are part of a regular checkup. Blood and urine tests can indicate unusual levels of hormones, cholesterol, or blood sugar, and help evaluate liver and kidney function, thyroid activity, and blood counts. The following general diagnostic tests are usually performed for diagnosing erectile dysfunction:

- Urine tests for protein (albumin) and sugar (glucose) can confirm the presence of diabetes and indicate the level of kidney function.
- Blood tests check the levels of several body chemicals that are potential factors in erectile dysfunction. For example, a high blood sugar level indicates diabetes; about 60 percent of men with diabetes experience erectile problems. A high cholesterol level may indicate the presence of atherosclerosis, which might slow the flow of blood into the penis. A lowered blood level of the male hormone testosterone or a high blood level of the hormone prolactin also can cause erectile dysfunction.
- Liver and kidney function tests look for hormonal imbalances that may be present in these organs when they are not properly removing waste from the body.

The following tests are performed less frequently to diagnose erectile dysfunction:

- A thyroid function test measures the levels of thyroid hormones. Thyroid hormones regulate body metabolism and the production of sex hormones.

- A complete blood cell count (CBC) measures the number of red blood cells and white blood cells. Too few red blood cells may indicate anemia, which can limit the amount of oxygen the body's cells receive. Increased white blood cell levels can indicate the presence of infection.

The following specialized tests can be used to more directly evaluate erectile function through examination of the blood vessels, nerves, muscles, and other tissues of the penis and surrounding areas:

- An evaluation of blood circulation to the penis is made by taking the pulse of the penis and surrounding pelvic area. This procedure tells the doctor whether the blood supply to the penis is sufficient to produce an erection.

  Other approaches to studying penile blood flow include measuring penile blood pressure with the use of a special cuff or with ultrasound. Special types of ultrasound testing, such as duplex ultrasound or Doppler ultrasound, provide motion pictures of penile blood flow while an erection is induced by injection of a drug.
- An assessment of secondary sex characteristics such as breast enlargement in a man (gynecomastia) may indicate testosterone deficiency or an excess of the female hormone estrogen, either of which can decrease erectile function.
- Penile nerve function tests can determine if there is sufficient sensation in the penis and surrounding area. In one such test, called the bulbocavernous reflex, the physician squeezes the glans (head) of the penis, which causes the anus to contract if nerve function is normal.
- An evaluation of nocturnal penile tumescence is made. A man normally has five to six erections during sleep, especially during rapid eye movement (REM) stages, which occur during the dream segments of sleep. Nocturnal erections occur about every 90 minutes and last for about 30 minutes each. Failure to have nocturnal erections may indicate a problem with nerve function or blood supply to the penis. Nocturnal erections can be measured at home using either of two methods:

  1. A *snap gauge* is a band that contains three plastic strips that are wrapped around the penis. These strips snap when they are stretched. Each of the strips has a different strength so that a rough measure of penile rigidity and the change in its circumference can be assessed during a nocturnal erection.
  2. A *strain gauge* is a circular device that measures the change in circumference at the base and at the tip of the penis during an erection.

- Biothesiometry uses vibration to measure the perception of sensation. A decreased perception of vibration may indicate nerve damage in the pelvic area, which can lead to erectile dysfunction.

- Injection of a vasoactive substance (a substance that affects the width of the blood vessels) into the penis may be used to cause an erection by dilating (widening) the blood vessels and erectile tissues. These erections may last about 20 minutes, during which time penile pressure is measured and X-ray films may be taken of the penile blood vessels using a special dye.
- Specific nerve tests are used for patients with suspected nerve damage as a result of diabetes or a history of nerve disease, or when a physical examination reveals a nervous system abnormality, suggesting neurological causes of erectile dysfunction.

Treatment

At least half of all men between 40 and 72 have at least occasional problems either getting or keeping an erection. Because it is often believed to be "all in your head" or due to aging, many men think that their case is hopeless and simply stop having sex. Men and women should recognize that sexual intercourse is just one form of sexual relations, albeit an important one; various types of sexual play, including oral sex, can keep a couple close.

About 95 percent of cases of erectile dysfunction are treatable. During the 1990s, the variety of treatment options expanded. A urologist (a physician who specializes in treating disorders of the urinary tract) can describe what methods are most appropriate for you. Regardless of the method you ultimately choose, consider the following important factors:

- *Motivation.* Honestly evaluate what is motivating you to seek treatment and try to understand your expectations about treatment. Unrealistic expectations may undermine the success of treatment. Be committed to the treatment you choose and do what is necessary to make the course of treatment successful.
- *Willingness to adapt.* All treatments for erectile dysfunction require active participation by the patient. Be willing to change your habits, learn new sexual techniques, and adapt to unanticipated events or circumstances to make the treatment work.
- *Partner's attitude.* Erectile dysfunction is often called a couple's problem for a variety of reasons. If a couple is having difficulty getting along, this may result in sexual problems. Also, some treatments for erectile dysfunction may require a man's partner to participate or administer medication. Since partners often experience similar emotional responses to the problem, some couples find that counseling can help them adjust to the treatment and reestablish a mutually satisfying sexual relationship. Either way, a partner's involvement in and commitment to treatment definitely help a man recover. Although the man might be reluctant or embarrassed to have his partner involved, most partners of men with erectile dysfunction want to be involved in the treatment process, because they both will benefit.

Sildenafil   Sildenafil is an oral medication for treatment of erectile dysfunction that has been available since 1998. Sildenafil does not produce erections, but it improves erections already produced by sexual stimulation. Foreplay is an essential component for the erection. Sildenafil works by inhibiting the enzyme responsible for relaxing an erection by breaking down a chemical called cyclic guanosine monophosphate (cGMP). The action of sildenafil in the body increases the levels of cGMP, relaxing the smooth muscles in the penis and increasing blood flow into the penis.

Sildenafil is absorbed and processed rapidly by the body. It must be taken a half hour to an hour before sexual intercourse and should not be used more than once a day.

Warning: Sildenafil must not be taken by men who are using nitrates, which are medications taken for chest pain and high blood pressure. Men who are using nitrates who then take sildenafil risk dangerously low blood pressure and stroke.

Overall, studies have shown that sildenafil is effective for about 50 to 75 percent of men being treated for erectile dysfunction. Effectiveness rates vary depending on the cause of the problem, but the drug has produced positive results for a range of men under treatment, including those with diabetes (57 percent) and spinal cord injuries (83 percent), as well as men who have had a radical prostatectomy (43 percent).

Sildenafil has few major side effects, but minor side effects include headaches, flushing, indigestion, and blue-green color vision deficiency. Sildenafil is available only with a doctor's prescription.

Is Sildenafil for You?

What it is

Sildenafil is a prescription medication that is used to treat erectile dysfunction. It is the first oral medication for this purpose approved by the US Food and Drug Administration.

What it is not

Sildenafil is not an aphrodisiac. It will not arouse or increase sexual desire. It is not a means to improve erections in men who do not have erectile dysfunction. It is not a chemical substitute for working on a relationship.

How it works

Sildenafil blocks an enzyme in the penis that naturally breaks down a chemical called cGMP, which is produced during sexual stimulation and plays an important role in creating and sustaining normal erections. cGMP allows smooth muscle in the penis to contract, allowing more blood to enter the penis and producing a firmer erection. The longer cGMP remains in the penis, the better the chance of reaching and maintaining an erection. Sildenafil allows more cGMP to remain in the penis, but it does not increase the body's production of the chemical. This is why sexual arousal is necessary in the first place—to produce some cGMP.

How sildenafil should be taken

Sildenafil comes in three dosages: 25-, 50-, and 100-milligram (mg) tablets. The medication can be taken on an empty stomach about 1 hour before sexual intercourse, although it may work from 30 minutes up to 4 hours after the tablet is swallowed. Physicians usually prescribe a home trial of 50-mg tablets. If side effects develop, a lower dosage may be tried. If the response is not adequate and there are no side effects, dosage may be increased to 100 mg. Older men and those with liver or kidney failure may begin with the 25-mg tablets.

Note: Only one tablet a day should be taken. Taking more than 100 mg a day will not significantly improve the erection response and will only increase the likelihood of having side effects.

What side effects are known?

Headache is the most common side effect (about 16 percent of men taking sildenafil). A drop in blood pressure and facial flushing occur in about 10 percent of men who are using the drug. Indigestion occurs in 7 percent and nasal congestion in 4 percent. About 3 percent report some visual disturbance (blurred vision, increased light sensitivity, or seeing a bluish tinge on objects). None of these side effects is severe, and most are described as mild. Very few men stop taking the medication because of the side effects.

What medications should not be taken with sildenafil?

Men taking any type of organic nitrate medication or medications containing nitrates should not take sildenafil. Nitrate-containing medications include a number of vasodilator drugs, such as nitroglycerin. Certain street drugs, such as amyl nitrate, also will cause problems if taken with sildenafil.

How much does sildenafil cost, and will insurance cover it?

The cost at most pharmacies is about $8 to $10 a pill. Some insurance prescription drug plans cover the cost, but others do not. Some insurance plans reimburse for only a few pills a month. Contact your insurance provider directly for details on coverage.

How do I obtain sildenafil?

Because of the side effects and contraindications of sildenafil, you should see your physician for an examination. If the doctor determines that the drug is likely to help you, he or she will write a prescription.

Warning: Because of the popularity of and demand for sildenafil, some Web sites are offering prescriptions to men without obtaining sufficient medical information about them. People who order the drug directly over the Internet, without a physician's examination or a review of their medical history, are putting themselves at risk for dangerous side effects or even death. Men who have other medical problems, especially heart disease, or who have not been sexually active should check with their physician before resuming sexual activity.

Self-Injection Therapy   Another method for treating erectile dysfunction is self-injection drug therapy. It requires that the man or his partner use a tiny needle to inject a small amount of medicine directly into the side of the penis. The injections are relatively painless and create an erection that begins about 5 to 15 minutes after the injection and lasts from 30 minutes to 2 hours. No foreplay is needed.

Drugs used for self-injection therapy include a prostaglandin (a synthetic fatty acid) called alprostadil, papaverine hydrochloride, and phentolamine in combination with papaverine. Each of these drugs creates an erection by relaxing smooth muscle tissue and widening the major artery to the penis, which enhances blood flow to the penis.

Originally, the US Food and Drug Administration (FDA) approved these drugs for other medical purposes, but only the prostaglandin drug has been approved specifically for treating erectile dysfunction. Papaverine and phentolamine have not yet been approved for treating erectile dysfunction, even though they were the first drugs used experimentally for injection therapy. However, they are available and prescribed for medical reasons other than the FDA-approved use. Urologists have gained considerable experience with all three of these drugs, and all are considered safe for self-injection therapy.

Not all men respond to this type of treatment. Apart from the fact that most men have trouble injecting a needle into their penis, self-injection therapy cannot be used by men with certain heart or liver diseases. Of those who can take the injections, some do not respond by developing good erections, while others may get erections that do not go away and require a counterinjection to soften them. Still, about 70 percent of men find that they achieve satisfactory erections after self-injections. Generally, a doctor can teach a person to do the injections in one or two office visits. The men are asked to return for follow-up visits, particularly at the beginning of the treatment process, to see if changes are needed in the type of drug used or its dosage.

All medications used in self-injection therapy have both potential risks and side effects. Some men have experienced dizziness, heart palpitations, or a flushed feeling when using these medications. And there is a small chance of infection and the possibility of bleeding or bruising during injection.

One of the risks of self-injection therapy is prolonged erection or priapism—an erection that lasts more than 4 hours. Priapism occurs in only a small percentage of men, but it requires a trip to a hospital emergency department to receive medication to counteract the self-injection and relieve the erection. Men should know that any erection that lasts more than 2 hours needs to be treated by a physician to prevent damage to the penis.

Another potential risk, particularly for those who use self-injected drugs often, is the possibility of permanent scarring inside the penis. For this reason, doctors advise that self-injection therapy be limited to once every 4 to 7 days, depending on what medication is used and how a man responds to the initial treatment.

Self-injection therapy has the following advantages:

- It can be used anytime and involves only a small amount of preparation.
- It creates an erection that is very similar to a natural erection.
- The erection generally lasts long enough for successful and satisfying intercourse.
- It does not interfere with orgasm or ejaculation.
- It does not involve surgery and is only minimally painful.
- The drug costs $8 to $10 per injection, which is much less than surgery. (Sildenafil currently costs about $8 to $10 per pill; see page 154.)

Urethral Suppositories   In 1997 the FDA approved an alternative form of the drug alprostadil. The product is a single-use applicator filled with the drug. The user inserts the applicator about an inch into the urethral opening of the penis, where the drug is released, absorbed by the urethra, and transported to the surrounding tissues. An erection begins within 8 to 10 minutes and may last as long as 30 to 60 minutes. These times vary from one person to another.

The most common side effects associated with urethral suppositories are aching in the penis, testicles, legs, and the area between the scrotum and the rectum; a warm or burning sensation in the urethra; redness of the penis due to increased blood flow; and minor urethral bleeding or spotting, usually caused by improper application.

Vacuum Devices   Vacuum devices are simple mechanical tools that allow a man to develop an erection suitable for sexual intercourse. The devices available work best for men who are able to achieve partial erections on their own. They can be harmful to men who have blood-clotting problems or who use blood-thinning medication.

Vacuum devices work by pulling blood into the penis and then trapping it. The man inserts his penis into the hollow plastic tube that is closed at one end and presses the tube against his body to form a seal. A vacuum is created in the tube using a small hand- or battery-driven pump, and this, in turn, draws blood into the penis, causing the penis to engorge, enlarge, and become rigid. After 1 to 3 minutes in the vacuum, an adequate erection develops and a soft rubber O-ring is then placed around the base of the penis to trap blood and maintain the erection. Sexual intercourse can occur anytime after the tube is removed. The rubber O-ring maintains the erection until removed. It can be left in place for 30 minutes only, or blood supply to the penis is compromised. It takes practice to use this device skillfully.

The vacuum device has the following advantages:

- It can be used anytime, at the user's convenience.
- It is safe—it has no side effects (unless left on longer than 30 minutes) and does not involve surgery or injections.
- It works for most types of erectile dysfunction.
- It costs less than surgery or ongoing self-injection therapy.

The vacuum device has the following disadvantages:

- Setup time can interfere with a couple's mood or foreplay.
- Devices may not fit all body shapes.
- Once the O-ring is applied, there is no erection between the rubber band and the body, making the penis somewhat floppy, so guidance is needed for insertion.
- In some men the O-ring inhibits ejaculation.
- Some men complain of a coldness or numbness of the penis after the O-ring has been put in place.
- O-rings must be removed after 30 minutes to allow return of normal blood flow to the penis.

Vacuum erection devices range in price from $300 to $500 and require a physician's prescription. Some insurance companies reimburse all or part of the costs associated with this type of treatment. This can be a useful treatment for some men who take nitrate medications for chest pain or high blood pressure and are therefore unable to use sildenafil.

Penile Implants   An implantable penile prosthesis (artificial device) is another treatment option that has improved in design in recent years. All penile implants place prosthetic tubes inside the penis to mimic the engorgement process and create an erection. Since the 1950s, thousands of men have been treated successfully with implants. These devices work best for men who can ejaculate and have orgasms even if they cannot achieve erections.

Implants are effective in treating most types of erectile dysfunction. They have a 90 percent success rate when both partners are informed about how they work and what their limitations are. Men with penile implants do not require intensive follow-up treatment after implantation, and no medications or injections are required. In addition, once the implant is in place and functioning, there are no additional costs. The newer prostheses are very reliable, with a chance of mechanical failure in the range of only 2 to 4 percent per year.

One drawback of the implantable penile prostheses is that their placement permanently changes the internal structure of the penis. If the prosthesis is ever removed, normal erections do not return. There is also a small (3 to 5 percent) chance of infection that could require removal of the implant. Some men develop surgical or anesthetic complications or experience numbness at the head of the penis and uncomfortable intercourse. Also, because the erection is not caused by increased blood flow to the penis, the head of the penis is not part of the erection, and this softness may bother some men.

There are three types of penile prostheses currently available:

- *Inflatable penile prostheses* are the most natural-feeling of the penile implants, because the penis can be either erect or flaccid. These two-piece or three-piece implants are made of soft tubes of silicone or similar material. The tubes are filled with a sterile liquid that comes from a small reservoir placed either under the muscles of the abdomen (three-piece implant) or in the scrotum (two-piece implant). A tiny pump in the scrotum is used to move the fluid from the reservoir to the tubes. The more fluid that is pumped into the tubes, the firmer and larger the erection. When the erection is no longer desired, the pump is deactivated and the fluid returns to the reservoir, leaving the penis soft again. The major advantage of an inflatable penile implant is that it provides a more natural erection that the user can control. One major disadvantage is that this type of device is slightly more complicated to implant and, because it has more mechanical parts, there is an increased risk of leaks, twisting of the tubes, or mechanical failure.
- *Self-contained inflatable implants* use paired silicone cylinders that have a pump at the tip of the prosthesis. A reservoir within the shaft of the device allows fluid to transfer in such a way that the cylinder becomes firm. The advantage of this device is that surgery is slightly simpler than that for a two- or three-piece inflatable prosthesis. The major disadvantage is that the inflatable portion does not significantly increase the girth of the penis. The penis is also not as soft or as easily concealed when deflated.

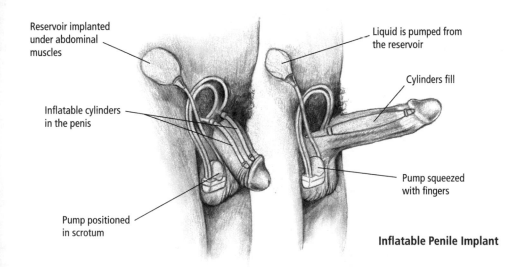

Reservoir implanted under abdominal muscles

Liquid is pumped from the reservoir

Cylinders fill

Inflatable cylinders in the penis

Pump squeezed with fingers

Pump positioned in scrotum

Inflatable Penile Implant

- *Semirigid prostheses* are made from silicone-covered bendable metal rods. They allow the penis to be rigid enough for penetration but flexible enough to be concealed in a curved position. They are the simplest and least expensive of all implants and have the least chance of mechanical failure. The major problem with semirigid implants is that the penis is always semierect. Even with bendable implants, concealment can be a problem with certain types of clothing. Another disadvantage is that the erection depends on the size and rigidity of the prosthesis. This type of prosthesis is not routinely used.

Vascular Reconstructive Surgery   A very small percentage of men may be candidates for reconstructive surgery to improve penile blood flow. Techniques being used on an experimental basis include revascularization (rerouting blood vessels to allow new, greater blood flow to the penis) and venous ligation (sealing off veins in the penis that leak blood during attempted erection).

Overall, the long-term experience with this type of surgery has been disappointing. Even the best results show that only one of 20 men can be helped with these procedures. Vascular reconstructive surgery is a very technical and expensive procedure. Complications include nerve damage, thrombosis (clotting of blood inside deep-lying veins, usually in the legs), and scar tissue formation. It is rarely used to treat men who do not have a specific vascular abnormality causing the erectile dysfunction.

CHAPTER 8

Disorders of the Reproductive System

The male reproductive organs are shown in the accompanying illustration. Sperm, which carry the man's genes, and testosterone, the primary male sex hormone, are made in the testicles. Each of the two testicles is about the size of a walnut, and they lie side by side inside the scrotum. (The left testicle usually hangs a little lower than the right.) The scrotum, a thin-skinned pouch, protects the testicles and acts as a climate-control system. Since the testicles need to be slightly cooler than body temperature for normal sperm development, the scrotum lies outside the body. The epididymis, which lies atop each testicle, is a coiled tube that collects sperm from the testicles and stores them until they are mature.

The vas deferens is a long duct that carries sperm from the epididymis past the prostate gland and into the seminal vesicle. The prostate gland and seminal vesicle produce fluids that support the sperm and make up 98 percent of the semen that is ejaculated through the urethra during orgasm. The urethra is also part of the urinary tract and transports urine from the bladder.

This chapter describes the most common disorders of the male reproductive system.

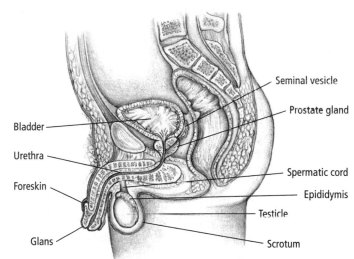

The Male Reproductive System
The most visible parts of the male reproductive system are the penis and the testicles. The two testicles are suspended in a pouch of skin called the scrotum. During sexual arousal, spongy tissue inside the penis becomes engorged with blood. The testicles produce sperm and the primary male sex hormone testosterone. From the testicles, sperm travel through a duct called the vas deferens into a pair of sacs called the seminal vesicles. The seminal vesicles produce a fluid that is added to the sperm to create semen—the whitish fluid that is ejaculated.

161

The Testicles and the Scrotum

The testicles are two male sex organs that produce sperm and the male sex hormone testosterone. The testicles are suspended in a pouch of skin called the scrotum. Each testicle hangs from a structure called the spermatic cord, which is made up of the vas deferens, nerves, and blood vessels. The vas deferens transports newly formed sperm to the urethra from a tube behind each testicle called the epididymis.

Testicular Injury

Having the scrotum hanging from the lower torso has its disadvantages. The legs help protect it from blows from the side, and the buttocks shield it from the back. But every man, at some time in his life, has gotten or will get a frontal blow to the groin and scrotum that causes excruciating pain. Despite the natural tendency to coil up in a fetal position, the blow usually is not as bad as it feels. The testicles are capable of moving about inside the scrotum in response to a blow. They usually bounce back with no lasting effects because the tissues within the scrotum are spongy and flexible and can absorb a great deal of shock without sustaining permanent damage.

Pain associated with testicular injury is very different from other types of pain. Testicles are organs that are located outside the body. Pain for them is similar to pain sensed by any other internal organ. It tends to be deeper, more intense, and more widespread than pain to the outside of the body. This is why a blow to the testicles can cause pain that is accompanied by sweating, nausea, and dizziness. It is the brain's way of acknowledging that a crucial organ has been hit and that the whole body must respond to this potential emergency.

The initial pain felt after an injury is caused by the swelling of the testicle within its protective pouch. The pressure caused by the swelling affects the surrounding nerves, causing pain to spread to the lower abdomen. An ice pack applied to the scrotum and anti-inflammatory drugs (such as aspirin or ibuprofen) can be used to reduce the swelling and the pain.

If pain and swelling persist after an hour, see a doctor immediately. The blow may have caused the testicle to rupture, or it may have twisted the spermatic cord that supports the testicle. Also, too much pressure from swelling within the scrotum can cause tissue damage that can lead to infertility, blood clots, or the loss of a testicle.

Undescended Testicles

The testicles are located inside the abdomen before birth. They normally descend into the scrotum about a month before birth. In 1 percent of males, for unknown reasons, one or both testicles may remain in the abdomen at birth. Usually this condition corrects itself within the next 3 months. If the testicles have not descended by 1 year of age, the infant should be examined by a physician to determine whether surgery is needed to bring them into position.

A male whose testicles remain undescended until puberty will be incapable of producing viable sperm. He is also at a significantly higher risk of developing testicular cancer. Surgery is usually performed while the child is a toddler, because critical emotional problems may arise when genital surgery is performed on an older child.

Testicular Torsion

Each testicle is suspended in the scrotum by a spermatic cord made up of blood vessels, nerves, and the vas deferens. On rare occasions, and for reasons not well understood, the cord becomes twisted and cuts off blood flow to and from the testicle. It is a very painful condition. Torsion usually occurs in children and teenagers, but it can occur in adults. Most cases have no identifiable cause. Torsion also can occur during sleep.

Signs and symptoms of testicular torsion may include sudden, severe pain in the groin; one testicle resting higher in the scrotum; one testicle lying horizontally in the scrotum; nausea and vomiting; swelling of the scrotum; and fever. Prompt treatment, usually surgery, is required to untwist the cord, fix both testicles in position, and prevent testicular strangulation. Permanent damage can result if the condition is not treated within 4 to 8 hours. If left twisted, the testicle will swell and then atrophy.

Epididymitis

Epididymitis, which is inflammation of the epididymis, can be caused by an infection. The condition may produce severe pain in the scrotum, fever, and a swollen area that may feel hot when touched. The doctor examines the testicle and tests a urine sample. He or she will prescribe antibiotics if the infection is bacterial. Additional treatment includes bed rest, over-the-counter painkillers, an ice pack applied to the scrotum, and a scrotal supporter if the infection is not bacterial. The condition usually does not cause permanent damage.

Orchitis

Orchitis, inflammation of the testicle, is a rare condition that is usually caused by mumps, or sometimes by an infection in the prostate gland or the epididymis. Symptoms include pain in the scrotum, swelling that usually occurs on only one side of the scrotum, and a feeling of "heaviness" in the scrotum. Diagnosis and treatment are the same as for epididymitis—the doctor performs a manual examination of the testicle and tests a urine sample. He or she will prescribe antibiotics for a bacterial infection or bed rest and pain relievers for a viral infection. Orchitis may cause permanent damage to one or both testicles and may lead to infertility.

Abnormal Fluid Accumulations

The suffix "-cele" refers to a swelling or noncancerous tumor within a body cavity. Sometimes fluids build up in the scrotum. For example, a *hydrocele* is a collection of watery fluid in the membrane covering the testicles. A *hematocele* is a collection of blood that may result after injury to or rupture of a testicle. A *spermatocele* is a cyst full of sperm that develops next to the epididymis. A *varicocele* is a mass of varicoselike veins caused by a malfunction of the valves within the veins of the spermatic cord. It has been described as feeling like a "bag of worms." Most often it causes a dull pain or a feeling of heaviness, usually on the left side of the scrotum.

Diagnosis of these conditions can be a simple matter. The doctor may use a special flashlight to shine light through the scrotum. If the light shines through the scrotum, it indicates a possible hydrocele. If light does not pass through the scrotum, it indicates a possible hematocele. A spermatocele lights up under a flashlight in a darkened room. The varicocele usually will not allow light from a flashlight to pass through the scrotum. Diagnosis is confirmed by manual examination or by an ultrasound examination of the scrotum.

These conditions are seldom serious or permanent and may even be painless. But if they continue to enlarge, they become very uncomfortable and may affect fertility. At this point, surgical removal is recommended.

Testicular Cancer

Testicular cancer is a growth of abnormal cells within a testicle. Doctors do not know the exact cause of testicular cancer. It accounts for only 1 percent of all cancers in men. However, it is the most common cancer in men aged 15 to 34. Testicular cancer is about four times more common in white men than in African American men, with rates for Hispanic, Native American, and Asian men between those two groups. Thanks to dramatic advances in therapeutic drugs, along with better diagnostic tests, survival rates for the cancer have been boosted significantly. Today, testicular cancer is frequently curable, especially with early diagnosis and treatment.

There are two different types of testicular cancer: seminomatous and nonseminomatous. Seminomas, which account for about 40 percent of all testicular cancers, are made up of a single type of immature germ cell (probably arising from the cells that produce sperm). Seminomas are usually slower growing and usually are found before they spread to other parts of the body.

Nonseminomas (also called teratomas) consist of a mix of different cell types. They account for about 55 percent of testicular cancers, tend to grow more rapidly, and often spread before they are discovered. An estimated 60 to 70 percent of men diagnosed with nonseminomas have cancer that has spread to nearby lymph nodes.

The risk of testicular cancer is three to 17 times higher than average for boys born with undescended testicles (see page 162)—a condition called cryptorchidism. The risk increases if the condition is not surgically corrected before puberty. Other conditions associated with testicular cancer include:

- Klinefelter syndrome—a chromosomal disorder in males characterized by small testicles, enlarged breasts, and a lack of secondary sex characteristics such as beard growth and voice change
- gonadal aplasia—failure of the testicles to develop
- hermaphroditism—development of both male and female sex characteristics
- low birth weight
- fetal alcohol syndrome (mother's use of alcohol during pregnancy)

Most testicular cancers are found by men themselves, either by chance or while performing a self-examination of the testicles (see page 91). Symptoms of testicular cancer include the following:

- a lump in either testicle
- enlargement of a testicle
- a feeling of heaviness in the scrotum
- a dull ache in the lower abdomen or in the groin area (where the thigh meets the abdomen)
- a sudden collection of fluid in the scrotum
- discomfort in a testicle or in the scrotum
- enlargement or tenderness of the breasts

If you notice any of these symptoms, see a doctor immediately. Cancer of the testicles usually *does not* cause pain, although some men may experience soreness or discomfort in the scrotum or in the groin area.

Men with suspected testicular cancer usually undergo a complete medical checkup, including a careful examination of the testicles. If the physical examination and laboratory tests do not show an infection or other disorder, additional tests will be conducted to find or rule out cancer. Various imaging methods are used to diagnose testicular cancer. One method is ultrasound, in which high-frequency sound waves are used to create images of the testicle. This procedure is painless and noninvasive.

The only way to determine whether a tumor is malignant (cancerous) is to examine a small sample of tissue from the testicle under a microscope. The tissue must be obtained by removing the entire affected testicle using a surgical procedure called a radical inguinal orchiectomy. The testicle is removed through a small incision in the lower abdomen.

The surgeon cannot simply cut through the scrotum or remove just part of the testicle because, if cancer is present, cutting through the outer layer of the testicle might cause the cancer to spread to surrounding tissues and lymph nodes. Removing the testicle can prevent the cancer from spreading to other parts of the body. Removal of one testicle does not interfere with fertility or the ability to have an erection.

Cancer Stages   Doctors measure the extent of the cancer by conducting tests that categorize, or "stage," the disease. These staging tests include blood analyses, imaging techniques, and, sometimes, additional surgery. Staging allows doctors to plan the most appropriate treatment.

There are three stages of testicular cancer:

* stage I—cancer of the testicle is confirmed
* stage II—cancer has spread to lymph nodes located toward the back of the abdomen below the diaphragm (the muscular wall separating the chest cavity from the abdomen)
* stage III—cancer has spread beyond the lymph nodes to sites away from the abdomen

Through blood tests, a doctor can check for tumor-associated markers, which are substances often present in abnormal amounts in people who have cancer. By comparing levels of these markers before and after surgical treatment, a doctor can determine if the cancer has spread beyond the testicles. Likewise, measuring marker levels before and after chemotherapy treatment can help show how well the treatment is working.

Treatment   Treatment of testicular cancer will depend on what cell type (seminomatous or nonseminomatous) is present, how advanced the cancer is, and the patient's age and overall health. If caught early enough, the initial removal of the testicle may also be the treatment for a seminoma. In some cases, radiation therapy directed to the lymph nodes is used to kill cancer cells that have spread there.

Surgery to remove the lymph nodes into which the testicles drain is often necessary for patients with testicular cancer. Doctors examine lymph tissue under a microscope to help determine the stage of the disease. Also, removing the tissue helps control further spread of the cancer.

Because *seminomas* tend to be slow growing and tend to stay in one area, they generally are diagnosed in stage I or II. Treatment is usually a combination of testicle removal, radiation, and chemotherapy. Surgical removal of lymph nodes usually is not necessary for patients with seminomas because this type of tumor responds very well to radiation treatment. Most stage III seminomas are treated with multidrug chemotherapy and radiation.

Even though *nonseminomas* grow more rapidly and often spread before they are caught, the cure rate is very high. Surgical removal of the lymph nodes is often necessary after the cancer has spread beyond the testicle, because nonseminomas do not respond as well to radiation therapy. Treatment of nonseminomas also can include chemotherapy with various drug combinations. Patients with stage II nonseminoma who have had a testicle and lymph nodes removed may need no further therapy, but some doctors recommend a short course of multidrug chemotherapy to reduce the risk of recurrence. Most stage III non-seminomas can be cured with drug combinations.

All men must be carefully monitored by their physician for at least 2 years after treatment for testicular cancer because about 10 percent experience recurrences, which are then treated with chemotherapy. Each method of treatment has different side effects, which can vary from one person to another. The loss of one testicle does not affect a man's ability to engage in sexual intercourse and does not cause infertility. A man with one healthy testicle can have a normal erection and produce sperm. Some men may choose to have an artificial testicle implanted into the scrotum for cosmetic purposes.

To be sure the cancer is completely gone, regular follow-up examinations are necessary. Testicular cancer seldom recurs after a man has been cancer-free for 3 years. Men who have been treated for cancer in one testicle have about a 1 percent chance of developing cancer in the remaining testicle. If cancer develops in the second testicle, it is almost always a new disease rather than the result of cells that have spread from the first tumor. These men should be conscientious about doing a testicular self-examination every month.

Side Effects Any kind of cancer treatment can cause undesirable side effects. However, not all people react the same way or to the same extent to any particular treatment. One of the main concerns of young men is how their treatment might affect their sexual or reproductive capabilities.

Removing one testicle does not impair fertility or sexual function. The remaining testicle can produce sperm and hormones adequate for reproduction. Removal of lymph nodes usually does not affect the ability to have erections or orgasms. It can, however, disrupt the nerve pathways that control ejaculation, causing infertility.

Modern "nerve-sparing" surgical techniques have increased the odds of retaining fertility. Many surgeons are abandoning procedures that involve total lymph node removal. By limiting the amount of surgery necessary to achieve a cure without disrupting the nerves, surgeons are now able to preserve the ejaculation function in as many as 90 percent of men.

Chemotherapy can cause increased risk of infection, nausea or vomiting, and

Self-Examination of the Testicles

Men of all ages, not just those at high risk for testicular cancer, should perform a testicular self-examination at least once a month. Most cases of testicular cancer can be caught in the early stages, when it is most curable, with a routine testicular self-examination. It is a simple procedure that takes only a few minutes. The best time to do a testicle self-examination is immediately after a warm bath or shower because the skin of the scrotum is relaxed, making it easier to find anything unusual. For how to perform a self-examination of your testicles, see page 91.

hair loss. Not all men experience these side effects. Some drugs may cause infertility, but many men recover their fertility within 2 to 3 years after therapy ends. Men who are receiving radiation therapy may experience fatigue or have lowered blood cell counts. Infertility also may result from radiation treatments, but it is temporary.

The Prostate Gland

Your prostate is a walnut-shaped gland that lies immediately beneath your bladder surrounding the urethra, the tube inside the penis that carries urine out of your body. It secretes a fluid that becomes part of semen. The gland can easily become inflamed during an infection, causing soreness, swelling, frequent urination, and a burning sensation while urinating. The prostate gland also can become enlarged, a condition called benign prostatic hyperplasia, which is a common problem in older men. An enlarged prostate gland can cause a number of bothersome problems when urinating, including hesitancy or straining to urinate; a weak stream of urine; dribbling; retention of urine; or the inability to control urination, also called incontinence. Other common symptoms include frequent urination, feeling an urgent need to urinate, and excessive urination at night.

If you have any of the symptoms of prostate enlargement, you should not feel embarrassed about talking them over with your doctor. You don't need to change your lifestyle to avoid situations, such as going to the movies, when it might be difficult to go for long periods without urinating. Effective surgical and drug treatments exist to help alleviate your symptoms.

The most feared prostate problem is prostate cancer, which now affects one in five men during his lifetime and is a leading cause of cancer death in American men. With early diagnosis and treatment, however, prostate cancer is curable.

Because the prostate lies in front of the rectum, the doctor can feel the prostate by inserting a gloved, lubricated finger into the rectum. This is called a digital rectal examination. It allows the doctor to determine whether the prostate is enlarged or has lumps or other areas of abnormal texture that he or she can feel.

Prostatitis

Prostatitis is inflammation of the prostate gland. There are three basic forms of prostatitis: bacterial prostatitis, nonbacterial prostatitis, and prostatodynia.

Bacterial prostatitis, also called infectious prostatitis, is divided into two types: acute and chronic. Acute bacterial prostatitis is a rare but serious disease caused by bacteria in the prostate gland. The bacteria may originate from an infection in another part of the body, such as infections in the sinuses or the ears, or from an infection in another part of the urinary tract. Chronic bacterial prostatitis is a recurring prostate infection that usually results when acute bacterial prostatitis has not been treated successfully. It tends to occur in older men who have an enlarged prostate gland. Nonbacterial prostatitis, the most common form of the disease, is similar to chronic bacterial prostatitis, except that no bacteria are present. Prostatodynia is pain in the prostate caused by inflammation, which is not accompanied by infection or swelling.

The symptoms of bacterial and nonbacterial prostatitis are similar. They include the following:

- discharge of fluid from the penis
- pain or itching deep within the penis or at the head of the penis
- discomfort during urination
- fever, pain in the groin area, lower-back pain, and difficult urination that is often accompanied by a burning or an itching sensation
- a frequent urge to urinate without passing much urine
- blood in the urine

A diagnosis of prostatitis is usually based on the symptoms, a urinalysis, and a physical examination. When the doctor performs a digital rectal examination, the prostate may feel swollen and tender to the touch. If there are symptoms of acute bacterial infection, the digital rectal examination may not be done because manipulation of the prostate may release bacteria into the bloodstream.

To diagnose chronic bacterial prostatitis, a urine culture is done. In this test, the doctor takes one routine urine sample and one midstream urine sample (the person urinates for several seconds before collecting the sample of urine). A digital rectal examination is performed, and the prostate gland is massaged to release prostatic fluid. Another urine sample, which contains the released prostatic fluid, is taken. The samples are then compared to see if the infection is in the prostate or in the urethra.

In a few cases, a cystoscopic examination may be performed to confirm a diagnosis. A cystoscope is a flexible, lighted viewing tube that is inserted into the urethra. Proper diagnosis is essential for treating prostatitis because the various forms of the disease require different treatments.

Bacterial prostatitis is treated with antibiotics, along with bed rest and painkillers, if symptoms are severe. Hospitalization may be required if the urethra becomes blocked, the fever leads to dehydration, or if bacteria spread to other parts of the body. It is difficult to rid the prostate gland of infection. Infections often seem to disappear shortly after treatment begins, but bacteria often hide within the soft tissues of the prostate. Therefore, antibiotic therapy may be required for up to a month.

For chronic infections, it is common to take antibiotics for several months. Surgical therapy is performed only as a last resort for chronic bacterial prostatitis—usually when the condition causes urinary retention (inability to urinate) or kidney problems.

Antibiotics are not effective for treating nonbacterial prostatitis. Prostatodynia is often treated with over-the-counter medications such as aspirin or ibuprofen.

Muscle relaxants are sometimes prescribed because prostatodynia is considered stress-related. The following steps may lessen the symptoms of nonbacterial prostatitis:

- Avoid coffee, alcohol, and spicy foods if they seem to aggravate the prostate gland.
- Cut back on excessive driving, cycling, heavy lifting, and vigorous exercise that may put stress on your prostate area.
- Practice relaxation techniques such as deep breathing exercises and meditation.
- Soak in a warm bath. The warm water increases blood flow, which decreases inflammation.

Benign Prostatic Hyperplasia

Benign prostatic hyperplasia (BPH) is a noncancerous enlargement of the prostate gland. As the prostate becomes larger, it can compress the urethra and obstruct the flow and release of urine. It is difficult to start urinating, and the stream of urine is weak. With such blockage, the bladder muscles enlarge and the bladder nerves become irritable, causing contractions of the bladder that result in a frequent urge to urinate. Eventually the muscles can no longer push urine past the blockage and urine backs up, leading to bladder problems, frequent urinary tract infections, and possible urinary retention (the inability to empty the bladder). Urinary retention requires immediate treatment. BPH usually does not affect sexual function.

By age 50, more than half of all American men show some signs of prostate enlargement, and by age 70, more than 40 percent have enlargement that can be felt on physical examination. No one is sure what causes BPH, but researchers know that it requires the presence of testosterone. BPH does not occur in men who have had their testicles surgically removed or in men who are unable to metabolize testosterone.

Recent studies point to a high-fat and high-cholesterol diet as a risk factor for BPH. Obesity also may be a risk factor. Men with a waist size of more than 43 inches are twice as likely to develop BPH as are men with a waist size of 35 inches or smaller. However, there is no conclusive evidence of a link between obesity and BPH.

Symptoms of BPH are generally described as irritative or obstructive. Irritative symptoms, which are related to bladder muscle failure, include the frequent need to urinate, numerous trips to the bathroom at night, and urgency (the frequent or constant urge to urinate). These are generally the first signs of a prostate problem, even though they might not be noticeable until years after the prostate has begun to enlarge.

Bladder outlet obstruction is a term used to describe a cluster of obstructive symptoms associated with BPH and related to problems with urine flow. They include decreased force and diameter of the urinary stream, the inability to urinate, trouble starting the flow of urine, a weak flow, double voiding (after urinating, a man is able to urinate again in 5 to 10 minutes), dribbling after urination, and overflow urinary incontinence. Other symptoms associated with BPH may include frequent urinary infections marked by a burning feeling during urination and strong-smelling urine. There may also be some blood in the urine, which occurs when blood vessels are stretched and broken by enlarging prostate tissue.

Men who have these symptoms should see their doctor. Other diseases, including cancer, can cause these symptoms. Although BPH is not cancerous, advanced stages can lead to complications related to kidney damage or kidney failure.

To diagnose BPH, a doctor takes a medical history and performs a physical examination, including a urinalysis, to rule out infection. The doctor examines the bladder by pressing down on the abdomen. He or she will perform a digital rectal examination by inserting a gloved, lubricated finger into the rectum to feel the prostate and determine whether it is enlarged.

Since the part of the prostate that usually obstructs urine flow is the tissue immediately surrounding the urethra, which cannot be felt during a rectal examination, a digital rectal examination is somewhat limited in diagnosing obstruction due to BPH. Therefore, the doctor may perform a test known as a urodynamic evaluation to measure urine flow. The amount of urine left in the bladder after urination also will be measured.

Blood tests may be done to rule out kidney dysfunction or to screen for prostate cancer. Ultrasound tests may be used to create an image of the prostate. Cystoscopy (examination with a viewing tube) also may be done to allow visual examination of the urinary tract. While none of these tests alone can diagnose BPH with certainty, as a group they can support a diagnosis.

BPH cannot be cured, but its symptoms can be relieved by various medications and surgical techniques. Initially, before symptoms become overly bothersome, a physician may suggest a "watchful waiting" approach that does not include any treatment. This involves asking the patient to keep track of symptoms to see if they lessen or stabilize on their own, or whether there are certain external factors that bring on the symptoms, such as intake of caffeine or alcohol, exercise, or stress.

As the problems associated with bladder outlet obstruction due to BPH become less tolerable or intolerable, more aggressive treatments may be used. There are two types of medication used to treat an enlarged prostate: alpha-blockers (which are medications to reduce high blood pressure) and drugs that shrink the prostate. Because symptoms return if medication is stopped, medication must be taken indefinitely.

Alpha-blockers work in about 75 percent of men who try them. These medications, such as terazosin, work by relaxing the muscular component of the prostate, which often allows urine to flow more freely. The problem with alpha-blockers is their side effects, which initially include low blood pressure and dizziness on standing. These symptoms typically lessen or disappear with continued use of the drugs. A newer alpha-blocker used to treat BPH, called tamsulosin, may be less likely to cause these side effects.

Finasteride is a drug that relieves symptoms by reducing the size of the prostate. Finasteride takes about 3 to 6 months before it starts to work, but it has been shown to reduce the size of the prostate by 30 percent. Up to 60 percent of men who use finasteride reported some relief of their symptoms. However, the relief comes with some serious possible side effects. In some cases, finasteride has been associated with a decreased sex drive and erection problems. There is also evidence that finasteride reduces the level of PSA (prostate-specific antigen; see page 174) in the bloodstream by approximately half. For this reason, doctors take this into account when measuring PSA levels for detecting prostate cancer in men who are taking finasteride.

A variety of surgical procedures are used to treat BPH by removing or reducing prostate tissue. A prostatectomy is the removal of part of the prostate gland. A prostatectomy can be either open or closed. In an open prostatectomy, the gland or excess tissue that is causing the obstruction is removed through an abdominal incision. In a closed prostatectomy, surgery is done through a cystoscope (viewing tube) that is inserted up the urethra. Although closed prostatectomies have largely replaced open prostatectomies, open procedures are still performed if the prostate gland is very large or if other procedures are performed at the same time.

Transurethral resection of the prostate (TURP) is a closed procedure. TURP involves passing a special cystoscope called a resectoscope into the urethra and inserting a tiny wire loop or cutting edge up through the scope to remove excess prostate tissue from around the urethra. TURP is one of the most commonly performed surgical procedures, with 300,000 to 400,000 done each year. One major benefit of this procedure is reduction of urinary problems associated with BPH. Approximately 90 percent of men who undergo this procedure show improvement in their urinary symptoms. However, approximately 1 percent of men who have this procedure experience subsequent problems with urinary incontinence. The procedure may need to be repeated if the tissue that was removed grows back.

Another closed procedure is known as transurethral incision of the prostate (TUIP). This procedure differs from TURP in that the surgeon makes tiny cuts in the prostate to lessen its grip on the urethra. TUIP reduces the chances of experiencing certain problems after surgery, such as retrograde ejaculation, which is ejaculation backward into the bladder during sexual intercourse. In some cases, repeated procedures may be necessary.

Other treatments for benign prostatic hyperplasia are currently being developed. Among them are microwave thermotherapy, intraurethral stents, laser therapy, and transurethral needle ablation (TUNA). Microwave thermotherapy uses heat generated by microwaves to eliminate excess prostate tissue. Intraurethral stents are small, tubelike structures that are inserted into the urethra to enlarge it and provide relief from urinary symptoms. Laser therapy uses laser energy to vaporize excess prostate tissue. TUNA uses microwave technology to cut away obstructing tissue. The long-term effectiveness of these techniques has not yet been determined. No matter which treatment you are considering, be sure to discuss the risks and the benefits with your doctor so that you can make an informed decision.

A man with an enlarged prostate may find that certain foods and medications may increase the intensity of BPH symptoms. Try the following lifestyle changes and keep track of your symptoms:

- Stick to a low-fat, low-cholesterol diet. Men who follow such a diet have a lower risk of BPH.
- Eat more vegetables. Men who do so have a lower rate of BPH than those who do not.
- Limit your fluid intake, particularly at bedtime. It may help reduce the number of times you have to get up to urinate in the middle of the night.
- Avoid caffeine and alcohol. They may irritate the prostate and increase the need for nighttime urination.
- Monitor your medications. Certain drugs—including oral bronchodilators, diuretics, tranquilizers, and antidepressants, as well as over-the-counter remedies such as antihistamines and decongestants—aggravate urinary problems. Check with your pharmacist.

Prostate Cancer

Prostate cancer is very common, although its exact cause is unknown. Each year more than 150,000 new cases of prostate cancer are diagnosed in the United States, and more than 30,000 deaths are caused by this disease. It is third after lung cancer and colon cancer as a cause of cancer death in men.

Your risk of getting prostate cancer escalates after age 50, and having a father or a brother with the disease triples your risk. You are also at increased risk if you are African American. Prostate cancer can grow slowly—so slowly that years can pass before the disease becomes evident. Most cancer of the prostate never becomes life-threatening because men tend to develop it later in life and often die of another cause. However, some cancers of the prostate may be more aggressive and shorten the person's life. In some men the cancer grows so gradually that it never produces any symptoms. In others, prostate cancer causes a weak or interrupted flow of urine, inability to urinate, difficulty in starting or stopping the flow of urine, frequent urination (especially at night), blood in the urine, pain or burning during urination, or persistent pain in the lower back, pelvis, or upper thighs.

Prostate cancer usually is discovered in one of three ways: as the result of a prostate-specific antigen (PSA) blood test (see box below); during a digital rectal examination; or during an operation called a transurethral resection of the prostate, done to treat an enlarged prostate. To promote early detection, every white male over age 50 with no family history of prostate cancer should have a digital rectal examination performed by his doctor. Every African American male over age 45 and every white male over 45 with a family history of prostate cancer also should have a digital rectal examination. See your doctor immediately if you experience any of the symptoms of prostate cancer. When discussing prostate problems with the doctor, men of any age should mention if they are sexually active.

The PSA Test

A blood test called the prostate-specific antigen (PSA) test has been developed to diagnose prostate disease, including cancer, enlargement, and inflammation. The PSA test measures the blood level of a protein called prostate-specific antigen that is produced only by the prostate gland and is normally not found in the blood. High levels of this protein in a man's blood suggest the possibility of prostate cancer but also may indicate less serious prostate problems, such as an enlarged prostate or inflammation. Because of this, the test results need to be confirmed by removing a tiny portion of the prostate gland and examining it under a microscope, a procedure known as a biopsy.

A considerable amount of controversy exists about whether the PSA test should become an annual part of the health checkup for men over age 40. The test is useful for detecting tumors that cannot be found during a digital rectal examination. On the other hand, the test results can be uncertain, resulting in unnecessary follow-up procedures that may include a biopsy or even surgery. Still, the PSA test is the best technique doctors currently have to discover tumors in the prostate gland while they remain small and are potentially curable.

If you are over 50 years of age (45 if you are African American), discuss with your doctor the pros and cons of having an annual PSA test and the possibility of follow-up procedures if elevated levels are found. Only by talking with your doctor about the test can you come to the decision that is best for you.

Various treatments for prostate cancer are available, including surgery, radiation therapy, hormone therapy, chemotherapy, and combinations of these. When determining a treatment plan for you, you and your doctor will evaluate the benefits and possible side effects or risks of the available therapies, taking into account your age, your feelings and preferences, any other health conditions you may have, and the stage of your cancer. If you are an older man and your cancer is at an early stage, your doctor may recommend nothing more than "watchful waiting." Watchful waiting means that you would have regular digital rectal examinations to monitor your prostate, PSA blood tests every 3 to 6 months, and, perhaps, a yearly biopsy of your prostate.

The most common surgical procedure for prostate cancer is a radical prostatectomy. Radical prostatectomies are performed when the cancer does not appear to have spread beyond the prostate. In a radical prostatectomy, the whole prostate gland and the seminal vesicles are removed, along with surrounding tissue and, often, pelvic lymph nodes. In some cases, a procedure called transurethral resection of the prostate (TURP) is used to relieve symptoms before other treatments are used. TURP is most often used to treat noncancerous enlargement of the prostate (see page 170). Cryosurgery (also known as cryotherapy) is occasionally used to treat prostate cancer that has not spread beyond the prostate. In cryosurgery, a surgeon destroys cancerous cells by freezing them with a metal probe. Cryosurgery is generally not used as a first-line therapy.

One of two types of radiation therapy may be used to treat prostate cancer: external radiation therapy and internal radiation therapy (also called brachytherapy). In external radiation therapy, the physician uses a machine to aim high-power rays (gamma rays or X rays) or particles (electrons, protons, or neutrons) from outside the body directly at the tumor and, in some cases, the surrounding lymph nodes. In brachytherapy, tiny (about the size of a grain of rice), low-level radioactive pellets are inserted (permanently or temporarily) into the prostate gland. The doctor uses an imaging method such as ultrasound or CT scanning to guide the placement of the pellets. The permanent pellets, which give off radiation for a period of weeks or months, are left in place. In some cases, pellets containing high doses of radiation are inserted for less than a day and removed. Brachytherapy and external radiation therapy are frequently used together.

Hormone therapy is usually used for men whose prostate cancer has spread to other parts of the body or whose cancer has returned after treatment. The goal of hormone therapy, which is not a cure, is to lower the levels of androgens (male hormones such as testosterone, which can stimulate the growth of cancer cells in the prostate), thereby shrinking the cancer or slowing its growth. The two most effective ways to lower androgen levels are to surgically remove the source of androgens, the testicles (in a procedure called orchiectomy), or to give injections of medications that block the production of testosterone. The injections are usually given monthly, every 3 months, or every 4 months at the doctor's office or at a cancer center. Hormone therapy probably works best if it is started as soon as possible after the cancer has reached an advanced stage.

Because the adrenal glands produce a small amount of androgens, drugs called antiandrogens are sometimes used in addition to orchiectomy and testosterone-lowering drugs to inhibit the body's ability to produce the hormones.

These medications are usually taken as pills one to three times a day. This treatment does not appear to be as effective as the other treatments for prostate cancer.

Chemotherapy is used for men whose prostate cancer has spread beyond the prostate gland and for whom hormone treatment has not been successful. Chemotherapy uses high doses of drugs, given intravenously or by mouth, to kill cancer cells. The treatment may help slow tumor growth and reduce pain. Because chemotherapy does not kill all the cancer cells, it is not recommended for treating early stages of the disease.

The side effects of the various cancer treatments include:

- problems with sexual function such as erectile dysfunction (inability to achieve or maintain an erection) or loss of sex drive
- problems with urination such as frequent urination, incontinence (leakage or dribbling of urine), blockage of urine flow, blood in the urine, or a burning sensation while urinating
- problems with bowel function such as diarrhea, blood in the stool, or irritation
- swelling of the penis, scrotum, or prostate
- bruising of, pain in, or damage to the treatment area or nearby tissues
- nausea, vomiting, or loss of appetite
- breast enlargement or tenderness, hot flashes, or osteoporosis (weakening of the bones)
- fatigue, infection, heart disease, hair loss, or sores in the mouth

Penile Disorders

The penis can be injured in a variety of ways. Blows to the groin, such as those that occur in sports, can result in excruciating pain or injury. Cuts that result from catching the penis in a pants zipper also are common, but they usually heal quickly. Less common are job-related accidents that sever the penis, either partially or fully. Reattachment may be possible, but full penile sensation and function are rarely fully recovered.

Several types of inflammation problems may involve the penis and the urethra. Balanitis occurs when the glans, or head, of the penis becomes red and sore. Usually the cause is unknown, but it is sometimes caused by urinary tract infection or allergic reactions to clothing or detergents. In uncircumcised men, the irritation may result when the foreskin is narrow or difficult to retract, and secretions become trapped beneath the foreskin.

A more severe form of chronic inflammation, called *balanitis xerotica obliterans,* produces a hardened, whitish area near the tip of the penis and over the opening of the urethra. The cause is often unknown but may be an infection or an allergy. Antibacterial creams may cure the inflammation, but often surgery is required to open the urethra.

Phimosis

Phimosis is shrinking or tightening of the foreskin. This is normal in a newborn or an infant, but the foreskin usually loosens up by puberty. In older men, the condition may result from prolonged irritation, and it may interfere with urination or sexual activity. Phimosis may be associated with penile cancer. The usual treatment is circumcision (surgical removal of the foreskin).

Paraphimosis

Paraphimosis is constriction of the head of the penis by an extremely tight, retracted (pulled back) foreskin. This often occurs as a result of phimosis (see above). Swelling and pain occur if the foreskin cannot be returned to its normal position over the head of the penis. The constriction also can cause loss of blood flow to the head of the penis, which is a medical emergency that is usually treated by circumcision.

Peyronie's Disease

In some men, the penis becomes curved during an erection. This condition is called Peyronie's disease. The cause is unknown, but fibrous or scar tissue forms inside the penis and causes it to bend at an angle during an erection. This painful condition makes sexual penetration difficult or impossible. The disease often resolves itself over several months. Vitamin E is the first-line treatment for this condition. Injections of corticosteroids into the affected area are sometimes helpful. Ultrasound therapy also has worked for some men. Surgery may cure the disease, but it can cause further scarring and make the condition worse or cause erectile dysfunction.

Priapism

Another rare and not well-understood disease is priapism, a painful, persistent erection not brought on by sexual desire or stimulation. The underlying cause (possibly drugs, blood clots, a tumor in the pelvis or the spine, infection of the genitals, sickle-cell disease, or leukemia) results in blood vessel and nerve abnormalities that trap blood in the penis during an erection. Immediate relief comes from draining excess blood from the penis with a needle and a syringe and irrigating the spongy tissue of the penis with an antihistamine fluid to wash out any clots or other blockage.

Penile Cancer

Penile cancer is the growth of cancerous cells on the skin and in the tissues of the penis. It is rare in the United States—about 1,000 cases are reported each year, accounting for fewer than 0.02 percent of all male cancers in the nation. However, 25 percent of those who develop the disease die of it. Penile cancer is linked to the human papillomavirus (HPV; see page 184), which also causes cervical cancer in women.

Penile cancer can occur anywhere on the penis, but the most common sites are the glans (the head of the penis) and the foreskin (the fold of skin covering the glans). These cancers are usually slow growing, so the penis can be saved in most cases when the cancer is diagnosed early.

Penile cancer is most common in older men and African Americans, and the incidence rises steadily after age 55. Poor hygiene may be a risk factor for penile cancer in men who are uncircumcised. The theory is that if the penis is not kept clean, smegma, which is a buildup of mucus and other secretions, can collect under the foreskin and cause irritation and inflammation of the glans. This chronic irritation may set the stage for the development of cancer. Almost all cases of penile cancer occur in men who were not circumcised at birth.

Symptoms of penile cancer include a red spot, crust, wartlike growth, or sore on the penis; discharge from the penis; pain; a lump in the groin; or bleeding during an erection or intercourse. If you have any of these symptoms, see your doctor.

For a definitive diagnosis of cancer, affected areas of the penis are biopsied (tiny bits of tissue are removed for examination under a microscope). If cancer is detected, more tests are ordered to see if the cancer has spread to other parts of the body. In one test, called lymph node dissection, a needle is used to draw cells out of a lymph node (a gland that is part of the immune system) in the groin area. The cells are then examined to see if the cancer has spread to the lymph nodes.

The most common treatment for penile cancer is surgery, using one of the following methods. Surgery may be followed by other treatments such as radiation or chemotherapy.

- *Wide local excision.* The cancer and some normal tissue on either side of the abnormal area are surgically removed.
- *Microsurgery.* The cancerous area, but little normal tissue, is removed. To do this, the doctor removes the cells while looking through the microscope.
- *Laser surgery.* The cancerous area is destroyed using a narrow, concentrated beam of light.
- *Penectomy.* The penis is partially or totally amputated. Although this is the most drastic method, amputation is the most common and most effective treatment for penile cancer. Lymph nodes also may be removed during this procedure. In partial penectomy, in which part of the penis is removed, some men remain capable of erection, orgasm, and ejaculation. Total penectomy leaves men significantly impaired sexually, but in some cases, stimulation of the remaining tissue can produce orgasms.
- *Radiation therapy and chemotherapy.* These treatments are used after surgery.

- *Biological therapy.* This relatively new treatment involves injections of the protein interferon to enhance the body's natural defenses against cancer. It is still considered experimental.

Other growths on the penis, such as warts, sores, and blisters, are almost always caused by infection (see chapter 9).

Sexually Transmitted Diseases

Sexually transmitted diseases (STDs) are infections that are passed from one person to another through sexual contact. Contact refers to the transfer from person to person of bodily fluids such as vaginal secretions, blood, and semen (including preejaculate, the few drops of semen that are released before ejaculation). The transfer of fluids takes place during vaginal intercourse, but it also takes place during oral and anal sex. Sometimes STDs can be transmitted by kissing or by close body contact. Some types of STDs also may be transmitted through needles shared by intravenous drug users. However, STDs are never acquired from toilet seats, towels, doorknobs, or other inanimate objects.

After colds and the flu, STDs are the most common infectious diseases in the United States, with more than 15 million new cases each year, 3 million of them among teenagers. By age 21, nearly one in five Americans requires treatment for a disease acquired through sexual contact.

The rapid spread of STDs is sometimes referred to as a "silent" epidemic because many of the diseases often have no noticeable symptoms in the early stages. But some of the potential consequences of STDs are serious: infertility, heart disease, liver and brain damage, blindness, cancer, and even death. Babies whose mothers are infected with STDs may have birth defects or developmental problems.

Researchers have identified about 50 STDs, including bacterial infections, which are curable, and viral infections, which are not. Among the 20 or so most common STDs, most are easily diagnosed by physicians using simple urine and blood tests, and many are easily treated with drugs that also help keep these diseases from spreading. But many STDs are never diagnosed, either because a person has no symptoms or because he or she is embarrassed to seek medical help.

If you have any reason to believe that you have been exposed to an STD, consult your physician without delay. Many STDs are highly contagious, and if you have sexual contact with someone who has an STD, you have a high risk of becoming infected. While having multiple sexual partners increases your risk of contracting an STD, even a person in a monogamous relationship can be at risk, since one partner might be harboring an infection acquired years earlier.

Another reason to seek medical help if you suspect you may have an STD is that it is possible to have more than one STD at a time. STDs weaken the body's immune system, making a person with one STD at greater risk of developing another.

Safer Sex

Note that the term is "safer" sex rather than "safe" sex because abstinence is the only guarantee against STDs. To help prevent the transmission of an STD, follow these precautions every time you have sex:

- Use a latex condom (see page 197) each and every time you have sex, including anal and oral sex. Never reuse a condom.
- Don't have sex with a stranger.
- Avoid having sex with multiple partners. Monogamy with an uninfected partner who is monogamous virtually nullifies the chances that you will contract an infection.
- Don't have sex if you or your partner have any symptoms of an STD.
- Use a spermicide containing nonoxynol-9, which may provide additional anti-STD protection.
- Use only water-based lubricants during sex. Lubricants containing oil, such as petroleum jelly, can damage latex, making holes in a condom.
- Do not use a condom after its expiration date or if it has been damaged in any way.
- Note that STDs can be transmitted during sex using sexual aids or body parts other than the penis, such as fingers.
- Avoid binge drinking, which lowers inhibitions and may lead to unsafe sex.
- If you have any doubts about your or a partner's health, get tested.

Keep in mind that birth control measures (see page 195) such as the pill, diaphragms, and IUDs (intrauterine devices) do not provide protection against STDs. Although contraceptive foams or jellies kill some infectious microorganisms along with sperm, they are meant to be used with condoms and not as substitutes.

Trichomoniasis

Trichomoniasis is an equal-opportunity STD, as likely to infect men as women, but much less likely to cause symptoms in men. However, even if you have no symptoms, if you are infected, you can infect your sexual partner.

Trichomonas vaginalis, a single-celled bacterium, can lodge in the urethra, the bladder, or, less often, the prostate. Sometimes it can cause a frothy or pus-like discharge and painful or frequent urination, especially early in the morning. Other symptoms may include mild irritation of the urethra and moisture at the opening of the penis. In rare cases, the epididymis, the cordlike structure behind each testicle, also may be infected with the bacterium, causing pain in the testicles.

If your doctor suspects that you may have trichomoniasis, he or she may want to examine secretions from your penis that you collect first thing in the morning before urinating. You may also be asked for a urine specimen.

Trichomoniasis in men will usually respond to treatment with antibiotics within a week. It is important to wait until the disease is cured before having sexual intercourse because this infection spreads easily.

How to Use a Condom

Condoms will not protect you against STDs unless you use them consistently and correctly. To use a condom correctly:

- Keep your penis away from your partner's genital area until the condom is on because drops of semen can leak out before ejaculation.
- With the lubricated side out, put the rolled-up condom over the tip of your erect penis and roll it all the way down toward the base. If you have not been circumcised, pull your foreskin back before putting on the condom. Leave about half an inch of space at the top to catch the ejaculated semen and to reduce the chance that an overly stretched condom will break.
- Withdraw your penis immediately after intercourse, holding the condom at the base to prevent it from slipping off as your erection subsides. Check the condom for signs of leakage.
- Throw the condom away after you use it; never reuse a condom.

If you don't have a condom, your partner may want to use a female condom, which is a soft, thin polyurethane sheath that fits inside the vagina and has a visible outer ring. A female condom doesn't protect against STDs as well as a male condom, but is better than no condom. It can be inserted up to 8 hours before sex and does not have to be removed immediately afterward.

Chlamydia

Chlamydia is the most common bacterial STD in the United States. The micro-organism *Chlamydia trachomatis* infects more than 3 million men and women each year. Chlamydia also is one of the most devastating STDs, because it often causes no symptoms and can lead to pelvic inflammatory disease (PID) in women. PID is responsible for up to 15 percent of cases of female infertility.

Among men, chlamydia is one of the leading causes of urethritis (inflammation of the urethra). If you experience pain during urination, burning or itching around the urethra, a discharge from the penis, or swelling in the testicles, you may have chlamydia. About 50 percent of infected men have none of these symptoms and do not get treatment, which puts their sexual partners at considerable risk.

Women are even less likely to have symptoms, but they are more likely to experience long-term consequences. In addition to developing PID, a woman with chlamydia can pass the infection to her baby during childbirth, causing pneumonia or conjunctivitis (inflammation of the membrane that covers the white of the eye and lines the inside of the eyelid).

The good news is that chlamydia is simple to diagnose and treat, thanks to new urine screening tests and antibiotics that can clear up the infection.

Genital Herpes

Genital herpes is caused by one of two types of herpes simplex virus: HSV-1 and HSV-2. Both viruses can infect the genitals and travel to other parts of the body, including the hands and the eyes. Usually, however, HSV-1 infects the mouth, causing small, painful blisters on the lips, while HSV-2 infects the genitals. If you have had one type of herpes infection, you can still get the other, although it is likely to be a less severe infection. Neither infection can be cured; they can only be controlled.

The symptoms of genital herpes usually appear within a week of infection in the form of itching, tingling, and soreness of a reddish patch on the skin in the groin area, which is followed shortly by small, red, painful blisters. In men these can occur on the penis, scrotum, buttocks, anus, or thighs. The blisters break, causing circular, open sores that develop a crust in a few days. During this time, walking may be painful and urination difficult. The person may develop a fever and feel ill. Within a week to 10 days the sores will scab over and heal—until the next outbreak.

Despite these painful symptoms, genital herpes must be diagnosed by examining (under the microscope) a sample taken from one of the sores. When the diagnosis is confirmed, the physician will prescribe an antiviral medication. Such drugs have two effects: if taken early enough, they can shorten an outbreak; if taken over time, they can reduce the number of recurrences. Recurrences often start with a sick feeling (flulike symptoms such as a cough, muscle pain, and headache) and a return of itching, tingling, or pain in the affected area.

Warning: If you have genital herpes, it is important to know that you can infect a sexual partner even between outbreaks, and even when you have no symptoms.

When herpes spreads, it can be life-threatening. It can infect the covering of the brain (the meninges) or the spinal cord. It can spread through the bloodstream to the liver, lungs, joints, or skin; babies and people with impaired immune systems are especially vulnerable. Even without spreading, the virus may affect the nerves in the pelvic area, causing pain, constipation, inability to urinate, and erectile dysfunction. However, these complications are rare.

Genital Warts

Genital warts, which are caused by the human papillomavirus (HPV), are one of the most common STDs. Some people who have been infected with HPV never get genital warts, but they can still spread the infection.

Typically, the warts first appear 1 to 6 months after exposure to the virus. The warts favor warm, moist places. In men this usually means the tip or the shaft of the penis, including beneath the foreskin in an uncircumcised male. Some men, particularly those who engage in anal sex, may develop warts inside the rectum or around the anus.

As with other kinds of warts elsewhere on the body, genital warts start small and soft and become hard and rough-surfaced, often developing stalks. Multiple warts often grow in the same area, creating a cauliflowerlike effect. The growth is rapid, especially in men with weakened immune systems—for example, men who have AIDS (acquired immunodeficiency syndrome).

The good news is that the warts usually disappear on their own after a few months. The bad news is that they tend to return, even if they have been removed. Genital warts can be treated (but not cured) with prescription creams or gels such as imiquimod or podofilox. These medications are applied directly to the affected area. The warts also can be removed with surgery, which is done using a local anesthetic, cryotherapy (freezing), or a laser. Warts in the urethra may be treated with anticancer drugs or removed surgically. Some doctors recommend removal more often than others. All doctors, however, will want to remove and examine a wart that is unusual in appearance or that lasts an unusually long time, to make sure it is not cancerous.

If you develop warts or have been exposed to sexually transmitted HPV, you must notify your sex partners so they can be examined and, if necessary, treated. (Certain types of genital warts in women are associated with cervical cancer.)

Molluscum Contagiosum

Molluscum contagiosum is a harmless viral infection that is more common among children than adults. It is easily transmitted by direct or nonsexual skin-to-skin contact and during sexual intercourse.

The infection produces tiny lumps (papules) that are shiny, pearly white, and circular. Each lump has a depression in the middle, which produces a cheesy fluid if squeezed. A crust forms before healing occurs. Papules may appear (in groups or alone) on the genitals, inside of the thighs, on the face, or other places.

Molluscum contagiosum usually clears up by itself in a few months but may require treatment that destroys the growths with heat, cold, or chemicals.

Gonorrhea

Gonorrhea is caused by the bacterium *Neisseria gonorrhoeae*. It is one of the most common infectious diseases in the world; after nongonococcal urethritis (see next page), it is the most common STD, infecting 1 million to 3 million Americans each year. Gonorrhea occurs most often among young adults with multiple sexual partners.

Following a short incubation period of 2 to 10 days, men who have been infected with gonorrhea typically develop discomfort in the urethra. This progresses to pain on urination and a discharge of pus from the penis; the urge to urinate is frequent and urgent, and the opening of the penis may become red and swollen. Gonorrhea acquired during oral or anal sex is not likely to produce symptoms. Symptoms that do occur include a sore throat (from oral sex) and pain in and discharge from the anus (from anal sex).

As a bacterial disease, gonorrhea can be treated with antibiotics, either with a single injection or a week-long course of oral medication. If gonorrhea has spread through the bloodstream, the antibiotics are given intravenously, which sometimes requires hospitalization. Many people with gonorrhea also have chlamydia (see page 183) so they should be tested for both.

Because gonorrhea is highly contagious, and because women who are exposed to it may not develop symptoms for weeks or months, it is important for people who are infected to identify and notify all previous sexual partners. Many clinics have special counselors, called contact tracers, who can help with this process.

Untreated gonorrhea may spread to other parts of the body, including the prostate and the testicles. Inflammation of either organ may cause infertility. (Like chlamydia, gonorrhea is a major cause of pelvic inflammatory disease in women, who may become infertile as a result.) If fluids infected with the bacterium come into contact with the eyes, the result may be gonorrheal conjunctivitis, an eye infection that, if left untreated, can lead to blindness. A different kind of eye infection may affect infants born to infected mothers.

Gonococcal arthritis, causing joint pain and swelling, can occur when gonorrhea spreads through the bloodstream. However, this condition is rare. Septicemia (commonly known as blood poisoning) is a potentially fatal disorder involving high fever, chills, headaches, and clouding of consciousness. It is another rare complication of bloodborne gonorrhea.

Nongonococcal Urethritis

Inflammation of the urethra that is not caused by gonorrhea (see previous page) is referred to as nongonococcal urethritis. It is the most common STD worldwide. About half of all cases of nongonococcal urethritis are a result of infection with chlamydia (see page 183) or genital herpes (see page 183); the other half have no known cause.

Regardless of its origin, nongonococcal urethritis generally follows the same course: an incubation period of 2 to 3 weeks followed by a discharge from the penis, which may be clear or contain pus, and a burning sensation during urination. When waking up in the morning, a man may find the opening of his penis to be red and stuck together with dried secretions. If symptoms recur, they may be severe or mild.

While a doctor can usually diagnose chlamydia by examining the discharge from the penis under a microscope, more elaborate laboratory tests may be required to identify other microorganisms. Antibiotics can be effective against nongonococcal urethritis but are less effective when the specific microorganism causing the problem cannot be identified. The cure rate is roughly 85 percent. Because recurrences are common, follow-up visits to the doctor are necessary for 3 months after treatment. If the infection returns, drug treatment is repeated for a longer period. Ideally, a man's sexual partners will be treated at the same time he is treated.

Left untreated, symptoms caused by chlamydia will most often disappear on their own in a month or so. However, the bacteria may cause epididymitis (painful swelling of the scrotum on one or both sides; see page 163).

Other complications of nongonococcal urethritis in men include prostatitis (inflammation of the prostate; see page 168) and urethral stricture (a narrowing of the urethra; see page 294). About 5 percent of men with nongonococcal urethritis develop Reiter's syndrome, which is a combination of arthritis, urethritis, and sometimes conjunctivitis.

HIV and AIDS

Acquired immunodeficiency syndrome (AIDS) is a fatal disease that was first reported in the United States in 1981 and has since become a major worldwide epidemic. By the end of 1999, more than 600,000 Americans had been diagnosed with AIDS, which began its spread among male homosexuals but is now more prevalent among minority populations.

Nearly a million Americans may be infected with the human immunodeficiency virus (HIV), which is the cause of AIDS. The progression from HIV infection to AIDS usually occurs within 10 years. With the development of new and more potent antiviral drugs, scientists hope that the time between HIV infection and the development of AIDS will lengthen.

HIV kills or impairs cells of the immune system, progressively destroying the body's ability to fight infections and certain cancers. It does this by multiplying within and ultimately destroying cells called T4 lymphocytes (T cells or CD4 cells), which are central to proper functioning of the body's immune defenses.

Blood, semen, saliva, tears, nervous system tissue, breast milk, and vaginal secretions can all harbor the virus. Most often, the virus enters the body through the lining of the vagina, vulva, penis, rectum, or mouth during homosexual or heterosexual sex. HIV is readily spread among drug users who share needles and syringes contaminated with infected blood. Rarely, HIV is transmitted to or from a healthcare worker through accidental sticks with contaminated needles. Before universal screening of blood donors and the introduction of reliable techniques to destroy HIV in blood products, HIV could be transmitted through blood transfusions. In the past, many people with hemophilia acquired AIDS through blood transfusions with infected blood products.

One quarter to one third of all untreated pregnant women who are infected with HIV transmit the virus to their fetuses during pregnancy or childbirth. Drug treatment during pregnancy and cesarean section can reduce this transmission rate to 1 percent.

People infected with HIV may experience a flulike illness within a month or two of exposure to the virus; many have no symptoms. This symptom-free period lasts from a few months to a decade, although the virus is actively multiplying, infecting, and killing immune system cells during this time. The only sign of this virulent activity may be a decline in blood levels of CD4 cells from a normal level of about 1,000. Once a person's CD4-cell count falls below 200, he or she is considered to have AIDS. By that time, other signs of the immune system's deterioration have appeared: swollen glands, lack of energy, weight loss, frequent fevers and sweats, persistent or frequent yeast infections, skin rashes, short-term memory loss, frequent and severe herpes infections, or a painful nerve disease called shingles.

Confirmation of HIV infection involves testing a blood sample for the presence of antibodies to fight the virus, which may not reach detectable levels for 1 to 3 months after exposure. A negative test result (meaning that no antibodies to the virus were detected in the blood) should be followed by repeated testing after 6 months if the person is still at risk or has symptoms.

Early diagnosis has become increasingly important as researchers have identified more effective drugs that, when used in combination, seem to delay development of the disease. These include drugs called nucleoside analog reverse transcriptase inhibitors (such as zidovudine, also called AZT), which interrupt an early stage of virus replication; and the more recent protease inhibitors, which interrupt the same process at a later stage. These "cocktail" drug regimens are not cures, and they typically cause unpleasant side effects such as nausea and diarrhea. However, when started early, they enable people infected with HIV to live relatively normal lives for longer periods.

AIDS

In addition to CD4-cell counts of less than 200, AIDS is defined by the presence of one or more of 26 conditions, most of which are "opportunistic" infections that a healthy person could easily fight off. These include highly aggressive forms of certain cancers such as lymphomas (cancers of the immune system) and a type of skin cancer called Kaposi's sarcoma. Other opportunistic infections are:

- *Pneumocystis carinii* pneumonia (PCP)
- severe cytomegalovirus infection
- toxoplasmosis
- diarrhea caused by *Cryptosporidium* or *Isospora* organisms
- candidiasis
- cryptococcosis
- chronic herpes simplex infection

People with opportunistic infections experience symptoms such as coughing, shortness of breath, seizures, severe and persistent diarrhea, fever, vision loss, severe headaches, weight loss, extreme fatigue, nausea, vomiting, lack of coordination, coma, abdominal cramps, difficult or painful swallowing, and mental changes such as confusion and forgetfulness.

In addition to treatment for such separate conditions, which can be very difficult to coordinate, adults with CD4-cell counts of less than 200 are given drug treatment to prevent the occurrence of PCP, which is one of the most common and deadly opportunistic infections associated with HIV. Regardless of CD4-cell counts, people who survive PCP must take these drugs for the rest of their lives.

The course of AIDS varies widely. Many people with AIDS are so debilitated by their symptoms that they are unable to hold a job or perform simple household chores. Others may go through periods of devastating illness followed by periods of normal functioning.

Despite years of research, there is still no vaccine for AIDS. Thus the only way to prevent infection by HIV is to avoid behaviors that allow transmission of the virus. This means not using intravenous drugs, not sharing needles if you use intravenous drugs, and not using anyone else's toothbrush, razor, or other implements that could be contaminated with blood. Also, of course, it means practicing safer sex (see page 181). People who have a history of other STDs are more vulnerable to infection with HIV, and should be treated immediately for any STD they may acquire.

It is not necessary to avoid normal contact with people infected with HIV, even if they have developed full-blown AIDS. That's because HIV is not spread through casual contact, including contact with:

- food utensils and food
- towels and bedding
- doorknobs
- swimming pools
- telephones
- toilet seats

HIV also is not spread by hugging, holding hands, or having other physical contact in which neither blood nor semen is exchanged.

If you do have to come into contact with the blood of someone whom you have reason to suspect may be infected with HIV, or if you are infected and there is any possibility of getting your blood on someone else, you should wear latex gloves or take other protective measures.

Researchers around the world are working to develop HIV vaccines and new therapies for AIDS and its associated conditions. Some vaccines and many drugs are in the testing stage. At the same time, researchers are trying to determine exactly how HIV damages the immune system so they can more precisely target their efforts. Of special interest to researchers are the 50 or so persons known to have been infected with HIV more than 10 years ago who have never developed AIDS. Do they have a less virulent form of the virus? Or does something in their genetic makeup protect them from AIDS? The answers may point the way toward a vaccine or, perhaps someday, a cure.

Syphilis

Syphilis is a bacterial infection that can be cured by antibiotics, usually penicillin, but that can cause serious problems if left untreated. The disease is much less common today than before the development of penicillin, and safer sex practices to curb HIV transmission also helped reduce the incidence of syphilis. Congenital (from birth) syphilis, which occurs in babies born to mothers with syphilis, is very rare today.

The spiral-shaped bacterium *Treponema pallidum,* which causes syphilis, enters the body through broken skin or through mucous membranes in the genitals, rectum, or mouth during sex. One intimate contact with someone who is infected—even if it's only kissing—can increase your chances of becoming infected by as much as 30 percent.

Left untreated, syphilis usually passes through four stages:

Primary stage. The first sign of the disease—a small, smooth, painless sore called a chancre—usually appears within 3 to 4 weeks of contact with an infected person. The sore grows on the penis but also may appear on the anus, rectum, mouth, or fingers. The sore does not bleed, but it may leak a clear fluid that is highly infectious. The surrounding lymph nodes may become enlarged and rubbery but are not tender. Since no pain is involved, about one third of infected men are not aware of the sore, which usually heals in 4 to 8 weeks.

Secondary stage. A skin rash usually introduces the secondary stage of syphilis, which begins 6 to 12 weeks after infection and may last up to a year. The rash may be short-lived, last for months, or disappear and then recur. Usually the lymph nodes are greatly enlarged at the same time, and the infected person may have one or more of the following symptoms:

- headaches
- bone aches
- loss of appetite
- anemia
- fever
- fatigue
- inflammation of the eyes, which can cause blurred vision
- inflammation of the kidneys, which can cause protein to leak into the urine
- inflammation of the liver, which may cause jaundice (a yellowing of the skin and the whites of the eyes)
- meningitis, which can cause headaches, neck stiffness, and sometimes deafness
- hair loss
- thick gray or pink patches on the skin (condylomata latum), which are highly infectious

Latent stage. During this stage, there are no symptoms, even though the infection is present. In some people, syphilis remains latent for the rest of their lives. But about one third of people who are untreated will enter the last (tertiary) stage.

Tertiary stage. There is no predicting when the tertiary stage will begin. It can be as early as 3 years into the infection or as long as 25 years later. Similarly, the effects are varied, from mild to severe. A process called gumma formation destroys tissues and organs—bones, brain, heart, blood vessels, liver, or skin. One consequence, called cardiovascular syphilis, affects the aorta and can lead to the formation of aneurysms (ballooning of an artery caused by blood pressing against a weakened area) and damage to the heart valve.

The active bacteria in the fluid from a chancre make primary syphilis easy to detect under a microscope. Blood tests can confirm the diagnosis at any stage.

Caught early, syphilis can be cured with a single high-dose injection (called a depot injection) of penicillin; later, a longer course of treatment is needed. However, more than half of those treated have an adverse reaction to the antibiotic within hours. In response to the sudden, massive death of bacteria, the body may produce a fever, headache, sweating, shaking, chills, or temporary worsening of the sores.

While organ damage caused by syphilis cannot be reversed, the prognoses for primary-, secondary-, and latent-stage syphilis are good. It is important to note, however, that infection does not confer immunity; once cured, you can become infected again.

Syphilis is infectious only during the primary and secondary stages, during which even practicing safer sex cannot provide complete protection. For this reason, abstinence is the best course early in the disease.

Neurosyphilis, syphilis of the nervous system, can occur during the tertiary stage of the disease but is rare in developed countries. Diagnosis may require testing a sample of cerebrospinal fluid. The outlook for recovery is poor. There are three major types of neurosyphilis:

- Meningovascular neurosyphilis is a chronic form of meningitis in which the linings of the brain and the spinal cord are inflamed.
- Paretic neurosyphilis causes behavioral changes and, ultimately, dementia.
- Tabetic neurosyphilis (tabes dorsalis) is a progressive disease of the spinal cord that begins with intense, stabbing pains in the legs and eventually affects walking and bladder control, among other symptoms. The person may develop tremors and spasms of pain in various organs.

Hepatitis B

Hepatitis is inflammation of the liver. Hepatitis is an umbrella term for infection with one of five different viruses—hepatitis A, B, C, D, or E—all of which cause different diseases but have one symptom in common: inflammation of the liver. Since the viruses are different, they cause different symptoms.

Hepatitis B, also called serum hepatitis, is spread by contact with infected blood, semen, and vaginal secretions, as well as by contaminated hypodermic needles and tools used for tattooing and body piercing. Newborns can acquire hepatitis B from their infected mother during delivery.

Those at risk for hepatitis B infection include:

- people who participate in any kind of sexual activity (anal, oral, or vaginal) with an infected partner
- people who have sex with multiple partners
- intravenous drug users
- emergency care personnel who are exposed to blood
- nurses and other healthcare workers
- people who are receiving hemodialysis

The pattern of infection for hepatitis B changed during the 1990s. Children in rural areas used to have the highest incidence. Today, young adults in urban settings are the most affected group.

Many people with the virus have no symptoms. Others may have mild to severe flulike symptoms, dark urine, light-colored stool, jaundice (a yellowing of the skin and the whites of the eyes), fatigue, and fever. If the disease goes untreated, the virus can cause liver damage, leading to cirrhosis or liver cancer.

More than 90 percent of those infected with hepatitis B get over their symptoms without lasting complications. A vaccine is now available for people such as healthcare workers who are at significant risk of being exposed to contaminated blood and other body fluids. The vaccine provides protection for up to 18 years. All American children are now vaccinated against hepatitis B during their first 18 months.

Chancroid

Once limited mainly to the tropics, chancroid, also called soft chancre or soft sore, is becoming more common in North America. Caused by the *Haemophilus ducreyi* bacterium, chancroid is characterized by painful, persistent ulcers on the genitals and enlarged lymph nodes in the groin.

Three to 7 days after infection, small blisters form on the genitals and around the anus. These quickly rupture to form shallow ulcers, which may enlarge and join together. At the same time, the lymph nodes in the groin may become tender, enlarged, and matted together, forming a shiny, red-surfaced abscess. Pus is discharged when the skin of the abscess breaks down. Left untreated, the abscess may leave deep scars.

The sores are the basis of the diagnosis of chancroid, but this may need to be confirmed by examining a sample of the pus under a microscope. The problem is that the chancroid does not always look like its textbook description and may be mistaken for an ulcer caused by syphilis or genital herpes. Chancroid, syphilis, and genital herpes are the most common causes of sexually transmitted skin lesions.

As with other bacterial STDs, antibiotics are the treatment of choice but, in this case, the drug must be injected every 6 hours for at least 7 days. It is sometimes necessary to remove pus from an abscess with a syringe. For at least 3 months after that, the person must be monitored by a doctor to make sure the infection is cured. It is important to find and examine the person's sexual partners so they can be treated if necessary.

A person with a chancroid ulcer who is exposed to HIV (human immunodeficiency virus) is more likely to become infected.

Pubic Lice

Pubic lice are not an infection but an infestation by small, wingless insects. Their scientific name is *Phthirus pubis,* but they are commonly called crabs, because of their crablike claws, which they use to grasp hair. Usually this is pubic hair, but crabs have been found in armpit hair and beards and may even attach to eyelashes. The lice may also settle around the anus and in the hair on the legs and trunk. The typical infestation involves fewer than a dozen lice.

An adult louse has a small, flat body up to 2 millimeters across. It is either grayish white or brown, colors that blend in with the surroundings and make the insect difficult to see. The lice lay shiny white eggs, called nits, at the bottom of the hair shafts, where they hatch 7 to 10 days later.

Sometimes pubic lice cause no symptoms. Most often, however, they cause small red sores and itching, which becomes worse at night. If lice infest eyebrows or eyelashes, they can cause the eyes to become inflamed.

While unaffected by ordinary soaps, pubic lice can be destroyed with a special shampoo or lotion containing malathion or carbaryl. Typically, the medication works in a single treatment, but it is important to follow the directions very carefully; if used incorrectly, the chemicals can be toxic. Itching may persist for a few days after successful treatment. Contact your physician, however, if you develop redness, swelling, tenderness, or drainage around the areas of infestation or if the lotion comes into contact with your eyes.

If you have pubic lice, it is not enough to kill only those that are attached to your body. You must also wash your clothes and bedding in water hotter than 140 degrees Fahrenheit, since the lice can survive without a human host for 1 to 2 days.

Since pubic lice are nearly always spread by close physical contact, the affected person's sexual partners also should be treated. They should avoid intimate contact with others until the lice are entirely gone.

CHAPTER 10

Birth Control

Birth control has several different meanings. When used as a synonym for family planning, it refers to control over the number or spacing of children using various methods to either prevent or control the frequency of pregnancy. When used as a synonym for contraception, birth control refers strictly to the prevention of pregnancy. Contraceptives are the means by which pregnancies are prevented.

Most polls on sexual behavior show that more than half of all American teenagers are sexually active by age 17. However, polls also show that only one third of all parents talk to their children about birth control, and two thirds of all sexually active teenagers never or rarely use contraceptives. This lack of communication may partly explain why there are about one million unwanted teenage pregnancies each year in the United States.

Taking Responsibility for Birth Control

Couples have attempted to control conception throughout the centuries using a variety of techniques, such as eating special herbs, performing religious rituals, or timing sexual intercourse with different phases of the moon. But safe and effective methods of contraception have been available only since 1930.

There is no such thing as an ideal method of contraception, and every method has its advantages and disadvantages. When choosing which method to use, you and your partner should weigh the advantages, disadvantages, and side effects of each method, taking into account your religious and moral values as well as personal and aesthetic factors.

Although most methods of contraception can be used without medical advice, you still should have a clear understanding of the female reproductive system and the menstrual cycle. Such knowledge not only increases the chances of success with the method you choose but also can enhance your sexual satisfaction. The method you choose will not be effective unless it is used correctly and consistently. Both partners need to share responsibility for birth control.

Methods of Birth Control

In choosing a method of birth control or contraception, you and your partner should understand the following:

- how the method works
- how and when to use it
- reasons for not using it
- undesirable side effects of the method and what, if anything, can be done about them
- the effectiveness rate of the method

There are many different birth control methods. They include oral contraceptives, hormone implants and injectable contraceptives, barrier methods, intrauterine devices, rhythm methods, and surgical sterilization.

Oral Contraceptives

The oral contraceptive, commonly called the pill, stops the ovaries from releasing eggs (ovulation) and blocks sperm from reaching an egg, or it prevents a fertilized egg from attaching to the wall of the uterus. Oral contraceptive pills contain either a combination of progestin (a synthetic form of the female hormone progesterone) and estrogen (the key female sex hormone) or progestin alone. The combination pills are taken daily for 3 weeks, stopped for a week to allow for the menstrual period, and then started again. They prevent the ripening and release of the egg.

A variation of the combination pill is the multiphasic pill. This newer version varies the amount of estrogen and progesterone throughout the menstrual cycle to more closely match the hormone changes that occur naturally. Simply put, the pill's hormones trick the body into thinking it is pregnant. After ovulation, elevated levels of estrogen and progesterone prevent the release of another egg during the menstrual cycle. The pill provides these hormones on a daily basis, suspending ovulation.

Progestin-only pills, also called minipills, are taken every day of the month, but they do not suspend ovulation. They work by making the mucus that lines the cervix (the opening into the uterus from the vagina) so thick that sperm cannot pass through it and reach the egg. Bleeding usually occurs during the last few days of the menstrual cycle.

When used properly, combination pills are as effective as the progestin-only pill and are more effective for long-term use. The progestin-only pill is usually prescribed only when estrogen might be harmful to the woman, such as when she is breast-feeding.

The pill can sometimes cause problems, such as fluid retention, weight gain, irritability, and a change in sex drive. Women over 35 who smoke and women with active liver disease such as hepatitis B, or who have advanced diabetes are advised not to take the pill as a precaution against possible complications.

Increasing evidence indicates that the pill provides health benefits in addition to preventing pregnancy. For example, the pill has beneficial effects on benign breast tumors and ovarian cysts, and significantly reduces the risk of ovarian and endometrial cancers, iron-deficiency anemia, pelvic inflammatory disease, and ectopic pregnancy. The longer a woman takes the pill, the greater the protective effects.

The so-called morning-after pill is a series of birth-control pills containing the female sex hormones estrogen and progestin. The first dose must be taken within 72 hours of the unprotected sexual intercourse. This inhibits growth of the lining of the uterus so it cannot sustain a fertilized egg. Morning-after pills are highly effective in preventing pregnancy when used correctly. Possible side effects include nausea, breast tenderness, and spotting (light vaginal bleeding).

Hormone Implants and Injectable Contraceptives

Hormone implants are soft capsules containing the hormone progestin. The capsules are inserted under the skin of a woman's upper arm by a doctor who has been trained in this procedure. For up to 5 years the capsules release a steady, low dose of progestin to block ovulation (release of an egg from an ovary). Hormone implants are a highly effective means of birth control. The most common side effect is irregular periods. Also, removing the implant may be difficult and painful.

Injectable contraceptives contain the female hormone progestin. They are injected by a physician at regular intervals, usually about every 3 months. Injectable contraceptives prevent sperm from reaching the uterus by thickening the mucus that covers the cervix. Some doctors consider this to be the most effective reversible contraceptive method available. The most common side effect is irregular menstrual periods. Injectable contraceptives also have positive health effects—an increase in blood iron levels as well as protection against pelvic inflammatory disease, ovarian cancer, and endometrial cancer.

Barrier Methods of Contraception

Barrier methods physically block access of sperm to the uterus. They include male and female condoms; diaphragms; cervical caps; and spermicidal foams, creams, gels, and suppositories.

A *male condom* is a thin, transparent, latex sheath that covers the erect penis and prevents sperm from entering the vagina. Male condoms are the most widely used nonprescription contraceptive, and they are 90 to 97 percent effective when used properly. Although there are no side effects from using condoms, some men claim that condoms dull the physical sensation and tend to interrupt sexual intercourse. Some of these complaints may only be a matter of becoming accustomed to using condoms. To learn how to use a condom correctly, see page 182.

A *female condom* was approved by the US Food and Drug Administration in 1992, but it has had limited appeal in the United States. The device is inserted into the vagina and held in place by a ring. However, because the female condom has a higher failure rate, the male condom is preferred.

A *diaphragm* is a dome-shaped, latex cup with a flexible rim that fits over the cervix to block sperm from entering the uterus. Diaphragms come in different sizes and must be fitted by a doctor or a nurse to be sure the diaphragm covers the entire cervix without causing discomfort. If properly fitted, neither the man

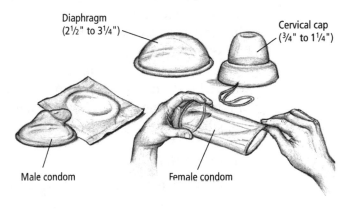

Barrier Contraceptives

nor the woman should notice its presence. A diaphragm should always be used with a spermicidal jelly or foam, which not only lubricates the diaphragm for insertion but also offers some protection against pregnancy if the diaphragm is dislodged during intercourse. The diaphragm should be left in place for 6 to 8 hours after intercourse. When used with spermicidal jelly or foam, the diaphragm is about 85 to 90 percent effective.

A *cervical cap* is similar to a diaphragm, only smaller and more rigid. It also is available in various sizes and must be fitted over the cervix. A cervical cap is more difficult to insert than a diaphragm; therefore a woman needs to be trained to insert it correctly. Although some women leave the cap in place for days or weeks, it must be removed during menstruation to allow menstrual blood to flow from the body.

A great variety of *spermicidal gels, foams, creams,* and *suppositories* are available in pharmacies without prescription. Basically they all work the same way—by killing sperm before they can reach the egg. No single type of spermicide has been found to be more effective than another. By themselves, however, spermicides are not as effective as other contraceptive products and may be only about 70 percent effective. To be effective, the product must be inserted into the vagina as close to the time of intercourse as possible, but no more than an hour before. After an hour, spermicides start to disintegrate. For best results, they should be used with a diaphragm or a condom. No serious side effects are associated with these products, but some people have experienced skin or vaginal irritation.

Intrauterine Devices

An intrauterine device (IUD) is a small plastic object that is placed inside the uterus by a physician, nurse, or midwife. How an IUD works to prevent pregnancy is not known for certain. In the United States, two types of IUDs are available. One type releases the female hormone progesterone and must be replaced every year. The other is made of copper and is effective for at least 10 years.

In rare cases, contractions of the uterus during menstruation can expel an IUD. If you can feel your partner's IUD with your penis during sexual intercourse, suggest that she see her doctor to check whether the IUD is being expelled.

Rhythm Methods

Rhythm methods (also called fertility awareness or the ovulation method) depend on avoiding sexual intercourse within 4 days before egg release. Most women release an egg from an ovary about 14 days before the start of their menstrual cycle. The unfertilized egg survives for only 24 hours, but sperm can survive for 2 to 7 days after intercourse, so fertilization may occur from intercourse that took place up to 7 days before release of the egg and 3 days after.

There are three variations of the rhythm method. In the *temperature method,* a woman determines her basal body temperature (her body temperature at rest) by taking her temperature before she gets out of bed each morning. This temperature drops slightly (about 0.2 degree Fahrenheit) just before ovulation. A day or so after the drop, a distinct rise (about 0.6 to 0.8 degree Fahrenheit) signals the beginning of ovulation. The couple avoids unprotected intercourse from the time the woman's temperature drops through the time it remains elevated for 3 consecutive days. The problem with this approach is that other factors, such as illness, can alter a woman's body temperature.

In the *mucus method,* a woman observes the changes in the consistency of her cervical mucus. Its consistency changes from dry immediately after menstruation to very slippery or watery shortly after an egg is released. The woman can have intercourse with a low risk of conception immediately after her menstrual period ends and up to the time she observes an increased amount of cervical mucus. When both the temperature and the mucus methods are used together, it is called the *symptothermal method.*

The *calendar-rhythm method* requires a woman to carefully keep track of her menstrual cycles over a year's time. She then subtracts 18 days from the shortest and 11 days from the longest of the previous 12 menstrual cycles. For example, if a woman's cycles last from 26 to 29 days, she must avoid intercourse from day 8 through day 18 of each cycle. This is the least reliable of the three rhythm methods. When it is used together with the symptothermal method, however, its effectiveness may reach the higher end of the estimated 53 to 86 percent range given for the rhythm methods. Note, however, that the low end of this range is little better than chance (50/50).

Surgical Sterilization

Sterilization is a procedure that makes a person incapable of reproducing. Surgical sterilization is the most common method of birth control among Americans. Surgical sterilization for a man is called *vasectomy*. This procedure involves cutting both vas deferens, the tubes that carry sperm from the testicles. This procedure can be performed on an outpatient basis in a hospital, clinic, or doctor's office. It takes about 20 minutes and requires only a local anesthetic. An incision is made on both sides near the base of the penis. On each side, the vas deferens is freed from the spermatic cord, pulled up through the incision, made into a loop, cut, and tied. (The vas deferens may also be cauterized, or sealed off, with an electric current.) The incision is closed with three or four sutures. When the local anesthetic wears off, the man may experience a mild, dull ache or pain for a few days. The man still ejaculates but the semen does not contain sperm.

The man is usually advised to rest in bed for 24 hours. Complications from vasectomy are rare (fewer than 5 percent of cases); the most common complications are bleeding and swelling of the scrotum. Most men return to work within a few days. Some doctors advise wearing tight-fitting underwear or a jock strap for 4 to 6 weeks to prevent swelling and pain in the scrotum.

It is important to remember that viable sperm may still be present in the seminal vesicles (the small sacs that store semen) after a vasectomy. For this reason, a man or his partner should continue to use some other form of contraception until those sperm are either ejaculated or die. The man is considered sterile only after a laboratory test confirms that two successive samples of ejaculate, collected 2 to 4 months after the procedure, are free of sperm.

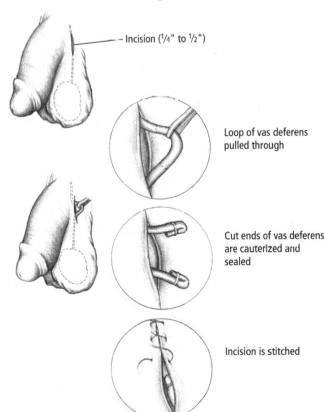

Incision (¹⁄₄" to ¹⁄₂")

Loop of vas deferens pulled through

Cut ends of vas deferens are cauterized and sealed

Incision is stitched

Contrary to what some men believe, vasectomy does not interfere with ejaculation, orgasm, or sex drive. In fact, several studies have shown that many men who have this procedure experience an increase in sexual desire. Vasectomy has been known occasionally to be associated with psychological problems or regrets about having the procedure. When these problems affect sexual performance, counseling is advised.

Women are sterilized by *tubal ligation*—the cutting and tying of the fallopian tubes, which carry the egg from the ovaries to the uterus. A variety of procedures are currently being used in the United States: abdominal tubal ligation, tubal coagulation by laparoscopy, and minilaparotomy. The first two methods require hospitalization and usually are performed under general anesthesia; the third can be performed on an outpatient basis.

Currently, the trend is for more tubal ligations done by laparoscopy. A thin tube (laparoscope) is inserted through a small incision in the woman's abdomen (usually through the navel). The doctor cuts the fallopian tubes and ties off the ends. (The ends of the tubes also may be cauterized.) The woman usually goes home the same day. Complication rates for this procedure are very low.

About a third of all married couples in the United States who use family planning methods choose sterilization of either partner. It is the method most often chosen by couples in which the woman is more than 30 years old. Vasectomy is more common than tubal ligation because it is simpler, just as effective, less expensive, and has fewer potential complications.

For couples who know that they do not want more children, sterilization is the most effective way to prevent pregnancy. Because the surgical procedures to reverse either vasectomy or tubal ligation are complicated and expensive, the results should be considered permanent. Although researchers are studying ways to easily reverse these procedures, they are not yet available.

If you have questions about any contraceptive method, ask your primary care doctor, a urologist (a physician who specializes in treating disorders of the urinary tract), or a gynecologist (a physician who specializes in treating disorders of the female reproductive system).

PART FOUR

COMMON HEALTH CONCERNS

CHAPTER 11

Heart, Blood, and Circulation

Adequate blood circulation is essential for life. The blood is kept in constant circulation by the pumping action of the heart, which sends blood to the lungs to pick up oxygen, and then pumps it to the rest of the body. The blood is pushed through a system of vessels, which branch repeatedly into increasingly smaller and thinner vessels, bringing life-sustaining blood to cells throughout the body.

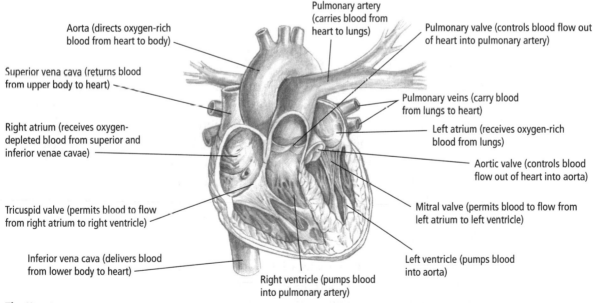

Aorta (directs oxygen-rich blood from heart to body)

Pulmonary artery (carries blood from heart to lungs)

Pulmonary valve (controls blood flow out of heart into pulmonary artery)

Superior vena cava (returns blood from upper body to heart)

Pulmonary veins (carry blood from lungs to heart)

Right atrium (receives oxygen-depleted blood from superior and inferior venae cavae)

Left atrium (receives oxygen-rich blood from lungs)

Aortic valve (controls blood flow out of heart into aorta)

Tricuspid valve (permits blood to flow from right atrium to right ventricle)

Mitral valve (permits blood to flow from left atrium to left ventricle)

Inferior vena cava (delivers blood from lower body to heart)

Left ventricle (pumps blood into aorta)

Right ventricle (pumps blood into pulmonary artery)

The Heart

The heart is a muscular organ about the size and shape of a fist and consists of two side-by-side pumps. The veins carry used, oxygen-depleted blood to the right side of the heart, which pumps it to the lungs for a fresh supply of oxygen. The oxygenated blood returns to the left side of the heart, which pumps it through the aorta. The aorta directs the fresh blood to a system of arteries, which carry it to tissues throughout the body. The veins return the used, oxygen-depleted blood to the heart, starting the process again.

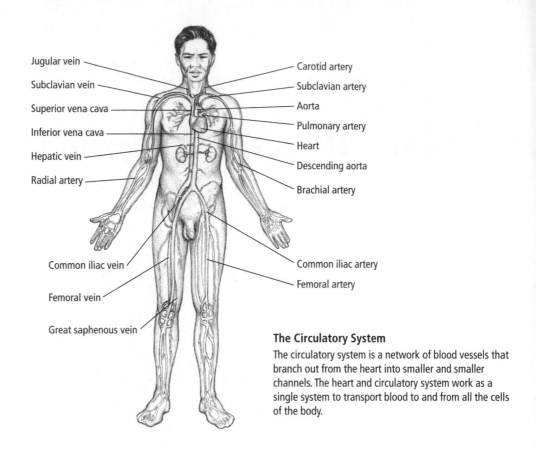

Jugular vein

Subclavian vein

Superior vena cava

Inferior vena cava

Hepatic vein

Radial artery

Common iliac vein

Femoral vein

Great saphenous vein

Carotid artery

Subclavian artery

Aorta

Pulmonary artery

Heart

Descending aorta

Brachial artery

Common iliac artery

Femoral artery

The Circulatory System
The circulatory system is a network of blood vessels that branch out from the heart into smaller and smaller channels. The heart and circulatory system work as a single system to transport blood to and from all the cells of the body.

Coronary Artery Disease

Coronary artery disease, also called simply heart disease, is a condition in which the coronary arteries (the blood vessels that supply blood to the heart muscle) become blocked, cutting off blood flow and, therefore, oxygen to the heart muscle. This damages the heart, causing it to malfunction. Coronary artery disease is the leading cause of death in the United States for both men and women. Nearly 20 percent of men aged 65 to 69 have had a heart attack, and nearly 30 percent of men aged 80 to 84 have had a heart attack. Nearly half of all men who die of coronary artery disease are not aware that they have the disease.

The following risk factors increase your risk of developing heart disease:

- *Family history.* Your chances of having coronary artery disease are much greater if either of your parents had heart disease before age 65.
- *High blood pressure.* This condition makes the heart pump harder, increasing the size of the heart muscle and, thereby, the chance of heart failure; it can directly damage coronary arteries.
- *Smoking.* Smokers have a 70 percent greater chance of developing coronary artery disease than nonsmokers.

- *High cholesterol levels.* High levels of cholesterol in the bloodstream lead to the formation of fatty deposits in the walls of the coronary arteries, causing them to narrow and obstruct blood flow.
- *Obesity.* Excess weight puts added strain on the heart, increases the risk of high blood pressure, and leads to higher levels of cholesterol in the blood.
- *Inactivity.* Regular exercise helps control cholesterol levels and weight. It also helps keep the heart strong and healthy.
- *Diabetes.* More than 80 percent of people with diabetes die of some form of blood vessel or heart disease.

Atherosclerosis

The heart receives its blood supply from the three coronary arteries that leave the aorta just outside the left ventricle. Like a tree, these three major arteries divide into smaller and smaller blood vessels until the entire heart wall is penetrated by hundreds of tiny blood vessels.

Coronary artery disease is caused by various gradual changes that occur in the coronary arteries. Collectively these changes are referred to as arteriosclerosis, which means hardening and thickening (literally "scarring") of the wall. Atherosclerosis is the most common type of arteriosclerosis. Atherosclerosis is the gradual thickening and hardening of an artery's inner wall by the formation of fatty deposits called plaques. These plaques cause narrowing of the artery's internal channel, thereby reducing the flow of blood (and oxygen) to the heart. This is similar to the way layers of minerals form a deposit inside a water pipe; as the minerals accumulate, the stream of water becomes steadily smaller.

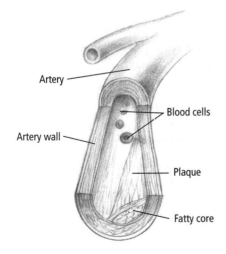

Artery

Blood cells

Artery wall

Plaque

Fatty core

Atherosclerosis
Atherosclerosis is the buildup of a cholesterol-containing substance called plaque inside arteries. Plaque often has a fatty core with a hard coating. The buildup of plaque can reduce or block the flow of blood to vital organs.

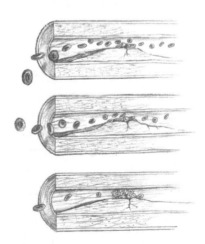

Plaque and Blood Clots
A buildup of plaque inside an artery is often the start of a blood clot. Plaque tends to crack (top). Your body interprets these cracks as injuries and forms blood clots around them to seal them and allow them to heal (center). If a clot inside a coronary artery grows large enough (bottom), it can block blood flow in the artery and cause a heart attack.

As the plaques become thicker, their surface becomes rougher. This encourages formation of blood clots within the artery. Small pieces of a blood clot can break off and travel through the bloodstream and block smaller blood vessels, causing a heart attack or stroke.

Atherosclerosis occurs more commonly in the coronary arteries than in other arteries of the body. The thickening of the artery wall progresses slowly until only a trickle of blood moves through the narrowed channel. The process may continue at the same rate until a small artery has been closed completely. As the artery gradually closes, the blood supply to the heart muscle becomes inadequate, causing heart damage.

Coronary artery disease is the most common result of an inadequate blood supply to the heart muscle. The most common symptom of coronary artery disease is angina (see below); the most serious consequence is a heart attack.

Angina

Angina is temporary moderate to severe pain or pressure in the chest. Sometimes the pain extends to the left shoulder and down the left arm or to the throat, jaw, and lower teeth. Occasionally it will reach the right side of the body. Many people describe their symptoms as discomfort rather than pain. Angina is caused by a lack of oxygen to the heart muscle.

Healthy coronary arteries can readily meet the heart's demands for oxygen. However, if the coronary arteries have become narrowed or hardened as a result of atherosclerosis, they cannot supply adequate blood to the heart muscle during times of increased demand, resulting in angina.

Angina associated with coronary artery disease usually occurs during times of exertion, emotional stress, or after a large meal, when the heart pumps faster and harder, trying to keep up with the body's increased oxygen demands. Often angina is worse when exertion follows a meal. Angina usually is worse in cold weather; walking into the wind or moving from a warm room to the cold air outdoors can trigger angina.

An episode of angina usually lasts fewer than 15 minutes and subsides with rest. Symptoms of angina that last longer than this may actually be a heart attack in progress, and you should seek immediate help. (See "Warning Signs of a Heart Attack," page 209.) Since heart disease develops unnoticed in many people, angina is considered to be a beneficial warning sign. If you experience angina, see your doctor as soon as possible.

Unstable angina refers to angina in which the established pattern of symptoms changes, or suddenly worsens. For example, angina pain usually remains constant and predictable from one episode to the next. But with unstable angina, the person may experience unpredictable changes, such as more severe pain, more frequent attacks, or attacks occurring with less exertion or during rest. These kinds of changes usually signal a rapid progression of coronary artery disease, with increasing blockage of the coronary artery, possibly because a blood clot has formed or a piece of plaque has broken away from the artery wall. The risk of heart attack is high. Unstable angina is a medical emergency that requires immediate treatment.

Although angina is most often caused by coronary artery disease, it also can result from other factors, such as defects in the aortic valve. Because the aortic valve is near the opening of the coronary arteries, these abnormalities may reduce blood flow into the coronary arteries and limit the amount of oxygen that goes to the heart. Another possible cause of angina is arterial spasm, in which, for reasons not fully understood, sudden temporary constriction or spasms occur in a coronary artery. Also, severe anemia (see page 238) may reduce the supply of oxygen to the heart, resulting in angina. Not everyone with an inadequate blood supply to the heart muscle experiences angina. Doctors do not yet understand why.

Angina is usually easy to recognize, but there are times when it mimics other conditions unrelated to the heart and blood vessels, such as indigestion and gastroesophageal reflux disease (GERD; see page 262). Diagnosis can often be made by a physical examination and an exercise stress test (which evaluates heart rate, blood pressure, electrical activity of the heart, and symptoms of angina and other problems related to inadequate blood supply to the heart while a person walks or runs on a treadmill or rides a stationary bicycle).

Treatment for angina includes learning to reduce and deal positively with stress, decreasing cholesterol intake, and losing weight if you are overweight. A wide variety of medications are available that reduce blood pressure, slow the heart rate, or widen the blood vessels. In addition, other medications are available that can help prevent the buildup of plaque in the arteries. If necessary, surgical procedures can be performed to bypass, clear, or widen the diseased coronary arteries.

Heart Attack

A heart attack is sudden death of a portion of the heart muscle that has been deprived of its blood supply. Most heart attacks are caused by blockage of a coronary artery. The blockage may be caused by a slow-growing plaque (fatty deposit) that blocks blood flow in the artery or by a quicker event, such as when a plaque ruptures or tears, causing a blood clot to form and clog the artery. Nearly 95 percent of sudden heart attacks are caused by a ruptured plaque and subsequent blood clot formation, which slows or prevents blood flow to the heart muscle.

When a blood clot forms on the rough surface of a plaque in the arterial wall, blocking an artery completely and suddenly, the result is often a sudden heart attack. Doctors also call this a "coronary thrombosis" or a "coronary occlusion." Heart damage occurs very quickly following blockage of a coronary artery. The affected heart tissue begins to deteriorate, and damage becomes permanent after about 6 minutes. This is why the speed of response to a heart attack is critical. The more quickly a person is treated, the better the chances of limiting damage to the heart.

For the heart muscle to function properly, it needs a continuous supply of oxygen-rich blood from the coronary arteries. The body has a remarkable ability to adapt to changing conditions—even narrowing of the coronary arteries—to ensure this continuous supply of blood. For example, if an artery starts to close gradually by thickening of its inner lining, and sometimes if it is closed by a blood clot, neighboring arteries gradually increase in size and send out new branches to supply adequate blood to the threatened area. This process is known as the formation of "collateral circulation."

In most cases, when a blood clot blocks a branch of the coronary artery, the symptoms appear suddenly, although it may take minutes, hours, or even days for the clot to grow large enough to block the artery. The time required for blockage to occur depends on the width of the channel inside the artery. If the artery is small and has narrowed gradually over a period of years, so that good collateral circulation is already present, blockage by a blood clot may cause mild symptoms or none at all. On the other hand, if the artery is large and there has been only slight narrowing, sudden obstruction by a blood clot may cause severe discomfort.

Rarely, a heart attack may occur when a clot from another part of the heart breaks away and lodges in the coronary artery. Another uncommon cause of a heart attack is a spasm in a coronary artery that stops blood flow. The causes of such spasms are usually unknown.

The symptoms and extent of a heart attack depend on factors such as the size of the blocked artery, the width of the channel inside the artery, the suddenness of the blockage, the extent to which an adequate collateral circulation has formed, and the general condition of the heart at the time of the attack.

The pain of a heart attack is usually, but not always, severe. Like angina, the pain occurs in the center of the chest and may spread to the back, left arm, or jaw; less often the pain spreads to the right arm. Because many people have strong denial capabilities ("It can't be happening to me!"), they may downgrade the severity of the pain and attribute it to some other cause, such as indigestion. Other symptoms of a heart attack include a heavy pounding of the heart, feeling faint or fainting, restlessness or anxiety, and sweating. The lips, hands, or feet may turn slightly blue. Older people may become disoriented or confused. Irregular heartbeats (arrhythmia) may seriously interfere with the heart's ability to pump effectively and may precede a heart attack.

Two of three people who have heart attacks experience intermittent chest pain, shortness of breath, or fatigue a few days beforehand. Some people may think these symptoms are nothing more than an angina episode. The key is to be able to recognize the difference between angina and the pain caused by a heart attack, which is usually more severe, lasts longer, and does not go away with rest or after taking nitroglycerin.

One of five people who have a heart attack has only mild symptoms or none at all. Such "silent" heart attacks are often diagnosed after the fact through a routine electrocardiogram (ECG; an examination of the electrical activity of the heart). Many of these silent attacks go unnoticed because they affect a less crucial part of the heart or because the person having the attack may have an unusually high tolerance for pain.

Warning Signs of a Heart Attack

Become familiar with the warning signs of a heart attack so you can seek immediate help if you or someone you know begins to experience them. The most common symptoms of a heart attack include:

- sudden, strong pain, pressure, fullness, or squeezing in the center of the chest that lasts more than just a few minutes and is not relieved by rest
- chest pain that spreads to the shoulders, neck, jaw, or arms
- chest discomfort accompanied by shortness of breath, light-headedness or fainting, sweating, cold or clammy skin, nausea or vomiting, or loss of consciousness

Less common heart attack symptoms are:

- other kinds of chest pain or stomach or abdominal pain
- unexplained anxiety, weakness, or fatigue
- palpitations, a cold sweat, or pale skin

A heart attack is a medical emergency. If you have any of the symptoms described above, call 911 or your local emergency number, or call an ambulance service, and ask for immediate transportation to a hospital emergency department. If you are with a person who has any of these symptoms, call 911 or your local emergency number, or take him or her to the nearest hospital emergency department without delay.

Other conditions may mimic a heart attack. These conditions include pneumonia, a blood clot in the lung (pulmonary embolism), inflammation of the membrane that surrounds the heart (pericarditis), fracture of a rib, spasm of the esophagus, indigestion, gastroesophageal reflux disease, and chest muscle tenderness after injury or exertion. An ECG and measurement of certain enzymes in the blood can confirm the diagnosis of a heart attack within a few hours. In many instances, an ECG can show when a person is having a heart attack. Several abnormalities may appear on the ECG, depending on the extent and the location of heart muscle damage. If a person has had a previous heart attack, however, the current heart muscle damage may be difficult to detect. If the results of a few

ECGs taken over the course of several hours are normal, the doctor usually considers a heart attack less likely but will wait for the results of blood enzyme tests before making a diagnosis.

The levels of certain enzymes in the blood can be measured to help diagnose a heart attack. For example, an elevated level of heart-muscle enzymes called troponins in the blood is an indication of damage to the heart muscle that results from a heart attack. The level of troponins increases about 4 to 6 hours after a heart attack, peaks 10 to 24 hours after the attack, and can be detected in the blood for about a week. Troponin levels are usually checked when a person is admitted to the hospital with chest pain and a possible heart attack and at 8-hour intervals for about 24 hours.

Another heart-muscle enzyme, called CK-MB, is also released into the blood when heart muscle is damaged. Elevated levels show up in the blood within 6 hours of a heart attack and they persist for 36 to 48 hours. Levels of CK-MB usually are checked when the person is admitted to the hospital and at 6- to 8-hour intervals over the next 24 hours.

If ECG and enzyme test results do not provide enough information to diagnose a heart attack, imaging techniques such as echocardiography (an ultrasound examination of the heart) or radionuclide scanning (see page 213) may be performed. An echocardiogram may show reduced motion in part of the wall of the left ventricle (the part of the heart that pumps blood to the body), suggesting damage from a heart attack. A radionuclide scan may show a persistent reduction in blood flow to a specific area of the heart muscle, suggesting a scar (dead tissue) caused by a heart attack.

Why You Should Take CPR Training

Cardiopulmonary resuscitation (CPR) is a critically important technique that could help you save the life of someone you love. CPR is used to revive a person when his or her breathing or heartbeat stops—a sign of sudden death. Sudden death can be caused by a number of events, including a heart attack, poisoning, drowning, choking, suffocation, electrocution, and smoke inhalation. The CPR procedures attempt to restart the person's breathing and heartbeat, employing techniques that keep the person's airway open, use rescue breathing to administer oxygen, and apply rhythmic pressure to the chest to force the heart to pump blood. Use CPR until emergency medical personnel arrive.

Your local hospital or fire department, the local chapters of the American Red Cross or the American Heart Association, or your employer all may offer CPR training courses. Ask your doctor about CPR classes in your community. Take advantage of these opportunities for training because your knowledge could make the difference between life and death for someone. Once you learn the CPR procedures, practice them often so you won't forget the correct procedures when you need them the most. CPR should be performed only by people trained in this procedure.

When dealing with a possible heart attack, speed is vital. Half of the deaths caused by heart attacks occur within the first 3 or 4 hours after symptoms begin. The faster a heart attack victim gets to a hospital emergency department, the better the chances of survival. Anyone experiencing symptoms of a possible heart attack (see "Warning Signs of a Heart Attack," page 209) should seek immediate medical attention. If aspirin is available, encourage the person to swallow one tablet. Aspirin helps reduce the blood's tendency to clot, thereby reducing the chances of dying of a heart attack by 20 percent.

A person suspected of having a heart attack is usually admitted to a hospital's cardiac care unit (CCU). In the CCU, a person's heart rhythm and blood pressure and the amount of oxygen in the blood are closely monitored to assess heart damage. Nurses in these units are specially trained to deal with cardiac emergencies. Upon arrival, the patient is immediately given a thrombolytic (clot-dissolving) medication such as tissue plasminogen activator (tPA), streptokinase, or urokinase. These drugs are most effective if given within 6 hours of the start of the heart attack symptoms. If a blocked coronary artery can be cleared quickly, damage to heart tissue may be prevented or limited. After 6 hours, restoring blood flow to the heart does not help very much. Early treatment with thrombolytic drugs can increase blood flow and limit heart tissue damage. Aspirin, which prevents platelets from forming blood clots, or heparin, which also stops clotting, may enhance the effectiveness of treatment with thrombolytic drugs.

A beta-blocker drug also is given to slow down the heart rate and make the heart work less hard to pump blood through the body. Reducing the heart's workload also helps limit damage to the heart. Oxygen is given through a face mask, or via a tube with prongs inserted into the nostrils. This therapy increases the oxygen content in the blood, which provides more oxygen to the heart and helps to keep heart tissue damage to a minimum. Some physicians recommend coronary angioplasty (see page 216) to open the coronary arteries or coronary artery bypass surgery (see page 216) after a heart attack instead of treatment with thrombolytic drugs.

Depending on the extent of the heart attack, you may be released from the hospital for home rest within days. Your doctor will probably advise you to stay in bed and rest for several days and to avoid excitement, physical exertion, and emotional stress. If you smoke, your doctor will tell you to quit immediately (see page 107); smoking is a major risk factor for coronary artery disease and heart attack.

It is normal to feel anxious and depressed after a heart attack. Because severe anxiety can stress the heart, the doctor may prescribe a mild tranquilizer. To deal with the depression and with denial of illness, which also is common after a heart attack, patients and their families are encouraged to talk about their feelings with doctors, nurses, and social workers. Many hospitals where cardiac surgery is performed offer support groups in which people who have recovered from heart attacks or cardiac surgery have been trained to work as peer counselors for recuperating inpatients.

In general, most people who survive for a few days after a heart attack can expect to recover fully. However, about 10 percent, usually those who continue to have angina, irregular heart rhythm, or heart failure, will die within a year. Most of those deaths will occur within the first 3 to 4 months. To promote recovery and to help avoid possible future heart attacks, survivors usually are prescribed heart medications, cholesterol-lowering drugs (see "Medications for Heart Disease," page 214), a low-fat diet, and regular sessions of aerobic exercise in a cardiac rehabilitation program.

Managing Heart Disease

Once you are released from the hospital after a heart attack, your treatment will focus on long-range preventive care. Your doctor will recommend that you make lifestyle changes such as eating a healthy diet, exercising regularly, losing weight if you are overweight, and quitting smoking if you smoke. In addition, your doctor will want to monitor your condition with regularly scheduled checkups and tests, and he or she may prescribe medication to reduce risk factors for heart disease such as high blood pressure or high cholesterol level.

Sex and Heart Disease

Men with heart disease face exceptional challenges to their sexuality. Distressing pain and other symptoms make it difficult to feel comfortable, much less sexually aroused. Many men with heart disease are afraid to have sex because they and their partner fear that the increased physical exertion could cause chest pain or even another heart attack. But most men with heart problems can have sex without causing any physical problems. Talking to your doctor about such a delicate subject can be uncomfortable, but you need to find out what your limits are. Even if your heart condition is so serious it restricts your ability to have intercourse, you still can be affectionate and intimate with your partner in other ways. For example, you could bring your partner to orgasm using your hand or mouth. Remember that heart disease should never prevent you from having a loving and caring relationship with your partner.

Tests for Heart Disease   Physicians use a number of procedures to evaluate a person's risk for heart problems, the progress a person is making after a heart attack or surgery, and the status of a person's heart and circulatory system. These procedures include:

- *Continuous ECG monitoring* of the heart's electrical activity with a Holter monitor. The monitor, which is worn around the neck or over the shoulder, records an ECG for 24 hours, so the doctor can monitor an arrhythmia (abnormal heartbeat) or episodes of silent ischemia (inadequate blood flow to the heart).
- *Exercise stress testing* is an evaluation of heart rate, blood pressure, electrical activity of the heart, and symptoms of angina and other problems related to

inadequate blood supply to the heart while a person walks or runs on a treadmill or rides a stationary bicycle. This test can help determine the severity of coronary artery disease and the ability of the heart to respond to a reduced blood supply. The test may be performed before or shortly after the person leaves the hospital to help determine how well he is doing after the heart attack and whether ischemia is continuing. If this test reveals an arrhythmia or ischemia, drug treatment may be recommended. If ischemia persists, a physician may recommend coronary arteriography to determine whether coronary angioplasty (see page 216) or coronary artery bypass surgery (see page 216) is needed to restore blood flow to the heart.

- *Radionuclide scanning* combined with exercise stress testing may provide a physician with information about the person's angina. This test involves injecting a radioactive substance that travels through the bloodstream to a target organ and using a special camera to produce an image of that organ. Radionuclide scanning not only confirms the presence of ischemia but also identifies the area and the amount of heart muscle affected.

- *Exercise echocardiography* is a procedure in which ultrasound images of the heart (echocardiograms) are obtained while a person walks or runs on a treadmill. The test is harmless and shows heart size, movement of the heart muscle, blood flow through the heart valves, and valve function. Echocardiography is performed while the person is at rest and at the peak of exercise. When ischemia is present, the pumping motion of the wall of the left ventricle appears abnormal.

- *Angiography* allows blood vessels to be seen on film. A catheter (a thin, flexible tube) is usually inserted into the femoral artery, a large blood vessel in the groin area, and moved up through the aorta (the main artery in the body) and into the coronary arteries. A contrast medium (dye) is injected through the catheter into the artery to be examined, and a series of rapid-sequence X rays (similar to a movie) are taken. Narrowing and blood flow inside the arteries are clearly visible, allowing the physician to determine whether the arteries can be treated by bypass surgery or angioplasty. Occasionally angiography is used to detect spasm in coronary arteries that do not have any plaques. Certain medications are given to stimulate a spasm during the procedure to help diagnose the condition.

- *Computed tomography (CT) scanning,* a diagnostic procedure in which a computer is used to construct

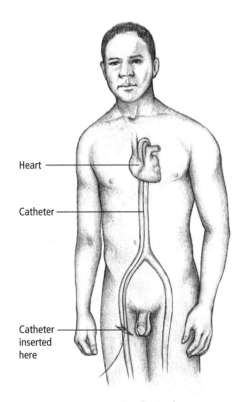

Heart

Catheter

Catheter inserted here

Angiography

cross-sectional X-ray images of the heart and coronary arteries, helps to detect calcification in the artery walls, which is associated with atherosclerosis. A faster version of CT scanning is used to examine artery walls for structural and functional abnormalities associated with a heart attack.

Medications for Heart Disease   Medications are available to improve blood flow and to minimize symptoms associated with coronary artery disease. The following four types of drugs are frequently used for treating heart disease:

- *Beta-blockers* interfere with the effects of epinephrinelike hormones in the body that normally increase heart rate and blood pressure. Beta-blockers reduce the resting heart rate. During exercise they limit the increase in heart rate, decreasing the body's demand for oxygen. Beta-blockers lower the risk of heart attacks and sudden death for people with coronary artery disease. Beta-blockers are estimated to reduce the risk of cardiac death by about 25 percent when taken by people who have had a heart attack. The more serious the heart attack, the more benefit these drugs provide. Possible side effects include slow heartbeat, fatigue, and erectile dysfunction. Some examples of beta-blockers are atenolol, metoprolol, and propranolol.
- *Nitrate drugs* such as nitroglycerin dilate (widen) the blood vessels, improving blood flow. Both short-acting and long-acting nitrates are available. A small tablet of nitroglycerin placed under the tongue usually relieves an episode of angina in 1 to 3 minutes. The effects of this short-acting nitrate drug last about 30 minutes. People with chronic stable angina are advised to carry nitroglycerin with them at all times. Some people learn through experience to take nitroglycerin just before reaching the level of exertion they know can induce their angina.

  Long-acting nitrate drugs are taken one to four times daily. They are available as skin patches or as a paste, which is absorbed through the skin over many hours. Over time, long-acting nitrates lose their ability to provide relief. Most doctors recommend that people try going 8- to 12-hour periods without taking the drug, to help maintain its effectiveness. Possible side effects include headache, flushing of the skin, and dizziness.
- *Calcium channel blockers* prevent blood vessels from constricting and interfering with blood flow. These drugs are also used to treat certain types of arrhythmias because they can slow the heart rate. Possible side effects include headache, flushing of the skin, and dizziness. Some examples of calcium channel blockers are amlodipine, diltiazem, and verapamil.
- *Anticlotting drugs* such as aspirin are helpful. Platelets are cell fragments circulating in the blood that are necessary for clot formation during a bleeding episode or when blood vessels are injured. But when platelets collect on the surface of a plaque on an artery wall, the resulting clot formation (thrombosis) can narrow or block the artery and cause a heart attack. Aspirin binds to

platelets and keeps them from clumping on blood vessel walls, reducing the risk of death from a blocked coronary artery. Regular aspirin use can reduce the risk of death and the risk of a second heart attack by 15 to 30 percent. People with a sensitivity to aspirin may take prescription medications that help prevent blood clots, such as dipyridamole and ticlopidine, as a substitute.

If you have heart disease and your cholesterol levels are high, your doctor may recommend that you take cholesterol-lowering medication. Different cholesterol-lowering drugs work in different ways. For example, some drugs decrease blood levels of LDL ("bad") cholesterol, while others increase levels of HDL ("good") cholesterol. Still others work by lowering triglyceride (another type of fat) levels in your blood. Your doctor will prescribe a particular medication for you, depending on your individual needs. You may need to take this medication for the rest of your life. Cholesterol-lowering medications include the following:

- *Bile acid-binding resins* prevent absorption of cholesterol into the blood and stimulate the liver to remove cholesterol from the bloodstream. Possible side effects include bloating, cramping, and diarrhea. Examples of bile acid-binding resins include cholestyramine and colestipol.
- *Fibrates* (also called fibric acid derivatives) decrease blood levels of triglycerides. These drugs also can decrease LDL cholesterol and moderately increase HDL cholesterol levels. People who take fibrates have a slightly increased risk of developing gallstones (see page 276) and gallbladder disease. Examples of fibrates include gemfibrozil and fenofibrate.
- *HMG CoA reductase inhibitors* (also called statin drugs) block the action of an enzyme (IIMG CoA reductase) in the liver, thereby significantly decreasing production of cholesterol in the liver. Possible side effects include occasional muscle aches and nausea. Very rarely, liver damage may occur. Examples of statin drugs include atorvastatin and simvastatin.
- *Niacin* (nicotinic acid) is a vitamin that decreases production of LDL cholesterol in the liver. Depending on the dosage, it also can increase HDL cholesterol levels. Possible side effects include bloating, cramping, and diarrhea. Very rarely, niacin may damage the liver. A variety of nonprescription versions of niacin are available over-the-counter.
- *Probucol* decreases blood levels of LDL cholesterol but also can decrease blood levels of HDL cholesterol. Diarrhea is the most common side effect of this medication.

You will need to watch for possible side effects while taking certain cholesterol-lowering medications and report them to your physician. Your doctor may ask you to try to live with some side effects for a few weeks to see if your body adjusts to it. Also, your doctor will carefully monitor your cholesterol levels and liver function regularly through blood tests.

Surgical Procedures for Heart Disease   Atherosclerosis and the resulting coronary artery disease are progressive. This means that once these problems develop, they will continue to worsen until they are successfully treated. When lifestyle changes or medication cannot control the progression of the disease, surgery may be necessary. Possible procedures performed to treat this condition include coronary artery bypass surgery, coronary angioplasty, and placement of a stent.

Coronary artery bypass surgery, commonly called bypass surgery, is highly effective for people who have angina and whose coronary artery disease is not widespread. Bypass surgery is the procedure most widely used to treat coronary artery disease due to atherosclerosis. It can improve exercise tolerance, reduce symptoms, and decrease the amount of medication needed. Bypass surgery is most likely to benefit people who have severe angina that cannot be controlled with medication, a normally functioning heart, and no previous heart attacks. About 85 percent of patients who undergo bypass surgery experience complete or significant relief of symptoms.

The procedure involves grafting (transplanting healthy tissue from one part of the body to another) veins or arteries onto the coronary artery to receive blood flow, thereby "bypassing" the obstructed area. Usually the bypass veins are taken from the leg. Most surgeons also use at least one artery as a graft. The bypass artery usually is taken from beneath the chest wall. These arteries rarely develop atherosclerosis, and more than 90 percent of them remain open and work properly 10 years after the bypass surgery. Vein grafts may become obstructed and, after 5 years, a third or more of them may be completely blocked. In such cases the procedure may need to be repeated.

Coronary angioplasty, also called balloon angioplasty, is performed to open a narrowed or blocked coronary artery. The procedure begins with insertion of a hollow needle into the femoral artery in the leg. A long guide wire is threaded

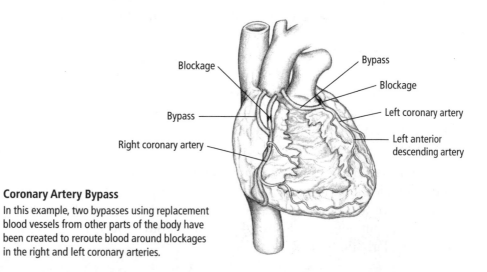

Blockage · Bypass · Blockage · Left coronary artery · Left anterior descending artery · Bypass · Right coronary artery

Coronary Artery Bypass
In this example, two bypasses using replacement blood vessels from other parts of the body have been created to reroute blood around blockages in the right and left coronary arteries.

through the needle and into the arterial system, through the aorta, and into the obstructed coronary artery. A catheter (a thin, flexible tube) with a balloon attached to its tip is threaded over the guide wire and into the obstructed artery. The catheter is positioned so the balloon is at the level of the obstruction. The balloon is then inflated and deflated several times, for several seconds each time. The inflated balloon compresses the plaque against the artery wall, widening the narrowed channel and restoring blood flow. The catheter and guide wire are then withdrawn.

Between 80 and 90 percent of arteries that are treated with angioplasty are opened. In about 20 to 30 percent of cases, the coronary artery becomes obstructed again (called restenosis) within 6 months, often within a few weeks after the procedure. Angioplasty is then repeated. This procedure may be used to successfully control coronary artery disease over the long term.

Stent placement is a newer procedure that has been performed more frequently in the past several years. Essentially it is angioplasty, with an additional step. Once the obstructed artery has been opened, a tiny metallic or plastic wire mesh (stent) is placed inside the artery to keep it open. This procedure may reduce the risk of restenosis by half.

Numerous studies have shown that success rates of angioplasty are about the same as those of bypass surgery. Most studies comparing these two procedures are now focusing on economics. Recent studies give the edge to bypass surgery in terms of the cost of treating patients over the long term.

High Blood Pressure

High blood pressure, or hypertension, increases your chances of developing heart disease or kidney disease and of having a stroke. About one in every four American adults has high blood pressure but may not be aware of it. It is often called "the silent killer" because it usually causes no symptoms. However, high blood pressure is easy to diagnose, and there are practical steps you can take to bring your blood pressure under control.

Blood pressure is the force of blood pushing against the walls of the arteries that carry blood throughout your body. It is measured in millimeters of mercury, or mm Hg, using an instrument called a sphygmomanometer (pronounced sfig'mo-mah-nom'e-ter). Blood pressure is highest when the heart contracts (beats) and pumps blood into the arteries. This is called the systolic pressure. Between beats, when the heart is resting, the pressure falls. This is called the diastolic pressure. A blood pressure reading is always given as a combination of these two pressures; the high (systolic) pressure is written above or before the low (diastolic) pressure. For example, if your blood pressure reading is 120 over 70, it is written as 120/70 mm Hg; 120 is the systolic pressure, and 70 is the diastolic pressure.

Different activities make your blood pressure rise or fall. For example, normally, blood pressure rises when you are exercising and falls when you are resting. A blood pressure reading of 140/90 mm Hg or lower is generally considered normal. High blood pressure is classified according to guidelines that reflect the levels at which blood pressure begins to pose significant health risks.

The guidelines for classifying blood pressure are shown in the following table:

Blood Pressure Classifications for People Age 18 and Older

Category	Systolic	Diastolic
Optimal blood pressure	Lower than 120 mm Hg	Lower than 80 mm Hg
Normal blood pressure	Lower than 130 mm Hg	Lower than 85 mm Hg
High-normal blood pressure	130 to 139 mm Hg	85 to 89 mm Hg
High blood pressure		
Stage I	140 to 159 mm Hg	90 to 99 mm Hg
Stage II	160 to 179 mm Hg	100 to 109 mm Hg
Stage III	180 mm Hg or more	100 mm Hg or more

A diagnosis of high blood pressure is based on two or more blood pressure readings taken at separate visits to the doctor's office. If your systolic pressure falls into one category and your diastolic pressure into another, the higher reading will be used to classify your blood pressure. For example, a blood pressure of 160/90 mm Hg would be classified as stage II. A reading of 170/120 mm Hg would be classified as stage III.

Because diastolic pressure represents the lower and more constant level of pressure in the arteries, physicians may emphasize it more, especially in younger people. However, the systolic blood pressure is more important for determining the risk of heart attack or stroke.

People with high blood pressure have elevated blood pressure most of the time. Their blood is pushing against the walls of their arteries with higher than normal force. If left untreated, high blood pressure can lead to:

- *Atherosclerosis.* Uncontrolled high blood pressure causes the artery walls to thicken and lose elasticity. This encourages formation of fatty deposits on the artery wall, which narrow the channel and interfere with blood flow throughout the body. In time, atherosclerosis can lead to a heart attack or a stroke.
- *Enlarged heart.* High blood pressure causes the heart to work harder. Over time this causes the heart muscle to thicken and stretch. The heart becomes less efficient and has to work harder and harder to pump blood throughout the body. Eventually this can result in heart failure.
- *Kidney damage.* The kidneys act as filters to rid the body of wastes. Over a number of years, high blood pressure can narrow and thicken the blood ves-

sels of the kidneys. The kidneys then filter less blood, and waste builds up in the bloodstream. This could lead to kidney failure. When kidney failure occurs, dialysis (a technique to remove waste products from the blood and excess fluids from the body) or a kidney transplant may be necessary.

- *Stroke.* High blood pressure can weaken the walls of the arteries or cause them to thicken. A weakened artery wall in the brain could break, causing a hemorrhage. If a blood clot blocks one of the narrowed arteries, a stroke may occur.

In most cases, the cause or causes of high blood pressure are unknown. This type is known as primary or essential hypertension. Primary hypertension cannot be cured, but it can be controlled. Secondary hypertension is caused by, or is "secondary" to, another disease. For example, some cases of high blood pressure can be traced to tumors of the adrenal gland, chronic kidney disease, or hormone abnormalities. Secondary hypertension can be cured by treating its underlying cause.

Preventing High Blood Pressure

Anyone, regardless of age, sex, race, or heredity, can lower his or her risk of developing high blood pressure or lower existing high blood pressure by taking the steps described here.

Maintain a healthy weight. As your body weight increases, your blood pressure rises. In fact, being overweight can make you two to six times more likely to develop high blood pressure than if you maintain a desirable weight (see the weight chart on page 69).

> ### Risk Factors for High Blood Pressure
>
> You are at increased risk for developing high blood pressure if you have one or more of the following risk factors:
>
> - You have close family members (parents, grandparents, or siblings) who have high blood pressure.
> - You are African American.
> - You are a male over age 35.
> - You are overweight.
> - You do not exercise regularly.
> - You use tobacco products (cigarettes, cigars, pipe, or smokeless tobacco).
> - You regularly consume more than two alcoholic drinks per day.

It's not just how much you weigh that is important; it also matters where your body stores excess fat. Your body shape is inherited from your parents, just like the color of your eyes and hair. Some people tend to store fat around their waists, while others store fat around the hips and thighs. "Apple-shaped" people who store extra fat at the waist appear to have higher health risks than "pear-shaped" people who store fat around the hips and thighs.

No matter where your extra weight is located, you can reduce your risk of developing high blood pressure by losing weight. Even a small weight loss can make a big difference. And if you are overweight and already have high blood pressure, losing weight can help you lower your blood pressure.

To lose weight, you need to consume fewer calories than you burn. But don't try to lose weight too quickly. The healthiest way to lose weight and keep it off is to do it gradually, by losing about a pound a week. By taking in 500 calories less per day and being more physically active, you should be able to lose about a pound (which equals 3,500 calories) a week.

Losing weight and keeping it off involves making permanent lifestyle changes. Here's how to eat healthfully and lose weight:

- Choose foods that are low in calories, sugar, and fat. Naturally, choosing low-calorie foods cuts calories. But choosing foods low in fat also can cut calories. Fat is a concentrated source of calories, so eating fewer fatty foods will help reduce your calorie intake. Cutting back on butter, margarine, fatty salad dressings, fatty meats, skin on poultry, full-fat dairy products such as milk and cheese, fried foods, and sweets will also improve your cholesterol profile.
- Choose foods that are high in fiber. These include fruits; vegetables; whole-grain foods such as cereal, pasta, and bread; and dried peas and beans. Foods high in fiber are excellent substitutes for foods high in fat. The former are lower in calories and are a good source of essential vitamins and minerals.
- Limit serving sizes. When trying to lose weight, it's not just the types of foods you eat, but how much you eat. To take in fewer calories, you need to limit your portion sizes. Try especially to take smaller helpings of high-calorie foods such as fatty meats and cheeses. And try not to go back for seconds. Today many restaurants take pride in serving large portions of food. This does not mean that you have to clean your plate. Choose the doggy-bag option; eat only half of what you are served and take the rest home for an excellent "free meal" the next day.
- Keep track of what you eat, when you eat, and why you eat. Write it down. Note whether you snack on high-calorie foods while watching television or if you skip breakfast and then eat a large lunch. Once you clearly see your eating habits, you can set goals for yourself—for example, cutting back on TV snacks or, when you do snack, having fresh fruit, low-fat or air-popped popcorn, or vegetables such as carrots and celery. If there's no time to eat breakfast at home, take fruit, a bagel (skip the cream cheese), or whole-grain cereal with you to eat at work. Changing your eating habits will help you change your weight (see page 73).

Exercise regularly. Another way to lose weight and control blood pressure is through regular physical activity. Cutting down on fat and calories combined with regular exercise can help you lose more weight and keep it off longer than with either diet or exercise alone.

Aerobic exercise provides added benefits. It helps improve the fitness of your heart, blood vessels, and lungs, which, in turn, protects you against heart disease. Activities such as stair climbing, bicycling, swimming, brisk walking, running, and jumping rope are called "aerobic," which means that the body uses oxygen to make the energy it needs during the activity. Aerobic activities provide health benefits if done at the right intensity for at least 20 to 30 minutes, three to four times per week. If you think you don't have time to exercise, try to exercise for two 15-minute periods or even three 10-minute periods during your day. You will still gain health benefits. (For more information on the health benefits of aerobic exercise, see page 56.)

You need to see your doctor before starting an exercise program if you:

- have a health problem such as high blood pressure
- have angina (chest pain)
- tend to feel dizzy or faint
- have difficulty breathing after a mild workout
- are middle-aged or older and have not been active
- are planning a vigorous exercise program

Otherwise, get up off the couch, get out, get active, and get fit.

Choose foods that are lower in salt. Most Americans take in more salt (sodium) than they need, which may help explain why the United States has higher rates of high blood pressure than countries where people eat less salt. Salt attracts water. Normally, if you have eaten too much salt, your kidneys eliminate the excess salt from your body along with a certain amount of water. But if your kidneys cannot get rid of the extra salt, your body retains the water that clings to the salt, which raises blood volume and, in some people, blood pressure.

Certain people appear to be salt-sensitive, which means that their blood pressure goes up when they eat salt. Researchers think that about half of all people with high blood pressure are salt-sensitive and that as many as 70 to 80 percent of blacks are salt-sensitive. Other groups that seem to have a high incidence of salt sensitivity are older people, people who have diabetes, and people who are overweight. There is a good chance that if you are a member of one or more of these groups, decreasing your salt intake would be beneficial to your health.

Research suggests that the average person needs only about 200 milligrams of sodium per day. Doctors recommend that people with high blood pressure take in no more than about 6 grams of salt per day, which equals about 2,400 milligrams of sodium, or about 1 teaspoon of table salt. A teaspoon of salt may seem like a lot to you, but remember that this refers to total salt intake for a day. This includes salt in processed and prepared foods, salt added during cooking, and salt sprinkled on food at the table. Americans eat an average of 4,000 to 6,000 milligrams of sodium each day, so many people could probably benefit from cutting back on their salt intake.

The key to cutting back on salt is in teaching your taste buds to enjoy less salty foods. Here are a few tips for cutting back on salt:

- Check food labels for the amount of salt in the foods you buy. Choose foods that are low in sodium. Look for labels that say "sodium-free," "very low in sodium," "low sodium," "light in sodium," "reduced sodium," "less sodium," or "unsalted." Then check the label for the amount of sodium per serving.

- Choose fresh or frozen vegetables, or canned vegetables labeled "no salt added." Choose fresh poultry, fish, and lean meat rather than canned, cured, smoked, or processed varieties.
- Use herbs, spices, salt-free seasoning blends, and lemon juice instead of salt to add flavor to your food.
- Cook rice, pasta, and hot cereals without salt. Avoid using instant or flavored rice, pasta, and cereal mixes because they usually have added salt.
- Choose "convenience" foods that are low in sodium. Cut back on frozen dinners, packaged dinners such as macaroni and cheese, packaged mixes, canned soups or broths, and salad dressings, which often contain large amounts of sodium.
- Buy low-sodium, reduced-sodium, or no-salt-added versions of canned soups, dried soup mixes, or bouillon; canned vegetables and vegetable juices; low-fat cheeses; margarine; condiments such as ketchup or soy sauce; crackers and baked goods; processed lean meats; and snack foods such as chips, pretzels, and nuts.
- Rinse canned foods, such as tuna, to remove excess sodium.

Drink alcoholic beverages only in moderation. Drinking too much alcohol can lead to the development of high blood pressure. To prevent high blood pressure, or if you already have high blood pressure, limit yourself to no more than two drinks per day. A drink is defined as $1\frac{1}{2}$ ounces of 80-proof distilled spirits, 5 ounces of wine, or 12 ounces of beer (regular or "lite").

Do not use tobacco. Although it is not a direct cause of high blood pressure, smoking puts you at risk of developing the disease. The chemicals in tobacco smoke can damage the artery walls, making them more susceptible to plaque formation. Plaques narrow the arteries and interfere with blood flow to the heart, brain, and other organs and tissues. Blood clots can form on the rough surface of a plaque. A blood clot or plaque can block an artery, causing a heart attack or a stroke.

The nicotine in tobacco is a powerful stimulant that causes the heart rate to increase, the arteries to constrict, and blood pressure to rise. Smoking also affects cholesterol levels in the blood: it can increase LDL ("bad" cholesterol) levels and decrease HDL ("good" cholesterol) levels. All of these tobacco-induced effects can contribute to the development of high blood pressure.

Although it is sometimes promoted as a smoke-free alternative to cigarettes and cigars, smokeless tobacco also puts you at risk of developing high blood pressure. The nicotine, sodium, and licorice contained in smokeless tobacco products all can raise blood pressure. Considering these health risks, it makes sense to give up your tobacco habit now.

Here are some other factors that may help prevent high blood pressure:

- *Potassium.* A certain amount of potassium is essential for proper body function. Eating foods rich in potassium may help protect some people from developing high blood pressure. Many people get enough potassium from eating fruits, vegetables, dairy products, and fish, so potassium supplements are rarely needed. Too much potassium can disturb your heart rhythm.

- *Calcium.* People with low calcium intake have higher rates of high blood pressure. It is best to get the calcium you need—1,000 to 1,500 milligrams per day for adult men (see page 303)—from the foods you eat. Low-fat and non-fat dairy products such as milk, yogurt, and cheese are excellent sources of calcium. It has not been proven that taking calcium supplements helps prevent high blood pressure.

- *Magnesium.* A diet low in magnesium may make your blood pressure rise. However, doctors do not recommend taking magnesium supplements to help prevent high blood pressure. The amount of magnesium you get in a healthy diet is enough. Magnesium is found in whole grains; green, leafy vegetables; nuts; seeds; and dried peas and beans.

- *Fish oils.* A type of fat called omega-3 fatty acids is found in fatty fish such as mackerel and salmon. Evidence suggests that eating fish at least twice a week can help reduce high blood pressure. Talk to your doctor if you are considering taking fish oil supplements. Most fish, if not fried or prepared with added fat, are low in saturated fat and calories and are a good source of essential nutrients.

- *Fats, carbohydrates, and protein.* Varying the amount and type of fats, carbohydrates, and protein in the diet has little if any effect on blood pressure. But for overall heart health, it is crucial to limit the amount of fat in your diet, especially the saturated fat found in foods such as fatty meats and full-fat dairy products. Saturated fats raise your blood cholesterol level, and a high cholesterol level is another risk factor for heart disease. Foods high in fat are usually also high in calories. Foods high in complex carbohydrates (starch and fiber) are often low in fat and calories—so eat these foods in moderate amounts instead of eating high-fat foods. Always check food labels (see page 7).

- *Caffeine.* The caffeine found in coffee, tea, and colas may cause blood pressure to rise, but only temporarily. In a short time your blood pressure will return to its previous level. Unless you are sensitive to caffeine, you do not have to limit caffeine intake to prevent high blood pressure.

- *Garlic and onions.* Increased amounts of garlic and onions have not been found to affect blood pressure. Of course, they are rich in antioxidants and are tasty substitutes for salty seasonings.

- *Stress management.* Stress can make blood pressure go up for a while and over time may contribute to high blood pressure. Stress management techniques such as biofeedback, meditation, and relaxation (see page 118) can help you to deal positively with the stress-producing events in your life, and may help you control your blood pressure.

Medications for High Blood Pressure

Medications are usually prescribed for people whose high blood pressure cannot be controlled through lifestyle changes, such as following a healthy diet and exercising regularly. In the past, many people with high blood pressure simply stopped taking their medications because of the unpleasant side effects. It used to be said that the treatment for high blood pressure was worse than the disease. This is no longer true. Newer and more effective drugs have been developed that have fewer side effects. Most people who take antihypertensive medications (drugs that lower blood pressure) feel better after they start taking them.

If you experience unpleasant effects from your antihypertensive medication, discuss these effects with your physician, but continue to take the medication until the doctor tells you to stop. He or she probably will prescribe a substitute medication that will not produce the side effects. Because so many drugs are now available, your doctor can work with you to fine-tune your drug regimen so that you can get the best treatment with the fewest side effects. This also applies in terms of drug costs, which can account for 70 to 80 percent of the cost of treating high blood pressure. If you are concerned about the cost of your medications, discuss it with your physician or pharmacist to see if less expensive alternatives are available.

There are eight categories of antihypertensive medications, each having a different method of action. Following is a summary of the types of medications used to treat high blood pressure:

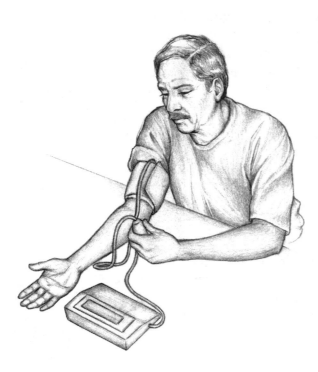

Monitor Your Blood Pressure

If you have been diagnosed with high blood pressure and your doctor has prescribed medication, he or she will ask you to measure your blood pressure regularly to see whether the medication is controlling it effectively. You can purchase a home blood pressure monitor at most pharmacies.

- *Diuretics* increase excretion of water and sodium by the kidneys, thereby reducing the volume of blood the heart has to pump. Diuretics are helpful to blacks, older adults, and people with heart failure or low renin activity. (Renin is an enzyme involved in maintaining the balance of water and sodium in the body.) Possible side effects include erectile dysfunction, decreased sexual desire, muscle cramps, and fatigue. Examples include chlorothiazide, furosemide, and amiloride.

- *Beta-blockers* slow the heart rate and block the output of renin by the kidneys. These drugs are helpful for people with high renin activity, a high resting heart rate, or coronary artery disease. Possible side effects include slow heartbeat, fatigue, and erectile dysfunction. Examples include atenolol, metoprolol, and propranolol.
- *Alpha-blockers* prevent arteries from constricting and block the effects of the stress hormone epinephrine, which increases blood pressure. These drugs are useful for people who have high cholesterol levels, diabetes, or poor circulation in the arms and legs (peripheral vascular disease). Possible side effects include headache, dizziness, and mild fluid retention. Examples include doxazosin, prazosin, and terazosin.
- *ACE (angiotensin-converting enzyme) inhibitors* block the activity of an enzyme (ACE) that forms a hormone that causes narrowing of blood vessels. These drugs are useful for people with diabetes, congestive heart failure, high renin activity, or certain kidney diseases. The most common side effect is an irritating, dry cough. Examples include benazepril, captopril, enalapril maleate, and lisinopril.
- *Angiotensin-receptor blockers* prevent the arteries from constricting and prevent the kidneys from retaining salt and water. They are useful primarily for people who cannot tolerate ACE inhibitors. Possible side effects are mild and include dizziness, fatigue, and stomach pain. Examples include losartan and valsartan.
- *Centrally acting drugs* act directly on the brain and the nervous system to lower heart rate and peripheral resistance by keeping the arteries from narrowing. These drugs are helpful to people with peripheral vascular disease. Possible side effects include drowsiness, dry mouth, fatigue, and dizziness. Examples include clonidine, guanfacine, and methyldopa.
- *Calcium channel blockers* prevent narrowing of the artery walls and also may slow or block the development of plaques. They are helpful for blacks, older adults, and people with unsteady heart rhythms, diabetes, angina, or pulmonary hypertension. Possible side effects include constipation, ankle swelling, headache, and dizziness. Examples include diltiazem, amlodipine, and verapamil.
- *Vasodilators* act directly on the smooth muscle of the arteries to widen artery walls. They are used only in emergencies and for people whose blood pressure cannot be controlled with other drugs. Possible side effects include an abnormally strong, rapid heartbeat (usually more than 100 beats per minute), increased fluid retention, and headache. Examples include hydralazine and minoxidil.

Heart Valve Disorders

The heart has four chambers—two small upper chambers (atria) and two larger lower chambers (ventricles). Each chamber is closed by a one-way valve. For various reasons these valves can malfunction, causing leakage (regurgitation) or failure to open properly (stenosis). The mitral valve, which allows blood to flow from the left atrium to the left ventricle (the main pumping chamber of the heart), and the aortic valve, which allows blood to flow from the left ventricle to the aorta (the main artery of the body), are the most common sites for valve disease. These valves are under great strain from the powerful contractions of the left ventricle, which pumps blood throughout most of the body.

Mitral Valve Prolapse

Mitral valve prolapse is the most common valve disorder. Usually it is an inherited structural defect. The two parts, or leaflets, of the mitral valve thicken, preventing them from coming together properly. The leaflets bulge back into the left atrium as the ventricle contracts, allowing small amounts of blood to leak back into the atrium. Prolapse is a term that means slippage out of position; in this case the valve leaflets have difficulty being in their correct position because they are too thick.

Most people with mitral valve prolapse experience no symptoms. Others may have a wide range of symptoms—such as chest pain, palpitations (an awareness of one's heartbeat), migraine headaches, dizziness, and fatigue—that cannot be explained by the valve problem alone.

Physicians diagnose mitral valve prolapse by using a stethoscope to listen to the characteristic clicking sound produced by the valves as they hit against one another. The condition also produces a heart murmur, or slight rushing sound, that the physician hears through the stethoscope when the heart contracts. Echocardiography (an ultrasound examination of the heart) allows a doctor to view the prolapse and determine its severity.

Most people with mitral valve prolapse do not need treatment. When symptoms such as extra heartbeats, a rapid heartbeat, or chest pain become bothersome, medications are prescribed to control them. In rare cases, when leakage becomes severe, surgical repair or valve replacement may be required. People with mitral valve prolapse are usually given antibiotics before dental or surgical procedures to decrease the risk that bloodborne bacteria will infect the heart valve.

Mitral Valve Regurgitation

Mitral valve regurgitation, also called mitral incompetence or mitral insufficiency, is leakage of blood back through the mitral valve into the left atrium each time the left ventricle contracts. This increases the volume and pressure in the left atrium, which, in turn, increases blood pressure in the vessels leading from the lungs to the heart. This results in lung congestion (fluid buildup).

In the past, rheumatic fever was the most common cause of this condition. But with the advent of antibiotics, rheumatic fever is now rare in the United States, and the few cases that are seen are primarily in older people who had rheumatic fever in childhood. A more common cause of mitral valve regurgitation today is a heart attack, which can damage the supporting structures of the mitral valve.

Mild cases of mitral valve regurgitation may not cause any symptoms. The condition may be recognized during a routine chest examination with a stethoscope, when a doctor hears a distinctive heart murmur caused by the blood leaking back into the left atrium when the left ventricle contracts. Diagnosis usually is confirmed by electrocardiography (ECG; an examination of the electrical activity of the heart) and chest X rays that indicate the left ventricle is enlarged. Echocardiography (an ultrasound examination of the heart) can produce an image of the faulty valve and indicate the severity of the problem.

Since the left ventricle has to pump more blood to make up for the blood leaking back into the atrium, it gradually enlarges to increase the force of each heartbeat. The enlarged ventricle may cause palpitations (awareness of one's heartbeat), which is particularly noticeable when the person lies on his left side.

The left atrium also tends to enlarge to accommodate the extra blood leaking back from the ventricle. A very enlarged atrium often beats rapidly in an irregular fashion (atrial fibrillation). This reduces the heart's pumping efficiency, and the lack of proper blood flow through the atrium allows blood clots to form. If a clot becomes detached, it may be pumped out of the heart and block a smaller artery elsewhere in the body, possibly causing a stroke or other damage. Finally, severe regurgitation reduces the forward flow of blood, causing heart failure, which may lead to coughing, swollen legs, or shortness of breath on exertion.

Treatment for this condition can take several forms. Repairing the valve can either eliminate or reduce the regurgitation enough to make the symptoms tolerable and prevent heart damage. Atrial fibrillation accompanying mitral valve regurgitation is usually treated with medications that slow the heart rate and help control the fibrillation. In severe cases, the valve may be replaced surgically.

Mitral Valve Stenosis

Mitral valve stenosis is a narrowing of the mitral valve opening that increases resistance to blood flow from the left atrium to the left ventricle. This resistance causes pressure to build up in the atrium; the pressure then backs up through the veins of the lungs, causing increased pressure and congestion in the lungs. The increased stress on the lungs can lead to shortness of breath and eventually to congestive heart failure. Typically, the valve leaflets fuse together. Surgery is needed to widen or replace the valve.

Mitral valve stenosis is almost always the result of rheumatic fever, which is rare today in the United States, where most cases occur in older people who had rheumatic fever during childhood. However, rheumatic fever can sometimes occur after an untreated "strep" throat infection (infection with streptococcal bacteria). Mitral valve stenosis also can be congenital (present from birth). Infants born with this condition rarely live beyond age 2 unless they have surgery to correct the condition.

If stenosis is severe, blood pressure increases in the left atrium and in the veins in the lungs, resulting in heart failure and an accumulation of fluid in the lungs (pulmonary edema). A person with heart failure easily becomes fatigued and short of breath. At first, shortness of breath may occur only during physical activity. Later the symptoms may occur even during rest. Some people find that they can breathe comfortably only when they are propped up with pillows or sitting upright.

Some people with mitral valve stenosis have a plum-colored flush in their cheeks. High blood pressure in the veins of the lungs may cause a small vein or tiny capillaries to burst and bleed slightly or massively into the lungs. Enlargement of the left atrium can result in atrial fibrillation (an abnormally fast heartbeat).

To diagnose mitral valve stenosis, a physician uses a stethoscope to listen for a characteristic heart murmur as blood rushes through the narrowed valve from the left atrium. Unlike a normal valve, which opens silently, a valve affected by mitral valve stenosis often makes a snapping sound as it opens to allow blood into the left ventricle. The diagnosis of mitral valve stenosis is usually confirmed by electrocardiography (ECG; an examination of the electrical activity of the heart), a chest X ray showing an enlarged atrium, or echocardiography (an ultrasound examination of the heart). Sometimes cardiac catheterization (a diagnostic test in which a thin, flexible tube is inserted into the heart through a blood vessel, to examine the heart) is performed to determine the extent and characteristics of the valve blockage.

Treatment for mitral valve stenosis may include a variety of drugs. Beta-blockers, digoxin, and verapamil are used to slow the heart rate and control atrial fibrillation. Digoxin also strengthens the heartbeat if heart failure occurs. Diuretics are often prescribed to reduce the blood pressure in the lungs by reducing the volume of circulating blood.

If medication does not reduce the symptoms adequately, surgical valve repair or replacement may be needed. People with mitral valve stenosis are given antibiotics before dental and surgical procedures to reduce the risk of a heart valve infection.

Aortic Stenosis

Aortic stenosis is an abnormal narrowing or stiffening of the aortic valve, which controls the flow of blood from the left ventricle to the aorta (the main artery of the body). As the valve narrows, the left ventricle has to beat harder to push the blood through the aorta and out into the body. The most common cause of aortic stenosis is the gradual buildup of calcium deposits on the valve, a natural consequence of aging. Although this condition may appear at about age 60, it usually does not produce symptoms until age 70 or 80. Aortic stenosis also may result from childhood rheumatic fever. When rheumatic fever is the cause, aortic stenosis usually is accompanied by mitral valve stenosis (see page 227), mitral valve regurgitation (see page 226), or both.

In aortic stenosis, as the ventricle attempts to pump enough blood through the narrowed aortic valve, the left ventricle wall thickens, and the enlarged heart muscle requires an increasing blood supply from the coronary arteries. Eventually the blood supply to the heart becomes insufficient, causing angina (chest pain) on exertion. An insufficient blood supply can damage the heart muscle, reducing its ability to pump blood through the body. This reduced functioning can lead to congestive heart failure (see page 233). A person with severe aortic stenosis may faint on exertion because the narrow valve prevents the ventricle from pumping enough blood out of the heart to the rest of the body.

In diagnosing aortic stenosis, a physician will listen for the characteristic heart murmur through a stethoscope, note abnormalities in the pulse and electrical activity of the heart, and look for an enlarged heart as revealed by a chest X ray. Electrocardiography (ECG; an examination of the electrical activity of the heart), echocardiography (an ultrasound examination of the heart), and cardiac catheterization (a diagnostic test in which a thin, flexible tube is inserted into the heart through a blood vessel, to examine the heart) may be used to determine the severity of the stenosis.

In adults with fainting, angina, and shortness of breath on exertion caused by aortic stenosis, the aortic valve is surgically replaced, preferably before the left ventricle is damaged beyond repair.

Heart Valve Replacement

In cases of a diseased or damaged valve, surgery may be required. Although it is sometimes possible to repair the valve, usually it is necessary to replace it. A replacement valve that is no longer working properly also must be replaced with a new valve.

Replacement valves can be made from human or animal tissue (biologic replacement valves) or from metal and plastic (mechanical replacement valves). Although mechanical valves last longer (20 years or more) than biological valves, they also can promote blood clot formation. This means that a person with a mechanical heart valve needs to take long-term therapy with blood-thinning medication to prevent blood clots from forming.

In valve replacement surgery, the person is given general anesthesia. The surgeon opens the chest cavity and exposes the heart (open heart surgery). The heart is temporarily stopped, and a heart-lung machine is used to pump blood throughout the body. The diseased or damaged valve is removed, and the replacement valve is put in position and attached with stitches. The surgeon then restarts the heart and disconnects the heart-lung machine. The chest cavity is closed and stitched together.

To prevent a heart valve infection, a person with a replacement valve must take antibiotics before all dental and surgical procedures.

Arrhythmia

When the heartbeat is abnormally fast or slow, or when it is irregular, the abnormality is referred to as an arrhythmia. A normal heart rate at rest is usually between 60 and 100 beats per minute. Heart rates slower than 60 beats per minute are called bradycardia. Heart rates faster than 100 beats per minute are called tachycardia. Some variation in heart rate is normal—for example, when the heart responds to exercise, to inactivity, or to other stimuli such as anger or pain. Only when the heart rate is unusually fast (tachycardia) or slow (bradycardia) or when the heart's electrical impulses travel in abnormal pathways is the heart rate considered abnormal. An arrhythmia may occur at unusual times and for no obvious reasons. This may signal an underlying cause of the abnormal heartbeat, such as coronary artery disease (see page 204).

The heartbeat originates in the heart's internal pacemaker (sinoatrial node), which sends out electrical signals that tell the heart muscle when to contract (beat). The heart rate also is influenced by external nerve impulses and by levels of hormones circulating in the bloodstream.

External nerve impulses that help regulate the heart rate come from the autonomic nervous system, which consists of the sympathetic and parasympathetic nervous systems. The sympathetic nervous system speeds up the heart rate, and the parasympathetic nervous system slows the heart rate. The sympathetic nervous system produces the hormones epinephrine and norepinephrine, which have a role in regulating heart rate and blood pressure. When something upsets the balance among these factors or interferes with the electrical signal from the sinoatrial node, an arrhythmia may result.

Various problems can arise to interrupt these electrical signals, resulting in arrhythmias that range from mild to severe. Factors that can increase the risk of arrhythmia include the following:

- excessive intake of alcohol
- excessive intake of caffeine
- smoking
- chemical imbalances in the body
- overactive or underactive thyroid gland
- illegal drugs such as cocaine and methamphetamine
- coronary artery disease
- heart valve disorders
- congestive heart failure

In some cases, however, arrhythmias occur without any detectable underlying cause. Even a person with a life-threatening arrhythmia may not be aware of it because some arrhythmias, regardless of their significance, may cause no symptoms. Other, relatively harmless arrhythmias, however, may cause a variety of symptoms. Although the symptoms of an arrhythmia may be disturbing, it is important to understand that an arrhythmia may also be a symptom of an underlying disease or condition that usually is more serious than the arrhythmia itself. Possible symptoms of arrhythmias include palpitations (awareness of one's own heartbeat), light-headedness, dizziness, fainting, chest pain, and shortness of breath.

If you have symptoms of a possible arrhythmia see your doctor. He or she will check your pulse and listen to your heart through a stethoscope to evaluate your heart rate. You may need to undergo additional testing to help the doctor make a diagnosis. Electrocardiography (ECG; an examination of the electrical activity of the heart) usually is used to diagnose an arrhythmia. However, when the abnormal heartbeats are intermittent, the ECG may not be able to detect them. In such cases the person may need to wear a Holter monitor for 24 hours. A Holter monitor is a portable ECG device that is worn around the neck or over the shoulder, with electrodes attached to certain areas of the chest. As the person goes about his or her daily routine, the device records the electrical activity of the heart on a special cassette tape. At the end of the 24-hour monitoring period, the physician analyzes the information on the tape. (People with severe arrhythmias are usually hospitalized for monitoring.) The doctor also may test your blood for a chemical imbalance or to determine if your thyroid gland is functioning properly. Chemical imbalances and thyroid problems can cause some arrhythmias.

While mild arrhythmias may not require treatment, more serious arrhythmias or those that produce intolerable symptoms may be treated with a variety of medications, such as beta-blockers and calcium channel blockers. Other drugs that control an abnormal heartbeat by slowing transmission of the heart's electrical impulses also may be prescribed. You may need to try several drugs before your doctor finds the medication that works best for you.

Electronic pacemakers also are often used to treat serious arrhythmias. A pacemaker is a battery-powered device that regulates the heartbeat with electrical impulses. Two types of pacemakers are available: temporary and permanent. A temporary pacemaker usually is inserted beneath the skin of the chest following a heart attack that has created a block of the heart's own electrical signal. The pacemaker produces electrical impulses that keep the heart beating at a normal rate. In most patients, the heart block usually corrects itself in a matter of days, and the temporary pacemaker is then removed.

A permanent pacemaker is implanted surgically just beneath the skin of the chest. Usually it is used to regulate an abnormally slow heart rate. When the heart rate slows to below a certain number of beats per minute, or when the heart misses a beat, the pacemaker produces electrical impulses that restore the normal heart rate. If necessary, the pacemaker can produce electrical impulses at a continuous, fixed rate. Less commonly, pacemakers are used to regulate an abnormally fast heart rate.

To implant a pacemaker, the surgeon numbs your chest with a local anesthetic and inserts a catheter (a thin, flexible tube) through a large vein (the subclavian vein) located just beneath the skin of your upper chest. He or she then threads one or more electrodes through the catheter and into one of the chambers of your heart. The electrodes, which will supply electrical impulses to your heart, are attached by fine wires to a small, battery-operated power source. The surgeon then creates a small pocket just beneath the skin of your chest below the collarbone, places the power source inside, and stitches the pocket closed.

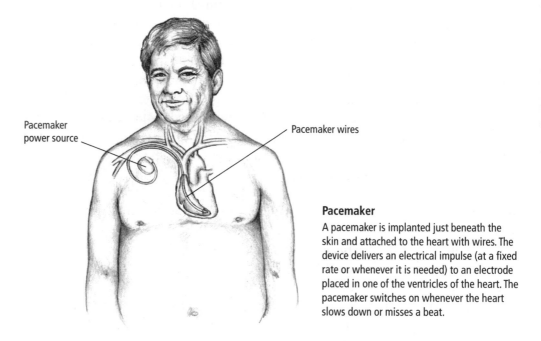

Pacemaker
power source

Pacemaker wires

Pacemaker
A pacemaker is implanted just beneath the skin and attached to the heart with wires. The device delivers an electrical impulse (at a fixed rate or whenever it is needed) to an electrode placed in one of the ventricles of the heart. The pacemaker switches on whenever the heart slows down or misses a beat.

You will be hospitalized for a day or two after surgery. For at least 8 weeks after surgery, you will need to limit movement, particularly on the side where the pacemaker is implanted, to prevent the wires from becoming disconnected. Your doctor will advise you to avoid making sudden, jerky arm movements and raising your arms above your head. You will also need to avoid all strenuous activities that involve use of your arms, such as tennis, swimming, bowling, sweeping, raking, scrubbing, vacuum cleaning, and lifting and carrying heavy or bulky objects. When the 8 weeks have passed, the wires will be set, and you can return to your normal routine.

Your doctor will examine your pacemaker about 2 weeks after surgery and again about 3 and 6 months after surgery. After that, he or she will continue to examine your pacemaker at regular intervals, at least once a year, to help ensure that it is functioning properly. The doctor can replace the battery in a minor surgical procedure. Pacemakers can remain implanted for 8 to 10 years before the battery needs to be replaced.

Interference from microwave ovens, high-voltage equipment, airport security devices, and radar are no longer problems with newer pacemakers, although their functioning still can be disrupted by magnetic resonance imaging (MRI) and diathermy (a physical therapy technique used to bring heat to muscles). Your doctor can tell you which devices and situations you need to avoid.

An implantable defibrillator may be used to treat ventricular fibrillation—a dangerously rapid, uncoordinated heartbeat that arises in the ventricles, the heart's pumping chambers, and prevents the heart from pumping an adequate amount of blood to the tissues. Uncontrolled ventricular fibrillation is a major cause of sudden death.

The procedure to implant a defibrillator is similar to the procedure for implanting a pacemaker. Two electrodes that monitor the electrical activity of the heart are inserted like pacemaker wires or attached to the surface of the heart and connected by fine wires to a small, battery-operated power source. These electrodes can supply an electrical impulse from the power source whenever the heart beats too rapidly, restoring the heartbeat to normal. The defibrillator's battery-operated power source is implanted in a pocket created by the surgeon under the skin of your abdomen.

You will be hospitalized for 1 or 2 days after the procedure, and you may have to wear a portable Holter monitor for 24 hours after surgery to monitor the electrical activity of your heart. Recovery at home will take about 6 to 8 weeks. The same precautions and restrictions that apply to pacemakers apply to implantable defibrillators. You cannot drive a car or operate heavy machinery if you have an implanted defibrillator, because there is a risk of briefly losing consciousness when it sends an electrical impulse to your heart.

Some serious arrhythmias are treated surgically. For example, catheter ablation (delivery of radiofrequency energy through a catheter inserted through an artery into the heart) often is used to destroy or remove the tiny area in the heart that is causing an arrhythmia. Coronary artery bypass surgery (see page 216) and coronary angioplasty (see page 216) are used to control arrhythmias caused by coronary artery disease (see page 204).

Congestive Heart Failure

Congestive heart failure (CHF) is a condition in which the heart is unable to pump an adequate amount of blood to the lungs and the rest of the body. CHF is often the result of failure to treat previously existing heart problems. It can be related to a variety of diseases and conditions, such as a heart attack, coronary artery disease, high blood pressure, heart valve defects, congenital (present from birth) heart disease, anemia, cardiomyopathy (degenerative disease of the heart muscle), or arrhythmia. All of these problems can cause the heart to pump inefficiently. When the heart cannot do its job, the body becomes overloaded with water and sodium, causing fluid backup and swelling in the lungs, liver, and legs and, eventually, fatigue, dizziness, and low blood pressure. If not treated, CHF can be fatal.

About 5 million Americans have congestive heart failure. Each year there are an estimated 400,000 new cases. Incidence of this chronic condition is reaching epidemic proportions in the United States. CHF is the most common health problem in hospital patients over age 65. Congestive heart failure affects equal numbers of men and women, and about a fourth of the 5 million people who have this condition are under age 60. CHF occurs in about 2 percent of Americans ages 40 to 59; in about 5 percent of Americans ages 60 to 69; and in about 10 percent of Americans age 70 or older. African Americans have a 25 percent greater chance than whites of developing CHF.

Symptoms of congestive heart failure include:

- shortness of breath, especially on exertion or while lying down
- wheezing
- fatigue
- swelling in the ankles and lower legs
- sudden large weight gain (20 pounds or more) due to fluid retention
- frequent urination at night

Heart failure affects either the left ventricle (called left-sided failure) or the right ventricle (called right-sided failure). In left-sided failure, the left ventricle must work harder to pump the same amount of blood throughout the body. This increased workload may cause the left ventricle to enlarge, the ventricle walls to thicken, and the heart rate to increase. These changes temporarily allow the heart to pump more blood, but gradually they lead to heart failure.

As the left side of the heart fails, the left ventricle does not completely empty of blood with each contraction. The retained blood creates back pressure on the lungs, causing them to become congested with blood. This in turn causes pulmonary edema (excess fluid in the lungs), which leads to breathing difficulties.

In right-sided heart failure, there is back pressure in the circulation from the heart into the veins. This is often caused by pulmonary hypertension (raised pressure and resistance to blood flow through the lungs), which leads to distended (enlarged) neck veins, enlarged liver, and edema (fluid retention and swelling) in the tissues.

Your doctor may perform echocardiography (an ultrasound examination of the heart) to determine the overall condition of your heart. You also may undergo an exercise stress test (see page 212) to evaluate how well your heart functions. Other diagnostic tests also may be performed to evaluate blood flow through the heart and to eliminate chronic lung disease as a possible cause of your symptoms.

Treatment for congestive heart failure includes dietary restrictions. Your doctor probably will recommend that you avoid caffeine, consume less sodium (salt), and eat smaller, more frequent meals. He or she also will advise you to decrease your level of physical activity to reduce the demands on your heart. Your doctor probably will prescribe a combination of three types of medications to strengthen the heartbeat and reduce the size of the heart (digitalis drugs), improve blood flow (vasodilators such as ACE inhibitors), and eliminate excess fluids and sodium from the body (diuretics). For people who have heart failure, beta-blockers are used to improve their symptoms and to prolong their life.

Once the heart failure has stabilized, attention is shifted to treating the underlying cause or causes of this condition. High blood pressure (see page 217) and arrhythmias (see page 230) usually are treated with medication. Heart valve defects, congenital heart defects, and coronary obstructions are corrected with surgery. When the cause of CHF is a long-term disease, such as emphysema (see page 247), the outlook is generally not as good. In severe cases of congestive heart failure, a heart transplant may be performed.

Studies are ongoing to better understand how the heart contracts normally and what goes wrong in CHF, to find new drug therapies and other innovative treatments, and to find better ways to detect the condition. Another approach is to develop devices to help a damaged heart function better. For example, a small mechanical pump called a left ventricular assist device (LVAD) can temporarily help the heart pump blood in people with severe CHF who are awaiting a heart transplant. After months of use, an LVAD often improves heart function in these people—so much so that a transplant is no longer needed. Efforts are under way to identify patients who may benefit from using a longer-term LVAD.

Vein Disorders

Veins are blood vessels that return deoxygenated (the oxygen content has been used up) blood to the heart from all parts of the body. The capillaries (tiny blood vessels) deliver deoxygenated blood from the tissues to the venules (small veins), which join together to form the veins. The veins carry the blood to the venae cavae (the two largest veins in the body), which deliver the blood to the right atrium of the heart. In the heart, the blood travels from the right atrium to the right ventricle, which pumps the blood through the pulmonary artery into the lungs. In the lungs, the blood is reoxygenated (gives up carbon dioxide and receives oxygen) and is returned through the pulmonary veins to the left atrium of the heart. The blood then travels from the left atrium to the left ventricle, which pumps the blood through the aorta (the body's main artery). From the aorta, the blood travels back to the tissues through the arteries, arterioles (tiny arterial branches), and capillaries.

Blood pressure in the veins is much lower than it is in the arteries. Also, the walls of the veins are thinner, weaker, and much less elastic than the walls of the arteries. Because of this, the veins need help to move the blood along. To keep blood flowing toward the heart, the linings of the veins have folds that work as one-way valves. Each valve has two halves (cusps) with edges that meet, like a pair of swinging doors. As blood travels through the veins back to the heart, it pushes these valves open. Surrounding muscles contract and press against the vessel walls, which helps keep blood flowing toward the heart.

Your legs contain two types of veins—superficial veins, which are located in the fatty layer beneath the skin, and deep veins, which are located in the muscles. Short veins connect the deep veins with the superficial veins. The leg veins depend on the powerful calf muscles to help move blood up toward the heart. Three common problems that can affect the leg veins are deep vein thrombosis, varicose veins, and superficial phlebitis.

Deep Vein Thrombosis

A clot that forms in a blood vessel is called a thrombus. Deep vein thrombosis is formation of blood clots in the deep veins in the legs. The condition is not always life-threatening. However, if a piece of blood clot breaks loose, it can travel through the bloodstream and lodge in an artery in the lung, obstructing blood flow. This is called a pulmonary embolism (see page 249), which is a potentially life-threatening condition. For this reason, all cases of deep vein thrombosis are considered serious.

Factors that contribute to deep vein thrombosis include:

- injury to the veins
- an increased tendency to form blood clots, which occurs, for example, after an injury or surgery
- sluggish blood flow in the veins, which occurs, for example, when a person is inactive or immobilized for long periods
- obesity

Occasionally, deep vein thrombosis occurs as a complication of superficial phlebitis (see page 238). Thrombosis also can occur in healthy people who sit for long periods while driving or flying.

Warning Signs of Deep Vein Thrombosis

About half of all people with deep vein thrombosis do not experience symptoms. Others may experience some or all of the following:

- inflammation of the calf, with swelling, warmth, and tenderness
- swelling of the ankle, foot, or thigh
- edema (fluid accumulation) in the ankles that is worse toward the end of the day
- brownish skin, usually above the ankle, that breaks open easily

If you experience any of these symptoms, talk to your doctor as soon as possible.

Imaging techniques such as radionuclide scanning (see page 213) and Doppler ultrasound (an imaging technique that provides motion pictures of blood flow) can be used to diagnose deep vein thrombosis. These tests can reveal important information about blood flow and the condition of the veins deep inside the legs.

Treatment may not be necessary if the blood clots are small and confined to the calf. If you walk a lot, the clots may dissolve on their own. People at risk for deep vein thrombosis (such as those recovering from surgery, and long-distance travelers) should flex and extend their ankles about 10 times every 30 minutes to keep the blood flowing. Support hosiery can help by putting pressure on the legs, causing the veins to narrow slightly, which makes the blood flow faster and clotting less likely. (**Warning:** If not worn correctly, support hose may aggravate the problem by obstructing blood flow in the legs. Ask your doctor or nurse to show you the correct way to wear support hose.) For more serious cases of thrombosis, a doctor may prescribe anticoagulant (blood-thinning) medication or thrombolytic (clot-dissolving) drugs to reduce the risk of pulmonary embolism. In some cases surgery to remove the clots may be necessary.

Varicose Veins

Varicose veins are enlarged, twisted veins just beneath the skin that result from weakening of the valves in the veins. Over time, the veins lose their elasticity and stretch, becoming longer and wider. Because of limited space, the elongated veins start to curve, form twisted, snakelike patterns, and bulge up into the skin. As the veins widen, the edges of the valves separate and the veins lose their ability to keep blood flowing toward the heart. Consequently, blood pools (collects) in the veins, causing them to enlarge even more. Although varicose veins are most common in the legs, they also can occur in the esophagus, and in the rectal area as hemorrhoids (see page 271).

Varicose veins appear blue and swollen, just beneath the skin, usually on the inside of the leg or the back of the calf. The affected area may ache, and your legs may feel tired. Your feet and ankles may swell, and your skin may become dry and itchy. However, many people, even those who have large varicose veins, have no discomfort. A small percentage of people have complications such as superficial phlebitis (see page 238), or bleeding, which can result from injury or scratching.

Treatment focuses on relieving symptoms, improving appearance, and preventing complications. Elevating your legs is one of the best ways to relieve symptoms. Treatment also includes wearing elastic support hose, taking regular walks, avoiding standing for long periods, and controlling your weight.

Very painful or unsightly veins may be surgically removed by a process called stripping. The procedure is performed using a local anesthetic and takes about half an hour per leg. Healthy veins take over the work of the veins that have been removed. After surgery, new varicose veins may develop elsewhere.

Although stripping relieves symptoms and prevents complications, the procedure also can leave scars.

Sclerotherapy is an alternative to stripping. An irritant solution is injected into the varicose vein, causing the vein's walls to stick together and block the blood flow through the vein. Other veins take over the work of the treated veins. After the procedure there is a chance that new varicose veins will develop.

Superficial Phlebitis

Superficial phlebitis (also called phlebitis or thrombophlebitis) is inflammation and thrombus (blood clot) formation in a superficial vein. This condition can affect any vein in the body but usually affects the leg veins. Phlebitis can occur after minor injury to a vein or as a complication of varicose veins. Although phlebitis occurs in people with varicose veins, most people with varicose veins do not develop phlebitis.

Symptoms include redness, swelling, and tenderness in the affected area. Some people may experience fever and a vague feeling of being ill. Deep vein thrombosis (see page 236) is a possible, though uncommon, complication.

Superficial phlebitis usually is treated by gently wrapping the leg with a compression bandage and by taking a nonsteroidal anti-inflammatory drug such as ibuprofen. The blood clot usually dissolves on its own. The affected area may remain tender for several weeks. In severe cases the doctor may inject a local anesthetic, make a small cut in the leg, and remove the thrombus. He or she will recommend wearing a compression bandage for several days and taking aspirin or ibuprofen to relieve pain and inflammation.

Blood Disorders

Blood disorders may occur when production of red blood cells cannot keep up with demand, when the composition of the blood changes, or when a disease affects the condition of the blood or blood vessels.

Anemia

Anemia is a reduction in the amount of hemoglobin (the oxygen-carrying protein in red blood cells) or in the number of red blood cells to below normal levels. Anemia reduces the blood's ability to supply oxygen to the tissues and remove carbon dioxide from the tissues. Anemia can result from excessive bleeding, decreased red blood cell production, or diseases that destroy red blood cells. Symptoms of anemia include paleness, weakness, fatigue, shortness of breath, and palpitations.

Excessive bleeding is the most common cause of anemia. When blood is lost, the body pulls water from the tissues outside the bloodstream in an attempt to keep the blood vessels filled. This extra water dilutes the blood and reduces the concentration of red blood cells in the blood. The body then increases red blood cell production in an attempt to correct the anemia. Before that occurs, however, the anemia may be so severe that blood pressure falls and the body's oxygen supply decreases to dangerous levels. Injuries, surgery, or a ruptured blood vessel are examples of possible causes of sudden blood loss that can lead quickly to a heart attack, stroke, or even death.

Chronic (continuous or repeated) internal bleeding is a more common cause of anemia than the sudden loss of blood. Possible causes of chronic internal bleeding include:

- nosebleeds
- hemorrhoids
- ulcers of the stomach or small intestine
- cancer or polyps in the gastrointestinal tract
- kidney or bladder tumors

Treatment depends on how rapidly blood is lost and the severity of the anemia. Transfusion of red blood cells is the only reliable treatment for rapid blood loss. Locating the source of blood loss and stopping the bleeding are the first steps in treating anemia caused by chronic bleeding. Depending on the cause, this could involve treatment with medication or surgery.

Iron deficiency is one of the most common causes of anemia. An adequate supply of iron is required for red blood cell production. In adults, blood loss is the most common cause of iron deficiency. In men, iron deficiency usually indicates bleeding in the gastrointestinal tract. Normal dietary iron intake usually is not enough to replace iron lost from chronic bleeding, since the body has a small iron reserve. Therefore, lost iron must be replaced with supplements. Iron deficiency anemia in men is cured by treating the underlying cause.

Anemia also can result from diseases, conditions, and genetic disorders that cause excess destruction of red blood cells, such as sickle-cell disease.

Sickle-Cell Disease

Sickle-cell disease is an inherited disorder characterized by sickle-shaped red blood cells. These cells contain an abnormal form of hemoglobin (the oxygen-carrying protein in red blood cells), which gives them their sickle shape.

Because these deformed blood cells are fragile, they break up as they travel through the blood vessels and have difficulty moving through the capillaries, the tiny blood vessels that deliver oxygen to tissues. The sickle-shaped cells block and damage the capillaries in the spleen, kidneys, liver, brain, bones, and other organs and reduce their oxygen supply. An inadequate supply of oxygen can cause significant damage to organs and tissues.

Sickle-cell disease affects mostly African Americans and people of Mediterranean ancestry. A child must inherit the defective gene from both parents to develop the disease. About 10 percent of African Americans have inherited one gene for sickle-cell disease. This means that they have the sickle-cell trait and will not develop the disease but will be carriers who can pass the disease to their children if their partners also are carriers. About 0.3 percent of African Americans have inherited two genes for sickle-cell disease, and they have the disease.

If you are African American or have a family member with sickle-cell disease and are planning to start a family, talk to your doctor about having a blood test to determine whether you are a carrier of the gene. If you are a carrier, your partner also must be tested. If you are not a carrier, you cannot pass the disease to your children. Both parents must carry the gene to pass the disease to their children.

Symptoms of sickle-cell disease may include headaches, breathlessness on exertion, fatigue, and jaundice (yellowing of the skin and the whites of the eyes). Bouts of severe pain, known as sickle-cell crises, can occur when dead or damaged red blood cells collect in the joints or in other parts of the body. A sickle-cell crisis also can result from an infection, dehydration, or prolonged exposure to cold weather. In addition, any activity that reduces the amount of oxygen in the blood, such as vigorous exercise, mountain climbing, or flying at high altitudes without sufficient oxygen, may result in a sickle-cell crisis. The crisis is characterized by a sudden worsening of the anemia, pain in the abdomen or long bones, fever, and sometimes shortness of breath. Abdominal pain may be severe and accompanied by nausea and vomiting.

Poor circulation to the skin may lead to sores on the legs, especially at the ankles. Damage to the nervous system may cause strokes. Older men may experience a decline in lung and kidney function. Younger men may develop persistent and often painful erections (priapism; see page 177).

Rarely, a person who carries the sickle-cell trait may have blood in the urine caused by bleeding from the kidneys. If a physician knows that this bleeding is related to the sickle-cell trait, exploratory surgery may be avoided.

Doctors usually recognize the combination of anemia, abdominal and bone pain, and nausea in young black men as signs of sickle-cell disease. The diagnosis usually is confirmed by electrophoresis, a blood test that can detect abnormal hemoglobin and indicate whether the person has the sickle-cell trait or sickle-cell disease.

In the recent past, people with sickle-cell disease were not expected to live into their 20s. Today, however, most live well past age 50. Deaths caused by exertion are rare. Because sickle-cell disease cannot be cured, treatment focuses on preventing crises, controlling the anemia, and relieving symptoms. Folic acid (one of the B vitamins) supplements help the body produce red blood cells to replace dead and damaged sickle cells. People with sickle-cell disease need to avoid activities that reduce the oxygen levels in their blood and should seek medical attention promptly, even for minor illnesses, such as a cold or other viral infection. Immunization against infectious diseases, such as pneumonia and influenza (see page 93), and use of antibiotics to fight infection are essential preventive measures for all people who have sickle-cell disease.

A person who is experiencing a sickle-cell crisis requires immediate treatment. He or she is usually given large amounts of fluids intravenously to prevent dehydration, antibiotics to treat infection, and painkillers to relieve the extreme pain. Blood transfusions may be given to increase the amount of normal hemoglobin in the blood. Supplemental oxygen also may be given to help provide more oxygen to the tissues.

Medications also are available to reduce the risks associated with a sickle-cell crisis. One such drug is hydroxyurea, which increases the amount of normal hemoglobin in the blood and thereby decreases the number of red blood cells that become sickle-shaped.

CHAPTER 12

Lungs

Without conscious effort, you breathe in and out 10 to 15 times each minute. When you are at rest and breathe normally, each breath lasts about 4 to 6 seconds and moves approximately 1.5 pints of air. During vigorous physical exertion you may take in as many as 5 or 6 pints of air per breath.

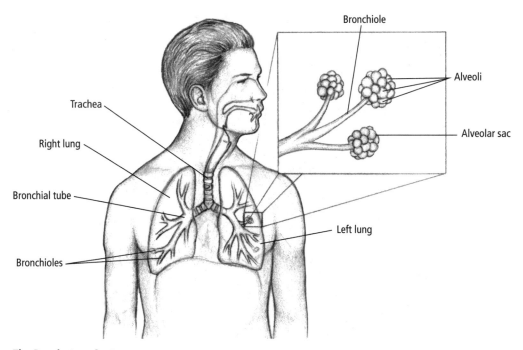

The Respiratory System

The air you breathe passes through your trachea (windpipe), which divides into two smaller tubes called bronchial tubes, each of which leads to one of the lungs. The bronchial tubes branch into smaller and smaller tubes called bronchioles. At the ends of the bronchioles are tiny clusters of air sacs called alveoli (inset), where oxygen is absorbed into the bloodstream and carbon dioxide is eliminated from the bloodstream.

Your diaphragm, the large muscle that forms the base of your chest cavity, does most of the work during normal breathing. It receives messages from your brain to contract, which expands the chest cavity and creates a negative pressure that results in inward air flow. Stretch receptors in the lungs inform your brain that enough air has been taken in, and the diaphragm is instructed to relax, allowing the air to move out. Your brain alters the rate and depth of respiration based on the levels of oxygen and carbon dioxide in your blood. Visual, auditory, or other stimuli, such as fear, also can alter the breathing pattern.

Your lungs are very spongelike. The right lung has three sections, or lobes, and is slightly larger than the left lung, which has only two lobes. Air enters the lungs through the trachea (windpipe) and is drawn through the two large bronchi (the main airways that lead into each lung) into smaller airways called bronchioles. The bronchi and the bronchioles are lined with tiny hairs called cilia that catch and sweep out large dust particles and mucus that is secreted by glands in the bronchioles and coats the airways.

Gases are exchanged (carbon dioxide is removed from the bloodstream, and oxygen enters the bloodstream) in the highly folded and moist surfaces of air sacs (also called alveolar sacs) at the end of each bronchiole. Each alveolar sac is made up of up to 30 tiny pouches called alveoli. Alveoli have walls that are only one cell thick and are richly supplied with capillaries (the smallest blood vessels in the body) to facilitate gas exchange. Healthy lungs provide approximately 850 square feet of surface area for this purpose. Only 10 percent of the lungs is solid tissue; the rest is air and blood.

Protecting Your Lungs

Lung cancer is the leading cause of cancer death among both men and women in the United States. Twice as many men as women die of chronic obstructive pulmonary disease (such as emphysema), and pneumonia is a more common cause of death among men than among women.

Lung disease is directly related to specific risk factors such as cigarette smoking and working in occupations that carry risks for developing lung disease. Plastics, wood, metal, and textile workers; bakers; millers; farmers; poultry handlers; miners; grain elevator workers; laboratory technicians; drug manufacturers; dry cleaners; and detergent manufacturers are all exposed to airborne agents that can cause occupational asthma, lung cancer, and other respiratory disorders.

Your lungs have a limited capacity to protect themselves against many different types of irritants. For example, foreign substances trapped by the mucus that lines the airways can be voluntarily expelled (coughed up) as needed. Also, macrophages—scavenging white blood cells—on the inner surface of the alveoli ingest and destroy dust, soot, and other foreign particles, including airborne bacteria.

You also can take steps on your own to protect your respiratory system. Not smoking and avoiding exposure to tobacco smoke are critical to protecting your lungs. Cigarette smoke is the major cause of lung cancer, chronic bronchitis, and emphysema. Exposure to cigarette smoke also increases your risk of respiratory infection, including colds. In the lungs, tobacco smoke increases the production of mucus, constricts air passages, and causes infections that break down the walls of alveoli, reducing the surface area for gas exchange. Cancer-causing substances (carcinogens) in tobacco smoke can cause abnormal cells to develop, which may eventually grow into malignant tumors that can spread to other parts of the body.

If your job exposes you to airborne irritants, be sure to wear a protective mask or, if needed, a respirator to prevent inhalation of those hazardous substances. Be familiar with the information and recommendations (such as precautions and first-aid measures) contained in the material safety data sheets for all of the hazardous substances you may be exposed to at work. Your employer should provide all necessary protective equipment, which should be in good working order. You should also monitor pollution warnings on television and radio before working or exercising outdoors.

Keep your home well ventilated to prevent the accumulation of carbon monoxide or other harmful gases and to prevent mold and fungi from growing inside. Clean air conditioners, humidifiers, dehumidifiers, and air purifiers regularly to reduce your exposure to dust, mold spores, and other irritants and allergens. Test your home for radon, a colorless, odorless radioactive gas that is the second most common cause of lung cancer in the United States. Install carbon monoxide detectors (which are available at hardware stores) on each floor of your home.

Symptoms of Lung Disease

Because you have plenty of reserve lung tissue, respiratory disorders may begin long before symptoms appear. Talk to your doctor about the following symptoms as soon as they occur:

- *Cough.* Pay particular attention to a cough that lasts more than a month, that brings up blood from your lungs, or that produces mucus (especially if it is yellowish, green, or brown).
- *Shortness of breath or difficulty breathing.* Except during physical exertion and at high altitude, breathing should not require noticeable effort or leave you feeling as though you cannot get enough air.
- *Chest pain.* You should not feel pain when taking deep breaths or coughing, nor should your lungs ache.
- *Abnormal breathing noises.* Wheezing or whistling noises that accompany breathing can indicate an obstruction of air flow.

Disorders That Obstruct Air Flow

The flow of air from the lungs can be limited or obstructed by a variety of structural changes in the lungs. Chronic obstructive pulmonary disease (COPD), a major cause of disability and death in men, refers to asthma, chronic bronchitis, and emphysema. With COPD the airway obstruction is generally irreversible. With asthma the obstruction is reversible with treatment, although the disease itself may not be cured.

Asthma

Asthma affects the lining of the bronchi and the bronchioles. These airways become inflamed and produce extra mucus. Smooth muscle tissue in the airways contracts, narrowing the passageways even further. Common symptoms of asthma include wheezing (a faint whistling noise that occurs with each breath), shortness of breath, chest tightness (feeling as if someone is squeezing your chest), and coughing. Signs of an asthma emergency include extreme difficulty breathing, bluish tinge (cyanosis) to the lips and face, severe anxiety, rapid pulse, and sweating.

People who do not manage their asthma carefully often miss work, frequently require treatment in hospital emergency departments, or may die of a severe attack. During acute (sudden) attacks, the airways become significantly constricted (narrowed), very little air passes through to the alveoli, and oxygen levels in the blood decrease. Without an adequate supply of oxygen, tissues in the body begin to die. However, the risks can be significantly reduced with careful management of the disease.

Triggers of Asthma Attacks

Specific substances, conditions, and circumstances can bring on an asthma attack in a person who has asthma. An important strategy for controlling your asthma is to know and to avoid your specific triggers:

- allergens—such as pollen, mold, animal dander (dead skin flakes) from household pets, and dust mite and cockroach droppings

- pollutants—such as tobacco smoke, wood smoke, smog, ozone, chemical fumes, dust, hair spray, perfume, and other sprays

- foods and food additives—such as beer, wine, shrimp, milk, eggs, nuts, soy, wheat, dried fruit, and processed foods

- weather changes—such as cold air, strong winds, and sudden changes in barometric pressure or humidity

- medications—such as aspirin, ibuprofen, and beta-blockers

- physical exertion

- viral infection or sinus infection

- gastroesophageal reflux disease (see page 262)

- anxiety

Controlling environmental factors that can trigger an asthma attack (see box on previous page) is only one step toward successful asthma management. Work closely with your doctor to establish an ongoing program to control your asthma. You will need to monitor your lung function daily with a peak flow meter (a device that measures the speed at which air can be forced from the lungs). This will help determine your response to treatment. Your physician also will check your lung function regularly with a device called a spirometer, which measures how much and how quickly air can be expelled after a deep breath, to monitor your condition and assess your response to treatment.

Medications used to treat asthma vary according to the individual and the timing of administration. Avoid relying exclusively on short-term rescue medications such as inhaled bronchodilators, which temporarily open up the bronchial tubes to increase air flow. Instead, work with your doctor to develop a long-term treatment plan that includes anti-inflammatory medications such as corticosteroids and antileukotrienes to prevent or reduce the severity of attacks.

Chronic Bronchitis

Bronchitis is inflammation of the lining of the bronchial tubes. The inflammation results in the production of extra mucus, which causes the person to cough regularly to clear the airways. Acute (short-term) bronchitis often occurs along with a severe cold (usually with a fever) and clears up completely on its own.

Chronic (long-term) bronchitis lasts for months but often goes unnoticed because of its gradual development. With chronic bronchitis, a mucus-producing cough lasts weeks after a cold apparently has cleared up. The coughing episodes become longer and longer after each subsequent cold. People with chronic bronchitis begin to accept the coughing and mucus production as "normal," especially if they smoke. Usually the cough is worse in the morning and in cold, damp weather.

People with chronic bronchitis often do not seek treatment because they consider the cough a nuisance rather than a symptom of a medical disorder. However, the chronic inflammation and accumulation of mucus provide an excellent environment for frequent infections. Lung tissue becomes permanently damaged, air flow is obstructed, and the reduced ability of the lungs to exchange gases forces the heart to work harder, increasing the person's risk for cardiovascular disease.

Treatment for chronic bronchitis focuses on reducing irritation and inflammation in the bronchial tubes. If you smoke, you must quit immediately (see page 107). If you work at a job that exposes you to irritating dust or fumes, you need to use protective equipment such as masks and respirators. You should avoid exposure to people with colds or the flu, and you need to have a flu shot each year at the beginning of the flu season (usually in October).

Your doctor will prescribe antibiotics if you have an active infection in your lungs, which may help but will not eliminate your cough. Sometimes bronchodilator drugs are prescribed as a temporary measure to help open up the airways. Corticosteroid medications also may be prescribed to reduce airway inflammation. Your doctor will discuss other treatment options with you, depending on the degree to which chronic bronchitis has affected your lungs and other body systems.

Emphysema

Unlike asthma and bronchitis, emphysema affects the air sacs (alveoli) rather than the airways. Like chronic bronchitis, emphysema develops gradually and therefore occurs mainly in adults over age 45. Often the two conditions occur together. Emphysema is more common in men than in women. Except in rare cases that result from a genetic disorder, emphysema usually develops after many years of smoking.

Chemicals in tobacco smoke cause cells in the lungs to produce too much of one protease (elastase) and too little of another protease (elastase inhibitor). (Protease, elastase, and elastase inhibitor are enzymes.) This imbalance damages the elastic tissue in the walls of the alveoli and the tiny bronchioles that lead to each alveolar sac. As a result, the overall surface area of the alveoli is reduced and the alveolar walls become thickened, which limits gas exchange (the exchange of carbon dioxide for oxygen). This reduces the amount of oxygen that the lungs transfer to the bloodstream, which can lead to heart and kidney failure. As more and more alveoli and bronchioles collapse and as the lungs lose their elasticity, breathing becomes labored, causing shortness of breath, and exhaling, in particular, becomes increasingly difficult.

Because the damage to lung tissue is permanent, treatment for emphysema focuses on providing relief of symptoms and preventing progression of the disease. If you smoke, you must quit immediately (see page 107). Your doctor may prescribe bronchodilators to help open your airways. Pulmonary rehabilitation, a comprehensive treatment program that strives to improve the comfort and functioning of a person with a chronic lung disease, can be helpful for some people. Other people may benefit by using supplemental oxygen supplied through a portable tank or a machine called a concentrator. For advanced cases of emphysema, lung transplantation or lung volume reduction surgery (removal of the most damaged portions of the lung) may be performed.

Lung Cancer

Changes in the structure of some of the many types of cells that make up the lungs may begin almost immediately upon exposure to carcinogens (cancer-causing substances). Some of the thousands of chemicals contained in tobacco smoke—both inhaled directly and released into the air through secondhand smoke—are known respiratory carcinogens. Substances such as radon, asbestos, arsenic, uranium, and certain petroleum products also can cause lung cancer.

Regular exposure to any of these substances can damage individual cells in the lungs, causing them to multiply into an abnormal mass of cells called a tumor. The tumor can be benign, which means that it will not spread to other parts of the body and usually will not grow back if it is removed. If the tumor is malignant, however, it can invade and destroy surrounding tissue and may spread to other parts of the body through the bloodstream, causing new tumors (called metastases) to form in other tissues. And because all blood flows through the lungs, cancer that begins elsewhere in the body may spread to the lungs.

A tumor in one of the bronchi can irritate the lining of the airway and cause a persistent cough, which may cause the tumor to bleed. As it grows, the tumor may block the airway, resulting in repeated bouts of pneumonia or other respiratory infections. A tumor located in the outer part of a lung may not produce any symptoms until it is large enough to press against the chest wall and cause pain. If you experience any of the warning signs of lung cancer (see box), see your doctor as soon as possible.

Tests for lung cancer include a chest X ray, a microscopic examination of mucus expelled from your lungs, and a computed tomography (CT) scan or magnetic resonance imaging (MRI) of your chest. If something resembling a tumor is seen on an X ray or a scan, your doctor may perform a bronchoscopy (see "Diagnostic Procedures," page 256) and a biopsy (removal of a small piece of tissue from the suspected tumor for examination under a microscope). Depending on the results, other tests and procedures may be performed to identify the type of cancer and the extent to which it has spread.

Two major types of cancer begin in the lungs. Non-small cell lung cancer generally grows and spreads slowly. This form of cancer accounts for about three fourths of all cases of lung cancer. The non-small cell cancers include squamous cell carcinoma, adenocarcinoma, and large cell carcinoma. The less common small cell lung cancer (sometimes called oat cell cancer) grows quickly and is more likely to spread to other parts of the body, such as the lymph nodes, brain, liver, and bones.

Treatment of lung cancer depends on the type of cancer cell involved, the size and location of the primary (or first) tumor, and the size and location of any

---

Warning Signs of Lung Cancer

If you smoke or are regularly exposed to tobacco smoke or other airborne carcinogens (cancer-causing substances), you are at significant risk for developing lung cancer. Contact your physician immediately if you experience any of the following symptoms:

- persistent cough
- chest pain
- unexplained weight loss
- loss of appetite
- shortness of breath, wheezing, or hoarseness
- coughing up blood or bloody mucus
- persistent fever
- recurrent respiratory infections such as pneumonia or bronchitis

secondary tumors (tumors that have spread from the primary tumor to another part of the body). Treatment options include surgical removal of the lung tumor, use of anticancer drugs (chemotherapy), use of radiation (radiation therapy), use of lasers (photodynamic therapy), or a combination of these treatments.

Although treatment is improving, the outlook for lung cancer is generally poor. If you smoke or are exposed to any known carcinogens, you should immediately take steps to prevent lung cancer.

Pulmonary Embolism

Deoxygenated blood travels through the veins from the rest of the body into the heart, which pumps it through the pulmonary arteries into the lungs for reoxygenation. Blood coming to the heart from the veins may contain large particles, such as pieces of blood clots or tissue, fat globules, or air bubbles. A sufficiently large particle (embolus) can block an artery that leads to the lung's network of capillaries (where gas exchange occurs). Pulmonary embolism refers to the sudden blockage of one or more of the pulmonary arteries.

Conditions that cause clots in the veins, such as deep vein thrombosis (see page 236), frequently lead to pulmonary embolism. Although they are a rare cause of pulmonary embolism, fat globules can form after bone fractures and lodge within the capillary network (rather than in the pulmonary arteries themselves).

The onset of symptoms of pulmonary embolism is sudden. As the level of oxygen in the blood decreases, the brain increases the respiratory rate, leading to hyperventilation (abnormally deep or rapid breathing). Even if the clot breaks up, a pulmonary embolism can lead to pulmonary hypertension, a condition in which high blood pressure in the pulmonary artery puts strain on the right side of the heart, which may cause it to fail. Over time, the left side of the heart also begins to fail. Heart disease that results from any pulmonary disease is called cor pulmonale. If you already have heart or lung disease, a pulmonary embolism that a healthy person could easily tolerate may be life-threatening or fatal.

Diagnosing pulmonary embolism requires one of two imaging procedures: a pulmonary arteriogram or a high-resolution CT scan. In both procedures, contrast medium (dye) is injected into the veins, and X rays are taken to locate the blockage. However, because symptoms of pulmonary embolism also can indicate a heart attack, your doctor probably will perform a chest X-ray examination, electrocardiography (an examination of

Warning Signs of Pulmonary Embolism

Pulmonary embolism occurs suddenly. If you have a condition that puts you at risk for pulmonary embolism—such as immobility, cancer, a leg injury, or heart failure—seek immediate medical care if you have any of the following warning signs:

- shortness of breath
- sharp chest pain
- rapid pulse
- sweating
- coughing up bloody mucus
- fainting

the electrical activity of the heart), blood tests, and possibly radionuclide scans (in which a radioactive substance is injected into the bloodstream to produce images of the pulmonary arteries) to help confirm the diagnosis.

In most cases the clot or embolus breaks up on its own and does not need to be removed surgically. Painkillers, oxygen, and blood thinners (to prevent further clots from forming and to help dissolve existing clots) are given while the artery is blocked. Treatment with thrombolytic (clot-dissolving) drugs also may be helpful. In rare cases, surgery to remove the clot may be required if it is very large.

The long-term goal of treatment for pulmonary embolism is to prevent the development of blood clots in the legs and other parts of the body. Usually this involves long-term use of anticoagulant (blood-thinning) drugs such as heparin or warfarin. This is especially important after hip surgery, elective neurosurgery, or a major injury. In cases of chronic, persistent clots, a filter may be installed in a major vein (location of the filter depends on the source of the clots) to prevent clots from traveling through the veins into the pulmonary artery.

Infectious Lung Disorders

Your lungs have built-in mechanisms for filtering out foreign substances that are inhaled with each breath. Despite these mechanisms, however, with repeated exposure to infectious agents such as viruses and bacteria, or with a change in your immune system, your risk of contracting a respiratory infection increases. This is especially true if your lungs have been damaged by smoking or exposure to environmental pollutants or if you have a chronic disease or take medications that decrease the effectiveness of your immune system. Some infectious microorganisms that enter the body through the lungs can affect many different organ systems. Others remain in the lungs, causing infection and inflammation.

Pneumonia

Pneumonia refers to an infection of the lungs. Lobar pneumonia is usually restricted to a single lobe of one lung (although more than one lobe may be involved), while bronchial pneumonia affects more widespread areas in both lungs. The specific type of pneumonia depends on the agent causing the infection. The three major microorganisms that cause pneumonia are viruses, bacteria, and mycoplasmas.

About half of all cases of pneumonia are caused by viruses. This type of pneumonia is most common in infants and children, older adults, and people whose immune systems are not working effectively. Viral pneumonia has symptoms similar to those of the flu: fever, headache, muscle pain, weakness, dry cough, and breathlessness. Medications are available to combat some of the viruses that can cause pneumonia, but antibiotics should not be prescribed, and would not be beneficial, unless bacteria are causing the infection.

Bacterial infection accounts for 30 to 50 percent of pneumonia cases in adults. *Streptococcus pneumoniae* (pneumococcus) is the most common bacterium involved, although many other microorganisms can cause bacterial pneumonia. The bacteria that cause pneumonia can spread throughout the body once they have entered the lungs. This can result in infection in the bloodstream (bacteremia or sepsis), the covering of the brain (meningitis), the lining of the heart (endocarditis), or the fluid in the joints (septic arthritis). Symptoms of pneumococcal pneumonia can appear either suddenly or gradually and include fever, pain on the affected side, shortness of breath, and a cough that produces mucus (the mucus is often blood-streaked).

Another type of bacterial pneumonia, called legionnaires' disease, is caused by the *Legionella pneumophila* bacterium. The natural habitats for these bacteria are bodies of water, but they also thrive in the evaporative condensers of air-conditioning systems and may be found in humidifiers and vaporizers as well. Legionnaires' disease is most common among middle-aged men. Risk factors include smoking, alcohol abuse, and a suppressed immune system (especially due to taking corticosteroid medications). The fever associated with legionnaires' disease is usually high, and other flulike symptoms occur, such as a vague sense of being ill, a cough, muscle pain, and a headache. The cough is initially dry but produces more mucus as the disease progresses. Antibiotics will eliminate the bacteria, but recovery may be slow.

Mycoplasmas are microorganisms that have characteristics of both bacteria and viruses. They tend to cause a mild but widespread form of pneumonia. Mycoplasma pneumonia is most common among children and young adults, especially those in closed communities such as schools, military barracks, and families. This microorganism acts by attaching to and destroying the cilia throughout the airways. Early symptoms (such as a vague sense of being ill, sore throat, and a dry cough) resemble the flu, but gradually, violent coughing bouts develop. Most people recover without treatment, although the use of certain antibiotics can speed recovery in some cases.

Pneumonia also can develop if bacteria, food, or other substances (including liquids or vomit) are inhaled (aspirated) directly into the lungs. This may occur when a person is choking or unconscious. The resultant infection is called aspiration pneumonia. Because aspiration pneumonia can cause severe damage to the lungs, it is treated in the hospital with intravenous antibiotics and supplemental oxygen. If food or other substances remain lodged in the lungs, the doctor may need to perform a bronchoscopy (see "Diagnostic Procedures," page 256) to remove them. If a toxic chemical has been inhaled, it is a medical emergency. Call 911 or your local emergency number, or take the person to the nearest hospital emergency department without delay.

Who Should Be Vaccinated against Pneumonia?

Pneumonia causes about 40,000 deaths in the United States each year. You should have a "pneumonia shot" if:

- you are age 65 or older
- you have diabetes
- you have chronic heart, lung, kidney, or liver disease
- you have sickle-cell disease
- your immune system is compromised (due to cancer, HIV, or AIDS, or from corticosteroid medication, radiation therapy, or chemotherapy)
- you have had your spleen removed or have a spleen dysfunction
- you have had an organ transplant or a bone marrow transplant
- you are a healthcare worker

The pneumococcal vaccine provides long-term immunity and can be given at any time of year. You should be revaccinated if you received the vaccine in childhood and have a chronic condition such as sickle-cell disease.

Tuberculosis

Tuberculosis (TB) was a leading cause of death in the United States until the 1940s, when antibiotics were developed that could effectively kill the bacteria that cause the disease *(Mycobacterium tuberculosis)*. However, since the early 1980s, strains of the bacteria that are resistant to available drugs have developed, and tuberculosis has again become a major public health problem.

Mycobacterium tuberculosis (or *M tuberculosis*) is easily spread by coughing, sneezing, laughing, or singing but generally does not cause disease without repeated exposure. However, you can be infected with tuberculosis without having the active disease. This type of infection produces no symptoms and is known as a latent infection. Infection, with or without the active disease, results in a positive TB (or tuberculin) skin test.

Although anyone can contract tuberculosis, certain groups of people are at higher risk. This includes homeless people, poor and medically underserved people, prisoners, nursing home residents, intravenous drug users, people with alcoholism, people with HIV infection, people with AIDS, and people with any disease that reduces the effectiveness of their immune system. People who are in regular contact with at-risk populations are also more likely to become infected. People from countries with high rates of tuberculosis may bring the infection with them when they emigrate.

Active tuberculosis disease may produce no signs or symptoms other than a vague feeling of being ill. Sometimes the infection causes a cough that persists for more than 2 weeks and may produce bloody mucus. Other symptoms may include chest pain, difficulty breathing, fever, night sweats, fatigue, loss of appetite, and weight loss.

Because a latent infection with tuberculosis produces no symptoms, a person may be infected for years without realizing it. The infection may be discovered only after the person is examined or treated for another disease or through a routine screening with the tuberculin skin test.

Active tuberculosis is diagnosed with a chest X ray and microscopic examination and cultures of sputum samples expelled from the lungs. The tuberculin skin test is used both to screen people at risk for active tuberculosis and to identify people with a latent infection.

Treatment depends on factors such as whether the TB is active or inactive, whether it has spread to other tissues, or whether the person has been treated for TB previously. Two or more antibiotics (such as isoniazid and rifampin) are given together daily for at least 6 to 9 months; some drug combinations can be given daily for the first month and then twice a week for an additional 8 months, although in some cases, treatment must continue for years. **Warning:** If the drug therapy is not strictly followed, the bacteria may mutate and become resistant to the drugs being used. If you do not take the drugs exactly as prescribed, you could have very serious problems.

Disorders of the Pleura

The outside of the lungs and the inside of the chest cavity are lined by a continuous membrane called the pleura (see Illustration). The portion of the pleura surrounding the lungs is called the visceral pleura, while the portion along the chest wall is called the parietal pleura. The pleural space is moistened with a small amount of fluid that allows the two sides of the lining to slide against each other easily during each breath. In a healthy person the two pleural surfaces are adjacent to each other and there is little space between the two pleural membranes.

Pleurisy

The pleura can become inflamed due to an infection of the underlying lung (such as pneumonia), an infectious

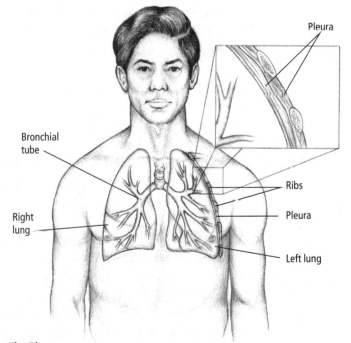

The Pleura

The pleura is a thin membrane with two layers that cover the lungs and chest cavity. Fluid between the two layers provides lubrication and allows smooth expansion and contraction of the lungs during breathing.

agent that enters the pleural space, injury (such as a rib fracture), and exposure to asbestos fibers. The pleura become swollen, and their surfaces may stick together rather than move freely when the person breathes. This causes chest pain that is aggravated by a deep breath or a cough. The pain may extend to the neck, shoulders, or abdomen on the affected side. Efforts to minimize the pain often lead to rapid, shallow breathing.

Because pleurisy is a symptom and not a disease or disorder, the only way to eliminate it is to treat the underlying cause. In the meantime, your doctor probably will recommend that you take a nonprescription painkiller such as aspirin, ibuprofen, or acetaminophen. Also, you might be more comfortable if you wrap your chest with elastic cloth bandages, or if you clutch a pillow to the affected side to minimize chest wall motion during breathing.

Pleural Effusion

Heart failure, cancer, pulmonary embolism, infection, and inflammation can cause fluid to accumulate in the pleural space. The presence of any excess fluid in the pleural space is known as pleural effusion. Fluid can accumulate due to changes in pressure in the lymphatic or blood circulation of the pleural space, or to changes in the permeability of the pleural membranes. If blood accumulates in the pleural space, the condition is known as hemothorax. If pus is involved, the condition is called empyema.

Sometimes a pleural effusion is discovered by chance on a chest X ray that was taken for another purpose. Common symptoms include chest pain and shortness of breath. Identifying the cause of and determining the appropriate treatment for pleural effusion require removing and examining some of the fluid using a procedure called thoracentesis (see "Diagnostic Procedures," page 256). A biopsy (removal of a small sample of tissue for examination under a microscope) of the pleural membranes also may be performed. To help the person's breathing and relieve the discomfort associated with pleural effusion, and to help make a diagnosis, some or all of the fluid is drained with a needle or a tube. Treatment depends on the underlying cause of the fluid buildup.

Pneumothorax

Pneumothorax refers to the accumulation of air in the pleural space. It can result from a penetrating injury such as a rib fracture, or from diseases—such as emphysema, asthma, tuberculosis, or cystic fibrosis—that cause an air leak from the lung into the pleural space. Spontaneous pneumothorax can occur for no apparent reason in tall men younger than 40 and among people who scuba dive or engage in high-altitude activities such as mountain climbing.

Symptoms of pneumothorax include acute (sudden) pain on one side accompanied by shortness of breath and, sometimes, a dry, hacking cough. However, you may experience less severe symptoms if only a small area of the pleural space is involved or if the condition develops slowly. As with pleurisy, the pain may extend to other areas, such as the shoulder or the abdomen.

Your doctor can diagnose pneumothorax based on changes in breath sounds, as detected with a stethoscope, and with a chest X ray. A small, spontaneous pneumothorax will usually clear up on its own in a few days as the air is absorbed into surrounding tissues. In emergency situations the air may need to be drawn out with a needle or a tube inserted into the chest cavity to relieve pressure. With a larger or recurrent pneumothorax, surgical repair may be required.

Other Lung Disorders

The following less common lung disorders can occur under specific environmental circumstances or as a result of another disease or an injury. You should watch for symptoms of these conditions if you are at risk.

- *Adult respiratory distress syndrome (ARDS).* This medical emergency often occurs within 24 to 48 hours after an acute respiratory illness or injury such as pneumonia, chest trauma, severe burns, near-drowning, or pulmonary embolism. The initial symptom is labored, shallow, rapid breathing. The skin may then turn blue due to lack of oxygen. ARDS usually occurs in a hospital setting and requires urgent attention including mechanical assistance to maintain breathing.
- *Occupational lung disease.* One type of occupational lung disease is black lung disease (anthracosis), which occurs among coal miners who have inhaled coal dust over the course of many years. Many other lung disorders can result from inhaling various substances (fumes or dusts) in the workplace. For example, silicosis, the oldest known occupational lung disease, results from repeated exposure to silica or quartz dust in occupations such as stone cutting, blasting, and mining. Berylliosis develops after exposure to beryllium, a metallic element used in the nuclear and aerospace industries and in the manufacture of electronics and chemicals. Irritant gases and fumes sometimes found in the workplace—including chlorine, phosgene, sulfur dioxide, hydrogen sulfide, nitrogen dioxide, and ammonia—can cause permanent damage to the respiratory system. Inhalation of asbestos fibers can lead to a chronic lung disease called asbestosis. Possible complications of asbestosis include lung cancer (see page 247), pleural effusion (see previous page), and respiratory failure (a condition in which there is too much carbon dioxide and too little oxygen in the blood). Typical symptoms of occupational lung disease include a chronic cough and shortness of breath. Measures to prevent occupational lung disease include the use of protective gear and clothing and the enforcement of dust control standards, along with regular screening tests. Since the 1970s, asbestos has been replaced by safer materials whenever possible.

- *Hypersensitivity disease.* This refers to allergic pulmonary disease that results from inhalation of organic dust or chemicals. Occupational exposure to potential allergens (substances that cause allergic responses) such as molds and dust from hay, birds, sugarcane, mushrooms, barley, malt, cheese, wheat flour, straw, sawdust, humidifiers, air conditioners, and a variety of chemical manufacturing processes can cause tumorlike granulomas to form inside the lungs. Once the lungs are sensitized to a specific allergen, the allergic response is rapid and severe. Symptoms include fever, chills, cough, shortness of breath, nausea, vomiting, and loss of appetite. The most effective treatment is to avoid all contact with the allergen, which will allow the granulomas to clear up on their own. If you are exposed to potential allergens at work, be sure to practice dust-control measures and wear appropriate protective gear such as a mask or a respirator.

- *High-altitude pulmonary edema.* If work or recreation takes you to high altitudes, watch for possible symptoms such as increasing shortness of breath, weakness, irregular heartbeat, rapid pulse, abnormal breathing sounds, dizziness, fatigue, and cough. Life-threatening high-altitude disorders can occur quickly after rapid ascents above 8,000 feet. Pulmonary embolism (see page 249) and pulmonary edema (fluid in the lungs) can occur if initial symptoms are ignored. The brain, heart, and muscles also can be affected by acute altitude sickness. A rapid descent to a lower altitude is the most effective treatment, but supplemental oxygen also should be used. To prevent this disorder, climbers should always make a gradual ascent, stop to rest at intermittent altitudes, and use supplemental oxygen as needed.

Diagnostic Procedures

The details about your symptoms of lung disease help your physician make an initial diagnosis. Tests of lung function and procedures to visualize your lungs are needed to confirm a diagnosis or to plan or monitor treatment. If your doctor thinks that you may have a lung disorder, you will likely undergo some of the following diagnostic procedures:

- *Spirometry.* This is the simplest and most commonly performed lung function test. Spirometry is used to check or to evaluate a lung disorder and to monitor a person's response to treatment. In this procedure the person takes a deep breath and exhales forcefully into the mouthpiece of a machine called a spirometer. The spirometer measures the total volume of air exhaled, which is the forced vital capacity (FVC), and the rate at which the air was exhaled, which is the forced expiratory volume in 1 second (FEV_1).

- *Arterial blood gases test.* This blood test is performed to determine the levels of oxygen and carbon dioxide in the blood and the acidity of the blood. Samples of blood are drawn from an artery. This procedure is useful for diagnosing and monitoring respiratory failure.

- *Thoracentesis.* If you have fluid in the pleural space, your doctor will insert a needle to draw some out. You will be awake, sitting upright, and leaning forward slightly. Your skin will be cleansed and anesthetized. The location at which the needle is inserted depends on where the fluid is located. This is determined by listening with a stethoscope, or by a chest X ray, ultrasound, or computed tomography (CT) scan.

- *Bronchoscopy.* Your doctor may want to look directly into your lungs with a bronchoscope, a thin, flexible tube with a light and video camera at its tip. Your doctor also can use the bronchoscope to take samples of mucus and tissue from the lungs. Bronchoscopy can be used for both diagnosis and treatment, such as removing foreign bodies and clearing unwanted fluids. The procedure is performed while you are awake and lying on your back. You will be sedated and given adequate pain medication. The doctor also will give you medication to keep you from gagging or coughing during the procedure. Oxygen is delivered to your lungs via a tube that has been passed through one nostril; the bronchoscope will be threaded through your mouth or the other nostril. Your doctor will watch the video display as the bronchoscope moves through the airway into your lungs. These images also will be recorded on videotape, and the most helpful images will be printed out.

- *Thoracotomy.* When a bronchoscopy is insufficient to make a diagnosis or shows problems that require more thorough evaluation, your doctor may recommend an endoscopic examination of the pleural space. During the examination, the doctor may perform either of two minor surgical procedures—a mediastinoscopy or a thoracoscopy. If the problem is more extensive, you may need to have a major surgical procedure called a thoracotomy. You will have general anesthesia for a thoracotomy, in which the chest cavity is opened and the lungs and surrounding tissues are examined. Pieces of tissue will be removed for laboratory analysis, and the overall state of the respiratory system will be assessed. Often this can be achieved through a small incision between the ribs. Sometimes a larger surgical opening must be created.

CHAPTER 13

Digestive System

Your digestive system starts with your mouth, where food enters and is broken down for processing. When you swallow, food passes through a narrow tube called the esophagus, which has muscles that squeeze food particles down toward the stomach.

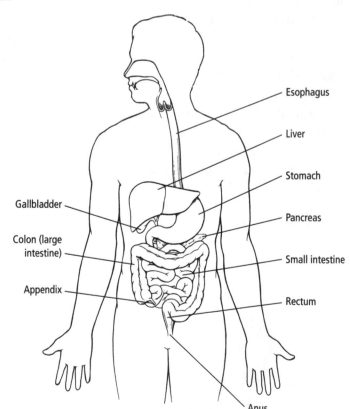

Esophagus

Liver

Stomach

Gallbladder

Pancreas

Colon (large intestine)

Small intestine

Appendix

Rectum

Anus

The Digestive System

Saliva secreted inside your mouth when you eat begins the digestive process of breaking down the food. Waves of muscular contractions move the food through the digestive tract—the esophagus, stomach, small intestine, colon, and rectum—to the anus, from which it is eliminated from the body. Along the way, other organs of the digestive system—the liver, gallbladder, and pancreas—secrete juices that promote digestion. The appendix, attached to the large intestine, has no known function.

The adult stomach has a capacity of 2.5 to 3 pints. When food enters the stomach it is held, churned, and released slowly into the small intestine at the rate required for proper digestion. The rate of release depends on the type of food. Carbohydrate-rich food passes through the stomach in a few hours, while foods high in protein and fat are retained much longer. The rate at which the stomach contracts and pushes food on to the small intestine is controlled by nerves and hormones released by the stomach, small intestine, and other digestive organs. A muscular valve called the pylorus keeps food in the stomach and prevents backflow from the small intestine into the stomach. Food held in the stomach is bathed in acidic gastric juices that begin breaking down proteins and killing bacteria.

The small intestine is a 21-foot coiled tube in the abdomen that is divided into three parts—the duodenum, the jejunum, and the ileum. The first foot or so is the duodenum, which receives food from the stomach. The duodenum releases hormones to ensure proper digestion of the food based on the amounts of carbohydrate, protein, and fat the food contains. Digestive juices from the pancreas and gallbladder enter the duodenum through the common bile duct. In the duodenum, iron, calcium, and folic acid are absorbed. All food looks the same once it has passed through the duodenum. This watery mixture of partially digested food, fat globules (known as micelles), enzymes, and other secretions is called chyme.

The next 8 feet of small intestine is the jejunum. Most of the digestion and absorption of water and nutrients occurs in this portion of the small intestine. Bile salts (used in breaking down fat for digestion) and vitamin B_{12} are absorbed in the ileum, which makes up the remaining 12 feet of small intestine.

Just as the lungs use air sacs to increase their surface area for gas exchange, so the small intestine uses villi (tiny, fingerlike projections) to ensure efficient nutrient absorption. The villi are further made up of microvilli, which provide a brush border with folds upon folds of membranes through which absorption of nutrients can take place. The total surface area of the small intestine is approximately 350 square yards, or 200 times the surface area of the skin. Each villus contains blood and lymph vessels to transport absorbed nutrients for use throughout the body.

When the chyme passes from the small intestine into the large intestine (colon) through the ileocecal valve (a muscle that prevents backflow of large-intestine contents into the small intestine), it is a watery mix of fibrous waste, indigestible carbohydrates (cellulose), some electrolytes (such as sodium and potassium), and other by-products of digestion. The 6-foot-long colon absorbs most of the remaining liquid and electrolytes. Harmless bacteria in the colon digest fermented, unabsorbed carbohydrates and produce gas as a by-product. These bacteria make up about 30 percent of the solid component of stool.

The cecum (a blind pouch) and its attached appendix (a narrow, worm-shaped tube) lie just below the junction of the small and large intestines. The large intestine is made up of four sections. The first three sections are the ascending colon (which connects with the ileum and ascends up the right side of the abdomen), the transverse colon (the longest portion, which stretches across the abdomen), and the descending colon (which descends along the left side of the abdomen). The sigmoid colon, the fourth and narrowest section of the large intestine, links the descending colon and the rectum. The rectum, about 8 inches in length, can expand considerably to permit storage of stool until it is expelled through the anal canal.

The digestive system uses both hormones (chemical messengers) and nerves to control digestion. The digestive nervous system, with more than 100 million nerve cells, is as large and as complex as the spinal cord. All of the more than 30 chemicals used to transmit instructions in the brain are found in the digestive nervous system. The digestive nervous system communicates with the brain through the vagus nerve, with messages from the digestive tract outnumbering those from the brain by about nine to one.

Common Symptoms of Gastrointestinal Diseases and Disorders

These common gastrointestinal symptoms may indicate an underlying health problem. If you frequently experience any of these symptoms or if they are persistent, talk to your doctor as soon as possible.

- *Vomiting.* Vomiting usually is preceded by nausea, sweating, and pallor (abnormally pale skin) and is accompanied by involuntary contractions of the abdominal muscles. Vomiting is a medical concern when the vomit contains blood (it may have reddish streaks or may resemble coffee grounds), when it is accompanied by sudden, severe abdominal pain, or when it lasts so long or occurs so frequently that it results in dehydration. Symptoms of dehydration include excessive thirst, infrequent urination, dry skin, fatigue, and light-headedness. Talk to your doctor if vomiting is persistent or if you experience any of these symptoms. Treatment will depend on the underlying cause of the vomiting.
- *Constipation.* Frequency of bowel movements varies widely; each person has his or her own usual pattern of bowel movements. Constipation refers to difficult, infrequent passing of hard, dry stool. It can be caused by a poor diet (especially a diet high in fat and sugar and low in fiber), long-distance travel, a sedentary lifestyle, poor bowel habits (such as frequently ignoring the urge to have a bowel movement), pregnancy, laxative abuse, certain medications, or specific diseases. You can prevent constipation by drinking plenty of fluids, eating a well-balanced diet that includes plenty of fiber, exercising regularly (such as taking a brisk walk every day), taking a psyllium-based fiber supple-

ment, responding promptly to the urge to have a bowel movement, and maintaining a regular routine for using the toilet. Talk to your doctor if the constipation is severe, occurs suddenly without an identifiable cause, lasts more than 10 days, or is accompanied by blood in the stool.

• *Diarrhea.* Diarrhea is frequent passage of loose, watery stool. Usually it results from consuming food or fluid contaminated by certain bacteria, parasites, or viruses. Certain medications also can cause diarrhea, as can anxiety, food allergy, and food intolerance. Diarrhea usually clears up on its own within 2 to 3 days. You can help manage the problem by drinking clear fluids and eating bland, low-fiber foods as your symptoms improve. Over-the-counter antidiarrheal drugs also are available. Contact your doctor if the diarrhea is accompanied by severe abdominal pain or a high fever (102 degrees Fahrenheit or higher), is bloody (it may be red-streaked or appear black and tarry), or lasts more than 3 days. You should also watch for symptoms of dehydration—excessive thirst, infrequent urination, dry skin, fatigue, or lightheadedness—and contact your doctor if you are unable to consume enough fluids to prevent these symptoms.

• *Gas.* Gas is a normal by-product of digestion. It is caused by the action of bacteria in the large intestine on carbohydrates and proteins in digested food. Air that is swallowed while eating may be belched back out through the mouth or passed along through the digestive tract until it is released through the rectum. The same is true for gases contained in carbonated beverages. Eating fatty meals can cause bloating and discomfort because the delayed emptying of the stomach that is caused by fatty foods allows gas to build up in the stomach. Persistent belching without an obvious cause may also indicate the presence of *Helicobacter pylori (H pylori),* a bacterium that is the most common cause of peptic ulcers (see page 264). Bloating and excess gas also may be symptoms of lactose intolerance (the inability to digest the milk sugar lactose due to a deficiency of an enzyme called lactase; see page 266). This condition can be controlled by taking over-the-counter lactase supplements, by eating only those dairy products that contain added lactase to aid digestion, or by following a dairy-free diet. Regular exercise, such as brisk walking, can help move gas along and prevent its buildup in the digestive tract, thereby eliminating cramping and bloating.

Disorders of the Esophagus

The esophagus is a narrow tube that permits the transfer of food from the mouth to the stomach. The upper third of the esophagus is composed of skeletal muscle, and the remaining two thirds is composed of smooth muscle. The upper portion works to propel food downward; the lower portion relaxes when food is propelled downward and then constricts (narrows) to ensure that nothing flows backward from the stomach. The esophagus is not meant to store or hold swallowed food or digestive juices, both of which can damage its delicate lining.

Common Symptoms

Difficulty swallowing is called dysphagia. It is a symptom of either an obstructive problem (such as cancer or scarring of the esophagus) or a muscular problem (such as megaesophagus, when the lower esophageal sphincter does not relax and allow food into the stomach).

Heartburn is another symptom of esophageal disorders. This burning pain rises in the chest and can be felt in the neck, throat, or face. Heartburn usually occurs after meals, after taking certain medications, or while lying down. Some people also may feel a burning pain or tightness when swallowing solids or liquids. Heartburn can indicate a problem with a medication or with the lower esophageal sphincter, the muscular valve that prevents stomach acid from rising up into the esophagus. (Heartburn also may be a symptom of coronary artery disease; see page 204.)

Some medications (especially aspirin, antibiotics, and quinidine) and vitamins and minerals (especially potassium chloride, vitamin C, and iron) may damage the esophagus if not taken properly. If you take a pill or a capsule without drinking enough water, it can release chemicals that irritate the lining of the esophagus and possibly cause ulcers, inflammation, or bleeding. If you are taking medications that can cause irritation on swallowing, be sure to drink plenty of fluid (at least 8 ounces) before and after taking them. Sit upright while taking the medication, and remain upright until you have drunk enough fluid to ensure that it has passed into the stomach. Be sure to tell your doctor if a certain pill or capsule continues to irritate your esophagus.

Gastroesophageal Reflux Disease

The most common disorder of the esophagus is gastroesophageal reflux disease (GERD). In GERD, the muscle at the bottom of the esophagus, the lower esophageal sphincter, does not close completely, allowing stomach acids and other irritants to flow backward (reflux) into the esophagus.

Certain medications can interfere with the action of this muscle, including nitrates, calcium channel blockers, theophylline, and anticholinergics. Smoking and diet also contribute to GERD. Excessive consumption of chocolate, peppermint, coffee, alcohol, and fried or fatty foods can weaken the lower esophageal sphincter.

Some people with GERD also have a hiatal hernia, in which a portion of the stomach protrudes through the diaphragm (the large muscle that separates the abdomen from the chest cavity) and allows stomach acid to remain trapped just beneath the sphincter muscle. Coughing, vomiting, straining, and sudden physical exertion can increase pressure in the abdomen, resulting in a hiatal hernia. This condition is common among pregnant women, obese adults, and many otherwise healthy people over age 50.

If you regularly experience heartburn, you should avoid the foods listed above as well as acidic foods that can cause additional irritation to the esophagus, such as citrus fruits and juices, tomatoes and tomato products, peppers, and onions. Eating smaller, more frequent meals may help. Also avoid lying down within 2 to 3 hours of eating. If you smoke, quit now (see page 107). If you are overweight, losing weight (see page 73) will help relieve gastroesophageal reflux disease symptoms. You can also try elevating the head of your bed on 6-inch blocks or sleeping on a specially designed foam wedge. Over-the-counter antacids may help, but if you find yourself taking them for longer than 3 weeks, talk to your doctor.

If changes to your diet and lifestyle do not improve GERD symptoms, your doctor may want to perform additional tests, such as an upper gastrointestinal (GI) series or an endoscopy (see "Diagnostic Procedures," page 282).

In cases of chronic heartburn and GERD, doctors usually prescribe medications to reduce the acid in the stomach and to hasten gastric emptying (moving food and acids out of the stomach and into the duodenum). In rare situations, surgery may be required to increase pressure on the lower esophagus. If the esophagus is badly scarred and narrowed, surgery also may be needed to widen the passageway.

Heartburn and GERD are more than painful and inconvenient. If left untreated, they can cause bleeding or ulcers in the esophagus and also may lead to frequent infections. The esophagus may become permanently narrowed due to scarring from the exposure to stomach acid. People who have had heartburn for 5 or more years are at increased risk for developing Barrett esophagus, a condition in which the cells that line the esophagus change from one type of cell to another. This condition cannot be cured and may lead to esophageal cancer.

Disorders of the Stomach and the Duodenum

Most digestion of food occurs in the stomach and duodenum. This portion of the digestive tract produces and receives from other organs a wide range of chemicals to break down food for nutrient absorption. The stomach uses both mechanical means and chemicals (such as hydrochloric acid and pepsin) to break down food. The duodenum releases hormones that stimulate the pancreas to ensure the proper release of enzymes to digest carbohydrates, proteins, and fats. The duodenum releases another hormone to stimulate the gallbladder to contract and release bile (which is made in the liver and stored in the gallbladder) into the duodenum to digest fats. This tremendous concentration of powerful chemicals accounts for many of the problems that can occur in the stomach and duodenum.

Common Symptoms

Almost everyone has experienced indigestion (also known as an upset stomach or dyspepsia). This painful, burning sensation in the upper abdomen is often accompanied by nausea, bloating, belching, and sometimes vomiting. Indigestion is usually a symptom of a digestive disorder, such as an ulcer. However, some people have persistent indigestion that has no identifiable cause; this is called functional indigestion or nonulcer indigestion. Smoking, drinking too much alcohol, taking certain medications, or being exhausted or stressed can cause or worsen indigestion.

If you frequently experience indigestion, see your doctor so that he or she can examine you, determine the cause of your symptoms, and provide treatment. Contact your doctor promptly if your indigestion is accompanied by vomiting, weight loss, lack of appetite, blood in vomit or stool, pain when you eat, or severe pain in the upper abdomen. Symptoms of indigestion accompanied by shortness of breath, sweating, or pain radiating to the jaw, neck, or left arm can be warning signs of heart disease or a heart attack (see page 207).

As with heartburn, you should not rely on antacids to treat indigestion. You may find that certain foods or situations (such as exercising too soon after eating) are related to your indigestion. Smoking, especially just before meals, often causes or aggravates indigestion.

Peptic Ulcer

A peptic ulcer is a hole or a break in the mucous membrane that lines the digestive tract, allowing digestive acids to come in contact with cells in the lining, injuring them. Peptic ulcers most often occur in the first few inches of the duodenum (duodenal ulcers) or in the stomach (gastric, or stomach, ulcers). While stomach ulcers occur more frequently in women than in men and generally develop after age 60, duodenal ulcers are the most common type of ulcer among both men and women and usually first occur between ages 30 and 50.

Many people who have a peptic ulcer have no symptoms, but most experience a burning or gnawing pain in the abdomen. Pain caused by a duodenal ulcer tends to follow a consistent pattern: pain is absent on awakening, appears by midmorning, is relieved by eating, recurs 2 to 3 hours after each meal, and wakes the person during the night. This pattern continues for a week or more, but the pain may disappear without treatment and then recur months or even years later. With gastric ulcers, eating causes rather than relieves the pain. Other symptoms of both types of peptic ulcers include feeling bloated, belching, nausea, vomiting, and weight loss. If the ulcer is bleeding, blood will appear in vomit or stool. Blood in vomit may appear as red streaks or brownish black and look like coffee grounds. Blood in feces causes black, sticky stool. Talk to your doctor immediately if you see signs of blood in your vomit or stool.

Contrary to popular belief, peptic ulcers are not caused by eating spicy foods or by stress. However, long-term use of painkillers such as aspirin or ibuprofen can interfere with the stomach's natural ability to protect itself against exposure to stomach acid and other digestive juices and can lead to ulcer formation. If you develop an ulcer from taking painkillers regularly, your doctor will recommend that you stop using them immediately and will probably prescribe ulcer-healing medication (such as cimetidine, famotidine, or ranitidine) to decrease the amount of acid in your stomach or medication (such as sucralfate) to protect the stomach lining from digestive juices. The ulcer should heal.

Over-the-counter antacids may provide temporary relief from symptoms of heartburn, indigestion, and excess stomach acid, but they also may mask symptoms of a more serious underlying disorder. Always use caution when self-medicating with over-the-counter antacids, and talk to your doctor if you use antacids regularly.

The most common cause of peptic ulcer is a bacterium called *Helicobacter pylori (H pylori)*. These corkscrew-shaped bacteria burrow into the protective lining of the stomach or small intestine and attach to underlying cells. The bacteria then release chemicals that further damage the mucous membrane and expose the cells to the damaging effects of hydrochloric acid and pepsin. This usually causes inflammation of the stomach (gastritis) and can lead to formation of an ulcer. *Helicobacter pylori* may be responsible for more than 80 percent of all stomach ulcers and more than 90 percent of all duodenal ulcers.

If you have symptoms of an ulcer, see your doctor. He or she will probably recommend an examination of your stomach and duodenum using either an upper gastrointestinal (GI) series or endoscopy (see "Diagnostic Procedures," page 282). If an ulcer is found, tissue collected during endoscopy will be examined for *H pylori*. Blood tests also can be used to detect *H pylori.*

If the ulcer is caused by *H pylori,* your doctor will probably recommend treatment for 2 to 3 weeks with antibiotics (usually two different drugs) and ulcer-healing medication to decrease the amount of acid in your stomach or medication to protect the stomach lining. This "triple therapy" kills the bacteria and promotes healing of the ulcer.

The following self-help measures can help you deal with a peptic ulcer:

- Quit smoking (see page 107).
- Avoid drinking alcohol, coffee, or tea.
- Avoid using nonsteroidal anti-inflammatory drugs such as aspirin or ibuprofen regularly.
- Try eating five or six small meals a day instead of three large meals.

If untreated, an ulcer can cause serious health problems. For example, as an ulcer eats away at the stomach or duodenal wall, blood vessels may be damaged and may bleed into the digestive tract. This can lead to anemia (see page 238), which causes symptoms such as dizziness, weakness, and fatigue. If a large blood vessel is damaged, the bleeding is life-threatening and requires immediate medical treatment. Symptoms of damage to a large blood vessel include weakness or dizziness when standing, vomiting blood, and fainting. The bleeding usually can be stopped in a procedure using an endoscope (viewing tube), but general surgery may be required.

Over time, an untreated ulcer may cause a perforation (hole) in the wall of the stomach or duodenum. This allows bacteria and partially digested food to leak into and infect the sterile abdominal cavity, which, in turn, can lead to peritonitis (inflammation of the peritoneum, the membrane that lines the wall of the abdominal cavity and covers the abdominal organs). A perforated ulcer causes sudden, sharp, severe abdominal pain. A peptic ulcer that has perforated, is bleeding, or has not responded to treatment with medication usually requires surgery to correct the problem. The type of surgery depends on the size and location of the ulcer and whether there are complications (such as perforation).

Disorders of the Small Intestine

Most of the nutrient absorption that takes place in the small intestine occurs in the jejunum and the ileum. Disorders of the small intestine are usually related to problems with breaking down and absorbing nutrients.

Malabsorption Disorders

Lactose intolerance is the inability to digest lactose, the sugar found in milk. It is caused by a deficiency of lactase, the enzyme needed to break down lactose during digestion. Symptoms of lactose intolerance include nausea, cramps, bloating, gas, and diarrhea. In general, symptoms appear about a half hour to 2 hours after a person eats or drinks food that contains lactose. Not all people with lactase deficiency experience symptoms, and the severity of symptoms varies from person to person. The disorder is especially common among adults of Asian, African, and Native American descent.

If you regularly experience symptoms of lactose intolerance when you consume dairy products, you may be lactose intolerant. To avoid these symptoms, your doctor may recommend that you consume smaller portions of your favorite dairy foods, eat only those dairy products that contain added lactase, or take over-the-counter lactase supplements (in liquid or tablets). He or she may recommend that you follow a dairy-free diet. Because not all dairy products cause symptoms in all people who are lactose intolerant, you may find some dairy foods easy to digest, and others intolerable.

Celiac disease is an allergy to gluten, a protein contained in most grains. In people with celiac disease, gluten damages the lining of the small intestine and interferes with its ability to absorb nutrients from food. Most cases of this rare disorder are diagnosed in infancy or early childhood. It is possible, however, for celiac disease to appear for the first time in an adult.

Gastrointestinal symptoms of celiac disease include recurring abdominal swelling and pain; fatty, yellow stools; and gas. Weight loss and unexplained anemia (characterized by fatigue and weakness) often occur. Other possible symptoms include bone or joint pain, muscle cramps, tooth discoloration, tingling and numbness in the legs, mouth sores, a painful skin rash, and behavior changes (such as depression). To diagnose celiac disease, doctors perform special blood tests and use an endoscope (viewing tube) to help remove tissue samples from the small intestine for microscopic examination.

Treatment for celiac disease is to follow a strict gluten-free diet. You will need to avoid wheat, rye, barley, and other grains that contain gluten. You also will need to watch for hidden gluten in foods such as pasta and beer. Rice and corn are safe to eat, and gluten-free flour and other food products also are available. Symptoms will begin to improve within a few days of beginning the diet, though full recovery may take up to 2 years. If left untreated, celiac disease can lead to intestinal cancer, osteoporosis (see page 301), and seizures.

Food Poisoning

Absorption of nutrients in the small intestine can be impaired by bacteria, viruses, parasites, and other microorganisms in food or fluids (including water). Symptoms of food poisoning usually come on suddenly and include vomiting, diarrhea, cramps, bloating, weakness, and loss of appetite. Symptoms also can occur 12 to 48 hours after consuming contaminated food or fluid, when the infectious microorganisms have multiplied to toxic levels in the digestive tract.

Treatment for food poisoning depends on the microorganism that is causing the problem. In most cases all that is needed is bed rest and plenty of clear fluids (such as water, a glucose-electrolyte solution, bouillon, or a sports drink). However, if you have diarrhea that contains blood or mucus or that lasts more than 3 days and a fever that lasts more than 2 days, see your doctor as soon as possible. Also, symptoms of dehydration—excessive thirst, infrequent urination, dry skin, fatigue, rapid heart rate, dizziness—require immediate medical treatment.

Keeping Your Digestive System Healthy

Most digestive system disorders can be prevented by following a healthy lifestyle. The following tips can help you keep your digestive system healthy:

- Consume at least 20 to 25 grams of fiber daily.
- Exercise regularly.
- Drink at least eight glasses of water (8 ounces each) every day.
- Avoid using laxatives except under your doctor's supervision.
- Reduce the amount of fat in your diet.
- Do not smoke or use other tobacco products.
- Use safe food handling and storage procedures.
- Avoid drinking, washing, or cooking with water that may be contaminated by microorganisms.

Crohn's Disease

Crohn's disease is a type of chronic inflammatory bowel disease that can occur anywhere in the gastrointestinal tract, although it most commonly occurs in the ileum. Crohn's disease causes inflammation that extends deep into the intestinal walls, causing pain in the lower right abdominal area (where the small intestine and the large intestine meet) and chronic diarrhea. There may be blood, mucus, or pus in the stool. Symptoms also may include rectal bleeding, weight loss, and fever. In some people with Crohn's disease, abnormal connecting channels called fistulas develop between the intestines and the skin in the genital area. If this happens, intestinal contents may leak through the skin. For reasons that are not known, symptoms also can occur in areas outside the gastrointestinal tract. For example, inflammation and redness may occur in the irises of the eyes, and inflammation and swelling may occur in the joints. An abnormal immune response may be the cause of these symptoms. Crohn's disease increases the risk of cancer and makes it more difficult to screen for cancer due to disease-related tissue changes. The cause of Crohn's disease is unknown, although it appears to run in families.

A doctor can confirm a diagnosis of Crohn's disease by examining the ileum and the colon with an endoscope (viewing tube) in a procedure called colonoscopy (see "Diagnostic Procedures," page 282). There is no cure for Crohn's disease. Medications such as cortisone and sulfasalazine are used to control the inflammation. Drugs also may be used to treat fistulas and the body's abnormal immune response. Your doctor may recommend that you avoid drinking milk or alcohol or eating spicy or high-fiber foods to help prevent worsening of your symptoms. If you are losing weight because your body is not absorbing enough nutrients, your doctor may recommend that you drink a high-calorie liquid nutritional supplement every day. This type of nutritional supplement is available in single-serving cans. In severe cases of weight loss, diarrhea, or bleeding, the doctor may recommend intravenous (directly into a vein) feeding in the hospital until the tissue has recovered sufficiently to permit normal absorption of nutrients. If treatment with medication is ineffective, surgery may be performed to repair a fistula or to remove severely damaged sections of the intestine. Surgery also may be required if the doctor finds precancerous changes in the cells in the intestine. However, surgery will not cure the disease or prevent recurrence of symptoms.

Disorders of the Large Intestine and Rectum

When partially digested food reaches the large intestine (colon), the nutrients have already been absorbed by the body. The colon is responsible for absorbing water and pushing out waste matter. The colon's work is made easier if you eat a healthy diet that includes plenty of fiber from fruits, vegetables, and whole grains. This helps the muscles in your colon push the waste along quickly and efficiently and reduces exposure of the intestinal tissues to carcinogens (cancer-causing substances) and other potentially harmful substances.

Ulcerative Colitis

Ulcerative colitis is a type of chronic inflammatory bowel disease. It is similar to Crohn's disease (see previous page), but it affects only the intestinal lining and is almost always restricted to the large intestine. Ulcerative colitis starts at the rectum and spreads upward through the large intestine. The disease causes chronic diarrhea that is usually bloody; as the intestinal lining dies and sloughs off, ulcers form that release mucus, pus, and blood into the colon. Other symptoms include abdominal pain, fatigue, weight loss, loss of appetite, and rectal bleeding. The nonintestinal symptoms that can occur with Crohn's disease also can occur with ulcerative colitis. People whose ulcerative colitis extends throughout the entire colon are at much greater risk of developing colon cancer than are those whose disease is limited to the rectum and the sigmoid (lower) colon.

Ulcerative colitis develops most frequently between ages 15 and 40. Most people with ulcerative colitis can control their symptoms by making simple dietary changes, such as avoiding raw fruits and vegetables or highly seasoned foods to minimize damage to the sensitive intestinal lining. Treatment for ulcerative colitis is generally the same as it is for Crohn's disease. Periods of remission (without symptoms) may last weeks, months, or even years. However, in most people, symptoms eventually return. During severe attacks (10 or more bouts of bloody diarrhea per day), a person must be hospitalized to receive intravenous drugs and feeding and to be monitored for perforation of the bowel. For some people, surgical removal of the rectum and all or part of the colon may be necessary.

Irritable Bowel Syndrome

Irritable bowel syndrome is a group of symptoms that includes cramping pain, gas, bloating, and alternating bouts of constipation and diarrhea. Sometimes people with irritable bowel syndrome pass mucus with their bowel movements. Irritable bowel syndrome is also called irritable colon, spastic colon, spastic bowel, mucous colitis, and functional bowel disease. Diagnosis of irritable bowel syndrome is usually made by ruling out other possible causes of the symptoms. Irritable bowel syndrome does not cause permanent damage to the intestines and does not increase the risk of colon cancer.

Stress and diet are the most common triggers for the symptoms of irritable bowel syndrome. Stress probably has a role in irritable bowel syndrome because the nervous system controls the colon and digestion. Contractions of the colon can begin as soon as the person starts eating, and the urge to have a bowel movement may come within 30 to 60 minutes after a meal. High-fat foods (such as red meats and dairy products), caffeine, and alcohol can bring on symptoms. Eating large meals can lead to cramping and diarrhea.

To control irritable bowel syndrome, avoid the foods that cause your symptoms. You also may find relief by eating smaller, more frequent meals and by eating less fat and more fruits, vegetables, and whole grains. Taking fiber supplements also may help. Stress management techniques (see page 118) will help you reduce or control stress. If self-help measures are ineffective, your doctor may prescribe anticholinergic or antispasmodic medication (such as atropine or dicyclomine) to help relieve spasms in the colon.

Diverticular Disease

Diverticula are small bulges or pouches that develop in the colon. These pouches form when the colon strains to move hard stool, and the increased pressure pushes through weak spots in the lining of the colon. This condition may result from eating a diet that is low in fiber. If there are no symptoms or mild symptoms, the condition is called diverticulosis. If the pouches become infected or inflamed—such as when stool or bacteria become trapped inside them—the condition is known as diverticulitis. Diverticular disease occurs mainly in developed countries such as the United States, where people regularly consume low-fiber processed foods.

Diverticulosis usually does not cause symptoms, although some people may experience tenderness or pain in the lower abdomen. Others may have mild cramps, bloating, and alternating bouts of constipation and diarrhea. Eating a well-balanced diet (see page 49) that is low in fat and high in fiber, taking fiber supplements, and taking antispasmodic medication will relieve the symptoms of diverticulosis and help prevent diverticulitis. If you have no symptoms, you do not need treatment.

The most common symptom of diverticulitis is abdominal pain, especially in the lower left abdomen. The pain may be accompanied by fever, nausea, vomiting, chills, cramping, and constipation. Diverticulitis is usually detected during a diagnostic examination such as a colonoscopy or a gastrointestinal (GI) series (see "Diagnostic Procedures," page 282).

Treatment for diverticulitis includes antibiotics, intravenous fluids, and bed rest. Surgery may be required if an infected diverticulum ruptures and produces an abscess (a pus-filled sac) or causes peritonitis (inflammation of the lining of the abdominal cavity), if a stricture (narrowing) develops in the colon, or if bleeding cannot be controlled. In most cases the affected portion of the colon is removed, and the remaining portions are rejoined. A colostomy (see box on page 275) also may be required.

Proctitis

Proctitis is inflammation of the lining of the rectum. Symptoms include bleeding, constipation, a feeling of fullness in the rectum, pain in the lower left abdomen or around the anus, and, sometimes, discharge of mucus and pus. Proctitis may occur after certain medical treatments, such as radiation therapy or antibiotic use. Inflammatory bowel disease, sexually transmitted diseases, injury to the rectum, and infection also may cause proctitis.

Diagnosis of proctitis is made by a proctoscopy (see "Diagnostic Procedures," page 282) and a biopsy (removal of a small piece of tissue for microscopic examination). Once the underlying cause of the inflammation has been determined, the doctor will recommend appropriate treatment. If inflammatory bowel disease is the underlying cause, the doctor probably will prescribe corticosteroid medication to relieve the symptoms.

Anal Abscess

An abscess is an infected cavity filled with pus. Abscesses can occur when bacteria penetrate and become trapped in the tissues of the anus or rectum. Anal abscesses that appear close to the tissue surface are very painful. Abscesses in deeper tissues tend to cause more general symptoms of infection such as fever, malaise (a vague feeling of being ill), and tenderness around the abscess. Your doctor will open and drain the abscess. When an anal abscess is drained, a fistula (an abnormal connecting channel between the intestines and the skin in the genital area) may develop spontaneously. Surgery is required to repair a fistula.

Hemorrhoids

Hemorrhoids are swollen (varicose) veins in the lining of the anus and rectum. Hemorrhoids may result from straining during bowel movements. Other possible causes include heredity, aging, and chronic constipation or diarrhea. In general, hemorrhoids can be irritating and painful but are considered normal and do not threaten your health.

Symptoms of hemorrhoids include persistent itching or discomfort around the anus and pain, especially during bowel movements. Hemorrhoids also can bleed. Be sure to tell your doctor if you see blood in your stool, on toilet paper, or in the toilet; bleeding can be a sign of colorectal cancer (see page 273).

A doctor can diagnose hemorrhoids by examining the anus and rectum with a gloved finger. To confirm the diagnosis, the doctor probably will perform a visual examination of the inside of the anus and rectum in a procedure called proctoscopy (see "Diagnostic Procedures," page 282). In some cases the doctor may perform a colonoscopy (see "Diagnostic Procedures," page 282) to examine the colon to rule out cancer and other possible causes of bleeding.

There are a number of steps you can take to relieve symptoms of hemorrhoids: eat a high-fiber diet that includes plenty of fruits, vegetables, and whole grains; drink at least eight 8-ounce glasses of water every day (but avoid alcohol and caffeine, which can irritate hemorrhoids); soak in a bath of plain warm water once or twice a day and cleanse the affected area with mild soap; apply ice packs to the area (to reduce swelling); and apply an over-the-counter hemorrhoidal cream to the affected area for a limited time (be sure to follow package directions). Outpatient procedures to remove hemorrhoids include rubber band ligation, in which rubber bands are placed around the base of a hemorrhoid to cut off its blood supply, causing it to shrink and fall off, and sclerotherapy, in which a chemical solution is injected directly into a hemorrhoid, causing it to shrink. In another procedure, heat is used to seal a hemorrhoid and stop it from bleeding. Some hemorrhoids must be removed surgically.

Appendicitis

The appendix is a small, finger-shaped organ with no known function that projects out from the large intestine. For reasons that are not fully understood, the appendix can become inflamed. Inflammation of the appendix is called appendicitis. Although appendicitis occurs most often in children and young adults, it can occur at any age. Symptoms occur in only about half of all people who have appendicitis, and many of those symptoms occur in other acute abdominal disorders. Because of the high risk of serious and potentially fatal infection associated with appendicitis, you should seek medical help immediately if you experience sudden, severe abdominal pain either with or without any of the following symptoms:

- pain that starts near the navel and moves to the lower right area of the abdomen
- pain that worsens when taking deep breaths, coughing, or sneezing
- pain that worsens when even slight pressure is applied to the area
- nausea or vomiting after the pain begins
- fever after the pain begins
- abdominal swelling
- inability to pass gas
- blood in the stools (they are red-streaked or look black and tarry)
- constipation

To diagnose appendicitis, a doctor examines your abdomen by gently pressing on it and listening through a stethoscope for sounds of normal digestion. (If you have a severe infection, there are no sounds.) Based on your symptoms and the examination, the doctor will admit you to the hospital for surgery to remove your appendix. He or she may perform a procedure called laparoscopy (see page 278) to confirm the diagnosis. If the appendix has not ruptured, the doctor can remove it through the laparoscope (viewing tube). In other cases, he or she may remove the appendix through a larger incision in the abdomen. Both types of surgery are performed in the hospital using general anesthesia. You will be in the hospital for 1 to 3 days, depending on the severity of your condition.

Polyps

A polyp is a growth of tissue in the lining of the wall of the colon. Polyps usually cause no symptoms and often are detected during a routine colonoscopy (see "Diagnostic Procedures," page 282). Research suggests that a high-fat, low-fiber diet may lead to the development of polyps in the colon. Heredity also may be a factor. A person who develops one polyp is likely to develop more polyps in the future and should be monitored by colonoscopy regularly.

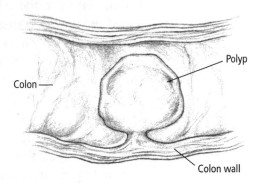

Small, benign (noncancerous) polyps are common in the colon and usually do not cause symptoms or affect your health. However, an adenomatous polyp (the most common type of polyp) is noncancerous but can become cancerous. Therefore your doctor will remove these polyps as soon as they are detected to prevent development of cancer. Small polyps can be removed through a colonoscope, but removal of larger polyps requires general surgery. Left untreated, small polyps will grow. The larger the polyp, the more likely that it is cancerous.

Colon Polyp

A polyp is a mushroom-shaped growth of tissue in the inner lining of the wall of the colon. The most common type of polyp, called an adenomatous polyp (shown here), is noncancerous, but it can grow and become cancerous.

Colorectal Cancer

Cancer of the colon and cancer of the rectum are two of the most common forms of cancer. The term "colorectal cancer" is often used to describe them. Colorectal cancer is the third most common type of cancer among men and also is the third leading cause of cancer death among men. But the rate of cure is high—up to 90 percent—when the disease is detected and treated early.

Nearly all cases of colorectal cancer arise from previously benign (noncancerous) adenomatous polyps. The risk of colorectal cancer increases with age (occurring most often after age 50) and may be higher among people who eat a high-fat, low-fiber diet. People with ulcerative colitis (see page 269) are more likely to develop colon cancer. Colorectal cancer can run in families: if you have a parent, sibling, or child who was diagnosed with colon cancer, your risk of developing colon cancer is greater than normal.

A doctor can detect cancers just inside the rectum during a digital rectal examination. Doctors recommend an annual digital rectal examination for all men 40 and older. The most common screening test to detect colon cancer is the fecal occult blood test, which checks for traces of blood in samples of stool. Doctors recommend that all men over age 50 have a fecal occult blood test every year.

A more accurate test, recommended every 5 years, is called a flexible sigmoidoscopy, a visual examination of the lower third of the colon and rectum that uses a probe with a light and a camera attached. The doctor inserts the instrument into the colon and looks through the viewing tube to check for polyps or signs of cancer. A colonoscopy is a similar procedure, but it examines the entire length of the colon. The doctor performing a sigmoidoscopy or colonoscopy may remove tissue for a biopsy during the test.

An alternative to these procedures is a barium enema. During this test, contrast medium (a dye) is inserted through the rectum into the colon, and X rays are taken of the colon to look for abnormalities. If a suspicious area is detected in the colon during a barium enema, the doctor will order a biopsy (microscopic examination of a small piece of tissue that has been removed from the colon) to confirm the diagnosis of cancer.

A tumor in the colon is classified by stages, according to whether it has affected only the top layer of the intestinal lining, penetrated farther down into the lining, involved the surrounding lymph nodes (part of the body's immune system that fights infection), or spread to other parts of the body.

Warning Signs of Colorectal Cancer

Colorectal cancer often has no warning signs. Because of this, your doctor will recommend regular screening with fecal occult blood tests (to check for blood in your stool) and colonoscopy (see "Diagnostic Procedures," page 282). However, if you experience any of the following symptoms, see your doctor immediately:

- changes in bowel movements—diarrhea or constipation that last for several days, stool that appears narrower than usual, or a feeling that your bowels are not completely empty after a bowel movement
- blood in the stool—red-streaked or black, tarry stools
- abdominal pain—persistent pain, cramps, or tenderness in the lower abdomen
- unexplained weight loss—losing weight without trying to
- fatigue—feeling tired without a specific cause, which may indicate internal bleeding or anemia

---

Treatment for colon cancer depends on how far the cancer has advanced and may include surgery, radiation therapy, chemotherapy (treatment with powerful anticancer drugs), or some combination of these. Surgical removal of the tumor and surrounding colon and lymph tissue is the most common treatment for colon cancer. After the cancerous section of the colon has been removed, the healthy sections are reconnected. In some cases the surgeon may perform a colostomy (see box on next page) to provide an outlet for feces. If the tumor is large, you may need to undergo radiation therapy before surgery to help shrink the tumor. Radiation therapy also may be used after surgery to ensure that all the cancerous cells have been killed.

If the surgeon is not sure that all the cancer has been removed, or if the cancer has spread to other parts of your body, you will need to undergo chemotherapy or possibly immunotherapy, in which your body's immune system is stimulated to destroy cancer cells.

Chemotherapy drugs may be given orally or intravenously. Several different types of drugs may be given simultaneously. You may need to be hospitalized during the first few days of treatment and then continue the treatment on your own at home. Chemotherapy usually is administered in cycles. For example, you may take the drugs for several weeks, stop taking the drugs for several weeks, and then repeat this cycle. Your doctor will explain the risks, advantages, and side effects of these therapies. Some people benefit from participating in a support group, which allows them to share information and experiences with others who are in a similar situation. Ask your doctor to recommend a support group in your area.

Colostomy and Ileostomy

Treatment of Crohn's disease, ulcerative colitis, polyps, and colorectal cancer sometimes requires removal of all or part of the large intestine. Depending on how much tissue must be removed, the surgeon may need to create a new path for stool to pass from the body. Surgery to create a new opening (called a stoma) through the abdominal wall when the rectum is removed is called a colostomy; if both the rectum and the colon must be removed, the procedure is known as an ileostomy.

The stoma is about the size of a quarter. A pouch is worn over the opening to collect waste and it must be emptied periodically. In some cases the surgeon can create an internal pouch made from a portion of the ileum, which the person periodically empties by inserting a tube through a tiny opening in the abdominal wall.

For some people a colostomy is temporary, and the surgeon performs a second operation to reconnect the healthy sections of the colon after the lower colon and the rectum have healed.

Ileoanal reservoir surgery is an alternative procedure that involves two separate operations. In the first operation, the colon and rectum are removed, and a temporary ileostomy is created. In the second operation, the ileostomy is closed, and part of the ileum is used to create an internal pouch to hold stool. This pouch is attached to the anus. The muscle of the rectum is left in place, so the stool in the pouch does not leak out. People who have this surgery are able to control their bowel movements, although the bowel movements may be more frequent and may be watery.

Disorders of the Gallbladder, the Pancreas, and the Liver

The gallbladder has a single, nonessential role in digestion: it stores bile produced by the liver until it is needed in the duodenum to digest fats. Both the pancreas and the liver help regulate metabolism (the chemical processes that take place in the body) and have essential roles in digestion. The pancreas releases hormones and enzymes critical to the breakdown of proteins, carbohydrates, and fats. The liver, one of the most complex organs in the body, performs more than

5,000 life-sustaining functions. It produces, monitors, recycles, and stores a wide range of chemicals that are essential for life. Everything that is absorbed by or injected into the body is filtered through the liver, which removes toxins and other potentially harmful substances from the blood. Unlike other organs, the liver receives blood from two sources: the hepatic artery, which supplies fresh, oxygenated blood, and the portal vein, which brings blood directly from the digestive tract for filtering before it goes on to the heart and the lungs. If the liver does not function properly, the consequences can be life-threatening.

Gallstones

The gallbladder is a small, pear-shaped sac beneath the liver where bile is stored and concentrated. Gallstones can form when an imbalance in its chemical composition causes the bile to harden into solid pieces. If the bile contains too much cholesterol, a tiny particle can gradually grow into a gallstone as more and more material hardens around it. Cholesterol stones are the most common type of gallstone. Another type of gallstone, a pigment stone, is small, dark, and made of bilirubin (the major pigment in bile). There may be one or more gallstones in various sizes, from the size of a grain of sand to the size of a golf ball.

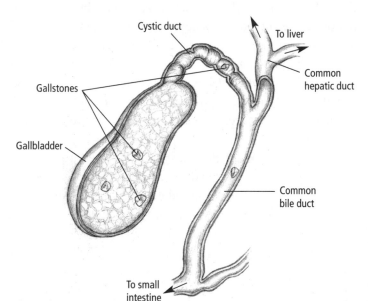

Gallstones

Gallstones are solid lumps, consisting mostly of cholesterol, that form in the gallbladder. In some cases, a small gallstone passes on its own out of the gallbladder through the bile duct and out of the body in stool, causing no pain. But if a large stone blocks the cystic duct, which causes intense pain, both the duct and the gallbladder are removed surgically.

The risk of developing gallstones increases with age. Obesity and frequent fasting also are risk factors. People who have diabetes or who take cholesterol-lowering drugs also may have an increased risk of developing gallstones.

A gallstone may block the normal flow of bile in the ducts that lead from the liver to the gallbladder and from the gallbladder to the small intestine. A backup of bile in these ducts can cause inflammation of the gallbladder, the ducts them-

selves, or (rarely) the liver. If a stone gets stuck in the common bile duct, digestive enzymes from the pancreas may flow backward and cause pancreatitis (see
below). Symptoms of a stone-related blockage include fever, jaundice (yellowing of the skin and the whites of the eyes), nausea or vomiting, and constant,
severe pain in the upper right abdomen. Pain also may occur in the chest or the
back or between the shoulder blades.

If your doctor suspects that you have gallstones, you probably will undergo an
ultrasound examination (see page 90), in which sound waves are used to create
images of the abdominal organs. Blood tests also may be performed. Specialized procedures performed to more closely examine the gallbladder include
cholecystogram (in which X rays are taken after a special iodine dye is injected
or swallowed) and endoscopic retrograde cholangiopancreatography (ERCP; see
"Diagnostic Procedures," page 282).

Surgery to remove the gallbladder is the most common treatment for gallstones that are causing symptoms. (Gallstones that are not causing symptoms
usually are discovered by chance during an examination for some other reason
and are usually left alone.) The surgery to remove the gallbladder is called a
laparoscopic cholecystectomy (see box on next page). After the gallbladder is
removed, bile flows directly from the liver to the duodenum. A medication
called ursodiol is sometimes used to slowly dissolve small cholesterol stones.
The drug is taken by mouth every day for 6 months to 2 years, until the stones
are dissolved. However, this treatment does not always dissolve the stones, and
it does not prevent their recurrence.

Pancreatitis

The pancreas is a large gland located behind the stomach and close to the duodenum. The disease most commonly associated with the pancreas is diabetes.
However, the pancreas can become inflamed when the digestive enzymes it produces become activated and attack its own tissues. This condition is known as
pancreatitis.

In acute pancreatitis, the pancreas suddenly becomes inflamed and then
returns to normal. Most people experience only one attack, but the condition can
recur. Acute pancreatitis usually is caused by alcohol abuse or by gallstones. An
attack usually lasts about 48 hours and begins with severe pain in the upper
abdomen. The pain may appear suddenly and be severe, or it may worsen gradually, especially after eating. The abdomen may be swollen and tender. The pain is
often accompanied by nausea, vomiting, fever, and a rapid heart rate.

These symptoms are often sufficient to diagnose acute pancreatitis, but a
blood test to check for high levels of amylase (an enzyme produced by the pancreas) can confirm the diagnosis. The doctor also may recommend a computed
tomography (CT) scan or an ultrasound of the abdomen. Unless complications
such as bleeding from the pancreas or infection in the abdomen occur, acute

Laparoscopic Surgery

A surgeon can examine the abdomen and perform certain surgical procedures using a laparoscope (a viewing tube). The laparoscope is equipped with a precision optical system that sends clear images to a video monitor. Laparoscopic surgery can be used to remove an inflamed appendix or a diseased gallbladder.

For laparoscopic surgery, the patient is given general anesthesia, a small incision is made in the abdomen, and the laparoscope is inserted. Other tiny incisions are made around the abdomen through which tiny surgical instruments are inserted through instrument tubes. The surgeon inflates the abdominal cavity with carbon dioxide gas to provide sufficient room in which to examine the tissues and manipulate the surgical instruments. For laparoscopic cholecystectomy, the surgeon uses tiny scissors to cut the cystic artery and the cystic duct and to separate the gallbladder from the liver. He or she then seals off the blood vessels to the gallbladder, draws the gallbladder out through the incision beneath the navel, and stitches up the incisions.

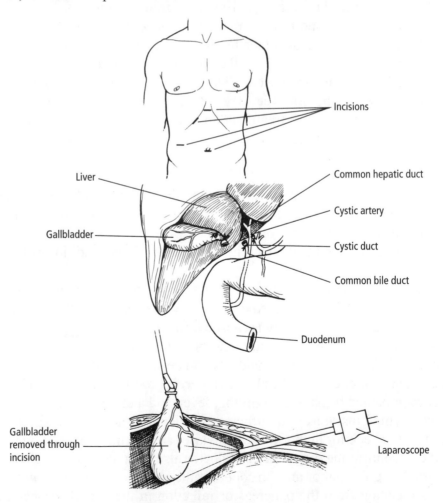

The surgeon performs the operation while viewing the inside of the abdomen on the video monitor. Usually the surgery is videotaped at the same time. The diseased tissue is removed through one of the instrument tubes. After surgery the patient will have only a small dressing over the incision. Often he or she can go home later that day and resume normal activities shortly thereafter.

pancreatitis usually will clear up on its own. However, most people with acute pancreatitis will need to be hospitalized to receive intravenous fluids and electrolytes to replace those lost through vomiting. Narcotic analgesics such as codeine are prescribed to relieve pain. Future attacks can be prevented by treating the underlying cause.

Chronic pancreatitis is more common in men than in women and usually develops after many years of alcohol abuse. Symptoms are usually the same as those of acute pancreatitis, but the attacks become more frequent as the disease progresses. People with chronic pancreatitis experience pain, weight loss (due to malabsorption of nutrients), and diabetes (due to insufficient production of insulin by the pancreas). Blood tests and other procedures such as ultrasound scanning, CT scanning, or endoscopic retrograde cholangiopancreatography (ERCP; see "Diagnostic Procedures," page 282) can be used to assess the condition of the pancreas. The disease is treated (but not cured) with pain medication, insulin (to control blood sugar levels), and pancreatic enzyme preparations (to correct enzyme deficiencies). In some cases, surgery to remove the pancreas (pancreatectomy) is required to relieve pain. All people with either acute or chronic pancreatitis must stop drinking alcohol.

Cirrhosis

Cirrhosis is a progressive liver disease that results from long-term damage to liver cells. The liver is continuously exposed to potential toxins, including drugs (over-the-counter, prescribed, or illegal) and alcohol—all of which can damage liver cells over time. Eventually the tissue becomes scarred, which blocks the flow of blood through the liver, causing liver failure and portal hypertension (high blood pressure in the veins from the intestines and spleen to the liver). In the United States, cirrhosis is among the leading causes of death. Men are more than twice as likely as women to die of chronic liver disease and cirrhosis.

Heavy alcohol consumption is the most common cause of cirrhosis. Other causes of the disease include viral hepatitis, hemochromatosis (excess iron in the body), Wilson's disease (excess copper in the body), cystic fibrosis, blocked bile ducts, and adverse drug reactions. Cirrhosis does not always cause symptoms and may be detected during a routine physical examination (the doctor may feel an enlarged liver) or blood test (the test may reveal abnormal liver function).

In the early stages of cirrhosis, some people may experience vague symptoms such as fatigue, weakness, exhaustion, loss of appetite, nausea, and weight loss. As the disease progresses, bile pigment builds up in the blood, causing jaundice (yellowing of the skin and the whites of the eyes).

Other common symptoms of cirrhosis include mental confusion due to a buildup of toxins in the brain, and hematemesis (vomiting blood) due to internal bleeding. In men, breast enlargement and hair loss may occur, possibly due to a sex hormone imbalance caused by liver failure. Possible complications of liver failure include ascites (accumulation of fluid in the abdominal cavity), malnutrition, and esophageal varices (enlarged veins in the wall of the esophagus), which can rupture and cause the person to vomit blood. Hepatoma, the most common form of liver cancer, is another possible complication.

The symptoms and signs of cirrhosis and the results of liver function tests (special tests of blood chemistry) are indicators of possible cirrhosis. However, a liver biopsy (removal of a small piece of tissue for microscopic examination) is required to confirm the diagnosis. To exclude rare causes of cirrhosis, special blood tests and cholangiography (X rays of the bile ducts) may be performed. Computed tomography (CT) scanning or magnetic resonance imaging (MRI) may be performed to evaluate the condition of the liver.

There is no cure for cirrhosis, so treatment focuses on slowing the progression of the disease and reducing the risk of complications. People with cirrhosis must not consume alcohol. Ascites may be treated with diuretics (drugs that increase urine production) and by restricting sodium (salt) intake. Portal hypertension may be treated with antihypertensive medication. Esophageal varices may be injected with a sclerosant (an irritant solution) to stop any bleeding. Mental confusion can be treated by reducing the levels of toxins in the bloodstream. This may require reducing the amount of protein in the diet, and taking antibiotics to reduce the number of bacteria in the intestinal tract. In cases of advanced cirrhosis, a liver transplant may be required.

Viral Hepatitis

Hepatitis is a contagious viral infection that causes inflammation of the liver. It is caused by one of the hepatitis viruses, A, B, C, or D. Most people with hepatitis recover on their own without treatment. Some people may experience mild recurrences over months or years. Still others may die of the infection. Hepatitis A and B are the most common types of viral hepatitis; hepatitis B, C, and D are the most dangerous. All donated blood and blood donors are routinely screened for all of the hepatitis viruses.

Many people with hepatitis experience no symptoms, and the disease may be detected during a routine physical examination because the liver feels enlarged or because a blood test shows abnormal liver function. A simple blood test is used to determine whether a person is infected with one of the hepatitis viruses.

Some people with hepatitis experience flulike symptoms such as fatigue, slight fever, nausea, vomiting, loss of appetite, weight loss, weakness, mild abdominal pain, muscle and joint aches, and diarrhea. People with chronic hepatitis often experience fatigue, joint aches, skin rashes, or memory loss.

Hepatitis A is spread through poor hygiene practices. It also is spread through contaminated food or water. The infection varies from mild to severe. Once you recover, you are immune to hepatitis A infection for life.

Hepatitis B is the most serious form of the disease. It is spread through unprotected sexual contact and sharing of contaminated needles by intravenous drug users. Many people who are infected with hepatitis B are carriers (they have the virus in their body but do not have symptoms) and can transmit the disease to other people. A woman can pass hepatitis B to her baby during childbirth. Vaccines are available to prevent hepatitis A and B. Your sexual partner should be vaccinated if you have hepatitis B.

Hepatitis C is spread primarily through sharing of contaminated needles by intravenous drug users. Symptoms of hepatitis C are similar to those of hepatitis B. In adults, the course of hepatitis C infection is influenced by several factors. In people who are older, the disease usually has a more rapid development. Many people infected with hepatitis C will develop severe liver disease, such as chronic hepatitis or cirrhosis, within 20 years of acquiring the infection. Rates of such disease are higher in people who are also infected with either hepatitis B or the human immunodeficiency virus (HIV). Even moderate long-term drinking of alcohol is associated with a higher likelihood of cirrhosis or liver cancer in people infected with hepatitis C. Certain forms of hepatitis C are not treatable. Other forms seem to be controlled with the use of antiviral drugs.

Your doctor will recommend that you be tested for hepatitis C if you:

- had a blood transfusion or organ transplant before July 1992
- were treated for clotting problems with a blood product before 1987
- have ever received long-term kidney dialysis
- had frequent ongoing exposure to blood products before 1987. (Recent exposure to blood products is not a risk because all blood products are screened for hepatitis C.)
- are a healthcare worker who was exposed to blood containing the hepatitis C virus
- are an intravenous (IV) drug user or former IV drug user

Hepatitis D usually is spread through sharing intravenous drug needles. It occurs only in conjunction with hepatitis B, and usually causes severe illness. There is no vaccine for hepatitis C or D.

Treatment of hepatitis focuses on controlling symptoms. Most people will recover within several weeks or months. Your doctor will want to know what medications you are taking (both prescription and nonprescription) to make sure they cannot damage your liver. Your doctor will recommend that you rest, eat a well-balanced diet, and avoid alcohol.

Other Gastrointestinal Disorders

The following less common disorders of the digestive system affect men far more frequently than women:

- *Primary sclerosing cholangitis.* Primary sclerosing cholangitis is a rare condition that occurs most often in young men and often is the result of inflammatory bowel disease such as ulcerative colitis. With this disease, the bile ducts (the tubes that carry bile from the liver) inside and outside the liver become narrowed due to inflammation and scarring. This causes bile to accumulate in the liver, which, in turn, damages liver cells. There are no initial symptoms, and the disease is usually detected by chance through a routine blood test for liver function. Symptoms develop between ages 30 and 50 and include fatigue, itching, and jaundice (yellowing of the skin and the whites of the eyes). Specialized tests are needed to confirm the diagnosis. No specific treatment exists for this progressive disease other than treating symptoms; cholestyramine may be prescribed to relieve itching.

- *Hemochromatosis.* Hemochromatosis is an inherited disease in which the body absorbs and stores too much dietary iron. The excess iron accumulates in the liver, pancreas, heart, testicles, and other organs, where it damages surrounding cells. The disease can result from excessive iron absorption (such as from having frequent blood transfusions) but usually is caused by a genetic error. Hemochromatosis is most common among men of northern European descent. The disease is diagnosed with blood tests to measure levels of iron in the blood and a liver biopsy. Symptoms usually appear during middle age and include weakness, weight loss, joint pain, and abdominal pain. The disease eventually causes changes in skin pigmentation (bronze coloration), liver damage, diabetes, and cardiac arrhythmia as it progresses. Liver failure or liver cancer may result. The disease cannot be cured, but its progression can be slowed through regular removal of blood (phlebotomy), such as by routine blood donation.

Diagnostic Procedures

If you have symptoms of a digestive disorder, your doctor may need to use one or more of the following diagnostic procedures to examine your gastrointestinal tract and determine the cause of your symptoms. Your digestive tract must be empty before undergoing any of these procedures. For an examination of your esophagus, stomach, or duodenum, you will need to fast (abstain from food and drink) after midnight the night before the procedure. For an examination of your ileum, colon, or rectum, you will need to follow a special liquid diet beginning at least 2 days before the procedure and then fast the night before the procedure. All of these examinations are usually performed on an outpatient basis.

- *Gastrointestinal series.* A gastrointestinal (GI) series is an examination that is used to diagnose or monitor problems in the digestive tract. An upper GI series examines the esophagus, stomach, and duodenum; a lower GI series examines the colon and rectum. These examinations are used to identify blockages, growths, ulcers, inflammation, and other structural abnormalities. Both procedures use barium sulfate to coat the lining of the digestive tract and provide clear images of the digestive tract on a fluoroscope (a special video monitor) or on X-ray film. For an upper GI series, you drink a barium mixture (a thick, white, chalky liquid called barium meal or barium swallow); for a lower GI series, a barium mixture (called a barium enema) is injected into the colon through the anus and rectum. You may be asked to change positions during the examination as the barium reaches different locations in your digestive tract. Usually you can go home immediately after the procedure and should experience no side effects other than constipation and white or gray stools until the barium is completely out of your system.
- *Endoscopy.* Endoscopy is a diagnostic examination in which a doctor uses a long, thin, flexible lighted tube called an endoscope to look inside the esophagus, stomach, and duodenum. You will be awake during this procedure, but before the examination begins, your throat will be sprayed with a numbing agent so you do not gag when the endoscope is passed down your throat. You also will receive pain medication and a sedative to help you relax. The endoscope has a precision optical system that works like a video camera, allowing the doctor to see inside each organ as it travels through the digestive tract. The endoscope also can blow air into the digestive tract to inflate it and make it easier to examine. Tiny surgical instruments then can be passed through the endoscope to remove tissue for microscopic examination. This procedure is usually brief—about 20 to 30 minutes—but you will need to lie quietly afterward at the doctor's office for an additional hour or two until the sedative wears off. You may have a sore throat after the procedure.
- *Endoscopic retrograde cholangiopancreatography (ERCP).* This diagnostic procedure allows your doctor to examine your liver, gallbladder, bile ducts, and pancreas using an endoscope. In ERCP, the initial steps are the same as those described for endoscopy. However, when the endoscope reaches your duodenum, the doctor injects contrast medium (a type of dye) through the endoscope and into your bile ducts. X rays are taken as soon as the contrast medium is injected. If the doctor sees a gallstone or narrowing of the ducts, he or she can pass tiny surgical instruments through the endoscope to remove the obstruction or widen the duct.

- *Colonoscopy.* Colonoscopy is a diagnostic examination of the entire length of the large intestine, from the rectum all the way up through the colon to the ileum. Colonoscopy can be used to look for polyps in the colon or to diagnose colon cancer. The procedure is performed with a special type of endoscope called a colonoscope. Before the procedure, you will receive pain medication and a sedative to help you relax. While you lie on your left side, your doctor will insert the colonoscope into your rectum and guide it up through the entire large intestine. As the doctor slowly withdraws the colonoscope, he or she examines your colon directly through the colonoscope or on a video monitor. Air can be blown through the colonoscope to inflate the colon and give the doctor a better view. Instruments can be passed through the colonoscope to take tissue samples or to remove polyps. If there is any blood in the colon, your doctor can use a special instrument or drug to stop the bleeding. Colonoscopy usually takes about 30 to 60 minutes, and you will need to lie quietly for an additional hour or two after the examination. Because of the medication you have been given, you should make arrangements in advance for someone to take you home after the procedure.
- *Sigmoidoscopy and proctoscopy.* As an alternative to a colonoscopy, your doctor may use a type of endoscope called a sigmoidoscope to examine only the rectum and the sigmoid (lower) colon. Or your doctor may use a type of endoscope called a proctoscope to examine only the anus and rectum. These procedures are similar to colonoscopy, but they examine only a limited portion of the gastrointestinal tract, and each procedure takes only about 10 to 20 minutes.

CHAPTER 14

Urinary Tract

Your kidneys are bean-shaped organs, each about the size of a fist, located near the middle of your back, just below your rib cage. Your kidneys help regulate blood pressure, maintain the proper balance of body fluids and electrolytes, eliminate waste products, control the body's acid-base balance, and stimulate bone marrow to produce red blood cells. Each day more than 200 quarts of blood pass through the kidneys to be filtered. Many by-products of the filtering process are reabsorbed and recycled. However, waste products from digestion, muscular activity, and routine metabolism must be removed from the body; otherwise they would accumulate to toxic levels. Excess water, urea (a by-product of protein breakdown), electrolytes, and other soluble waste products are removed from the blood by the kidneys and excreted as urine.

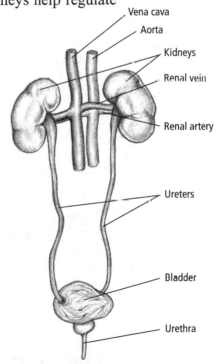

Blood to be filtered enters the kidneys through the renal artery. Each kidney contains about 1 million individual filtering units called nephrons. The kidney is divided into two major sections: the cortex, where blood is first filtered and all material is removed; and the medulla, where essential chemicals and fluids are reabsorbed into the blood and waste products are concentrated into urine. Urine created by the nephrons drains into the funnel-like renal pelvis before traveling down the ureter for storage in the urinary bladder. The renal vein carries filtered blood away from the kidney.

Urine is transported from the kidneys to the bladder via two 8- to 10-inch-long tubes called ureters; one ureter connects each kidney to the bladder. Muscles in the walls of the ureters constantly tighten and relax to force urine downward away from the kidneys. Small amounts of urine are emptied into the bladder from the ureters about every 10 to 15 seconds. If urine becomes stagnant or backs up, a kidney infection or a kidney stone can develop.

Your bladder is a hollow, muscular organ shaped like a balloon that stores up to a pint of urine. Circular muscles called sphincters close tightly around the meeting point of the bladder and the urethra, the tube that allows urine to pass outside the body. As the bladder fills with urine, nerves in the bladder signal your brain that you need to urinate. The sensation to urinate becomes stronger as the bladder becomes fuller. When you decide to urinate, your brain tells the bladder muscles to tighten, squeezing urine out, and the sphincter muscles to relax, allowing urine to flow through the urethra.

Warning Signs of Urinary Tract Disease

Many symptoms of urinary tract disease are vague—fever, weight loss, a vague feeling of being ill, fatigue, and vomiting—but others clearly indicate problems with the urinary tract. If you experience any of these symptoms, talk to your doctor:

- *Frequent urination.* If you are not drinking more fluids than usual but are urinating more, this could indicate that your kidneys or bladder are not working efficiently.
- *Painful urination.* A burning sensation while urinating suggests inflammation, infection, or obstruction of the urinary tract.
- *Hesitancy or straining during urination.* Any change in the force and diameter of the stream of urine, especially in men, suggests an obstruction of the urethra.
- *Unusual appearance of urine.* Urine is normally clear and ranges from colorless to deep yellow. Urine that appears red, brown, milky, or cloudy may indicate a urinary tract disorder.
- *Pain.* Pain in the side or the back between the rib cage and the hip can be a sign of inflammation, infection, or obstruction of the kidney.
- *Fluid retention.* When the kidneys are not functioning efficiently they do not maintain a good balance of water and sodium in the body, which can lead to fluid retention. This usually appears as facial puffiness but can progress until fluid collects in the lungs, the abdominal cavity, and elsewhere in the body.

Urinary Tract Infections: Urethritis, Cystitis, and Pyelonephritis

The structure of the urinary tract reduces the likelihood of infection by preventing urine from flowing backward toward the kidneys and by washing bacteria out of the body with the normal flow of urine. In men, the prostate gland also produces secretions that slow bacterial growth. Urine is normally sterile.

However, urinary tract infections are common, especially among women. An obstruction of the urinary tract (such as a kidney stone or an enlarged prostate gland) also increases the risk of infection. People with diabetes, immune disorders, or conditions that require regular use of a urinary catheter (a tube inserted through the urethra into the bladder to drain urine from the body) also are at greater risk.

An infection can begin when microorganisms, usually bacteria from the digestive tract (such as *Escherichia coli,* also called *E coli*), accumulate at the opening of the urethra. An infection that affects only the urethra is called urethritis. From the urethra, bacteria often move up to the bladder, causing a bladder infection (cystitis). Sexually transmitted microorganisms, such as those that cause gonorrhea and chlamydia, also can infect the urinary tract.

If a bladder infection is not treated promptly, bacteria may move up the ureters, causing a kidney infection (pyelonephritis), which can be serious. Kidney infections also can occur when bacteria or other microorganisms are carried to the kidneys through the bloodstream. When this happens, an obstruction in a ureter can trap infectious agents in the kidneys.

Urinary tract infections do not always cause symptoms. However, most men with a urinary tract infection will experience at least one or two of the following symptoms, especially upon waking in the morning:

- frequent urination
- painful urination
- reduced volume during urination
- fatigue
- fever
- a feeling of fullness in the rectum
- milky or cloudy urine
- reddish or brownish urine
- discharge from the penis
- itching around the urethral opening

A high fever may indicate that the infection has spread to the kidneys. Other symptoms of a kidney infection include pain in the back or side below the ribs, nausea, and vomiting.

A urinary tract infection is diagnosed through a urinalysis and a urine culture. First you provide a "clean catch" urine sample by washing the urethral opening with a disinfecting wipe and collecting a midstream sample (urinate for several seconds before collecting the sample of urine) in a sterile container. The sample is examined under a microscope for blood cells and bacteria. The bacteria will then be grown as a culture to confirm that an infection is present and to identify the bacteria and determine the best antibiotic to kill them. Some bacteria, especially those that are sexually transmitted, can be detected only by using special bacterial cultures.

For pyelonephritis, antibiotic treatment may last up to 6 weeks. If the infection does not improve within 3 days of starting treatment, you will need to undergo additional tests to determine whether an obstruction is present or whether an abscess (a cavity filled with pus) has developed. If kidney infections recur frequently, you may develop chronic pyelonephritis, a condition in which a kidney that has been infected several times or damaged by other disease becomes scarred, shrunken, and misshapen.

If the prescribed antibiotics do not eliminate the infection, your doctor probably will perform additional tests, such as intravenous urography or a computed tomography (CT) scan (see "Diagnostic Procedures," page 297) to check for another disorder or an anatomical abnormality.

If you are diagnosed with urethritis caused by a sexually transmitted microorganism, you will need to take measures to protect your sexual partner from infection. Your sexual partner also should be tested and, if necessary, treated for urethritis or any other urinary tract infection that is present. Otherwise you will risk passing the same infection back and forth between you or causing a worse and longer-lasting infection in your partner. You will need to continue using preventive measures such as latex condoms until the infection has been eliminated, not just until the symptoms disappear. Your doctor will tell you when the infection has completely cleared up.

Disorders of the Kidney

Your kidneys have tremendous excess capacity to do their job. In fact, you can lose more than 50 percent of your renal (kidney) function and remain healthy. However, serious health problems occur when renal function drops to 20 percent, and either a kidney transplant or dialysis (see box on page 292) is required if renal function drops below 10 to 15 percent. Once nephrons (the filtering units of the kidneys) have been destroyed, either suddenly through injury or poisoning or gradually after years of kidney disease, they can never be regenerated or repaired.

Diabetes and hypertension (high blood pressure) are the two leading causes of kidney disease. In diabetes, blood flow through the kidneys increases, causing the kidneys to enlarge, and the excess sugar in the blood damages the glomeruli (tiny blood vessels that are part of the nephrons). High blood pressure can cause kidney disease by damaging the small blood vessels needed for filtering and reabsorption of fluids. Conversely, hypertension can result from kidney disease if blood flow through the kidneys is obstructed or slowed, resulting in the release of hormones that cause blood pressure to rise. See page 365 for more information about diabetes and page 217 for more information about hypertension.

A healthy kidney removes extra electrolytes and other minerals from the blood. Normally the chemical composition of urine and prompt urination prevent these electrolytes and minerals from forming crystals and building up on the inner surfaces of the kidney. Some crystals that form may pass through the urinary tract unnoticed. However, others may accumulate until they have formed kidney stones.

Why kidney stones form in some people and not in others remains unknown. Men, especially white men, develop kidney stones more frequently than women. Kidney stones usually develop between ages 20 and 40, and once one stone has been diagnosed, more are likely to develop. A family history of kidney stones increases the risk, as do certain disorders of the kidney and recurrent kidney infections. Other diseases (such as gout and chronic inflammatory disorders) and certain medications (such as diuretics and calcium-based antacids) also can cause kidney stones.

The warning signs of kidney stones are unmistakable. Stones that are not causing symptoms may be found by chance on an X-ray or ultrasound image. Most kidney stones can be passed through the urinary system by drinking plenty of water (2 to 3 quarts per day), and taking over-the-counter pain medication as needed. If you ever pass a kidney stone, be sure to save it for testing: knowing the composition of the stone will help your doctor determine the appropriate treatment and recommend steps to prevent future stones.

Surgery is rarely needed to remove or to break up kidney stones. However, if a stone does not pass through the ureter and blocks urine flow, or if a stone causes ongoing urinary tract infection, medical treatment will be required. Extracorporeal shockwave lithotripsy (ESWL) passes shock waves through the body until they strike the stones and reduce them to the consistency of sand so they can be excreted in the urine. Lithotripsy usually is done on an outpatient basis. The procedure is performed using either intravenous sedation or epidural (spinal) anesthesia. Some lithotripsy devices require the patient to be in a water bath during the procedure, while others require that the patient lie on a soft cushion or pad.

A procedure called percutaneous nephrolithotomy may be performed when stones are especially large or when they are in tissues that make lithotripsy

---

Warning Signs of Kidney Stones

Some kidney stones do not cause symptoms. Others may cause sudden, severe pain when they move into the ureter and cause an obstruction. As the stone moves toward the bladder, you may feel a strong urge to urinate, or you may feel a burning sensation. Fever and chills in addition to these symptoms may indicate a urinary tract infection. Contact your doctor immediately if you experience these symptoms:

- sudden, severe pain in your back or lower side
- fever and chills
- weakness
- nausea and vomiting
- cloudy or foul-smelling urine
- blood in your urine
- a frequent need to urinate in small amounts
- a burning sensation during urination
- an inability to urinate although your bladder feels full

ineffective. In this procedure the surgeon makes a tiny incision in the patient's back and inserts a nephroscope (a special type of viewing tube) to locate and remove the stone. For stones that are lower in the ureter, a thin, flexible viewing tube (called a ureteroscope) is passed up through the urethra and the bladder to the stone; the stone is then either removed or shattered. Both of these procedures are performed using general or epidural anesthesia, and both require either a short hospital stay or are done on an outpatient basis.

Additional kidney stones are likely to develop unless preventive measures are taken. The chemical composition of the first stone must be analyzed so the doctor can determine appropriate dietary changes and prescribe appropriate medications. Often the person is asked to collect a couple of 24-hour urine samples for analysis (see "Diagnostic Procedures," Creatinine clearance, page 298). The doctor also will advise the person to drink plenty of fluids (at least eight 8-ounce glasses per day), especially water. Additional treatment will be required if an underlying cause for the stones is diagnosed. Regular urinalysis will be important for monitoring the effectiveness of preventive measures and treatment.

Glomerular Diseases

Blood enters the kidneys through arteries that branch off inside the kidneys into tiny clusters of looping blood vessels called glomeruli. The glomerulus is part of the nephron, the basic filtering unit of the kidney. When the glomeruli are damaged, protein and, in some cases, red blood cells leak into the urine. When a certain type of protein called albumin is lost in the urine, the body is less able to remove excess fluid; the excess fluid causes edema (swelling) in the face, hands, feet, or ankles. Diseases that affect kidney function by damaging these filtering clusters of blood vessels are called glomerular diseases. When the attached renal tubules are affected, a condition known as nephrotic syndrome develops.

In glomerulonephritis, the membranous tissue in the kidney that serves as a filter becomes inflamed. In glomerulosclerosis, the tiny blood vessels that form the clusters become hardened or scarred. Signs of a glomerular disease include facial puffiness, hematuria (blood in the urine; see box on next page), or foamy urine caused by excretion of extra protein. Nephrotic syndrome is marked by very high levels of protein in the urine, low levels of protein in the blood, swelling (usually of the face, hands, or feet), and high levels of cholesterol in the blood. Blood tests, urinalysis, and other specialized tests can determine the type and the location of damage.

Glomerular diseases also can result from infection in other parts of the body, such as "strep" throat, endocarditis (inflammation of the lining of the heart), and human immunodeficiency virus (HIV) infection. Treatment varies according to the underlying cause and the tissues affected.

Hematuria

Hematuria refers to excess red blood cells in the urine. In some cases of hematuria, the urine looks normal and the blood is visible only under a microscope; this is called microscopic hematuria. In other cases, the blood is visible to the naked eye and the urine looks red or cola-colored; this is called gross hematuria. (Note that some foods and food dyes also can cause the urine to look red or brown.) Usually the causes of hematuria are not serious, but all cases should be evaluated so the doctor can determine the cause and treat it appropriately. Symptoms such as pain or fever also can provide clues to the cause of hematuria, as does the timing of the blood's appearance in the urine (at the beginning, end, or throughout urination). Possible causes of hematuria include the following:

- urinary tract infection or obstruction
- enlarged prostate
- kidney stones or bladder stones
- kidney cancer or bladder cancer
- injury to the urinary tract
- overexercising
- sickle-cell disease
- certain medications (including painkillers, blood-thinning drugs, and antibiotics)
- IgA nephropathy

Kidney Failure

During acute renal failure, the kidneys may suddenly lose their ability to remove wastes, concentrate urine, and conserve water and essential nutrients. Urine production decreases or stops completely. Often there is blood in the urine. Protein waste products quickly accumulate in the blood, damaging tissues and reducing organ function throughout the body. This condition, known as uremia, can be fatal if kidney function is not restored promptly and if the blood is not filtered and cleansed. Symptoms of this toxic reaction include drowsiness, confusion, loss of appetite, nausea and vomiting, and seizures. The onset of symptoms is rapid, often occurring within days, but the condition can be reversed if diagnosed and treated quickly.

Disorders of the kidney itself also can lead to acute renal failure. These disorders include direct injury to the kidney, a urinary tract infection such as acute pyelonephritis (see page 286), kidney stones (see page 289), renal cell cancer (see "Kidney Cancer," page 293), and any obstruction of the urinary tract. Acute renal failure also can be caused by reduced blood flow, which can occur after an injury, during complicated surgery, when there is uncontrolled bleeding elsewhere in the body, following severe burns, or as a result of another serious illness. Exposure to poisons, solvents, certain medications, or a blood transfusion can cause injury to the kidney tubules and, in turn, acute renal failure. Severe infections, autoimmune diseases, and uncontrolled high blood pressure are other possible causes of renal failure.

Both kidney failure and its underlying cause must be treated promptly. Dialysis (see box) may be required to cleanse the blood mechanically and prevent complications such as congestive heart failure (see page 233). If you experience acute kidney failure, you will be placed on a diet that is low in protein, potassium, and sodium, and your fluid intake will be closely matched to your fluid output. You may recover adequate kidney function within 2 months, although your kidneys will not return to full normal function for much longer, perhaps a year.

Dialysis

With kidney failure, when the kidneys can no longer remove waste and excess water and acid from the blood and maintain the body's chemical balance, a person must undergo kidney dialysis. In this procedure, blood from an artery in the person's arm or leg flows through a tube and into a machine called a dialysis unit that works as an artificial kidney. The blood is filtered and cleansed in the dialysis unit and returned through another tube inserted into a vein in the same arm or leg. Usually dialysis is performed at a dialysis center (although it can be done at home) three times per week. The person can sleep, read, write, talk, or watch television during the 3 to 4 hours of each treatment.

In another type of dialysis (called peritoneal dialysis), a cleansing fluid (called dialysate) is placed in the abdomen through a permanently implanted catheter (tube) to filter and cleanse the blood. To begin treatment, the person attaches a bag containing dialysate to the catheter and allows the fluid to drip into his or her abdominal cavity. The dialysate is left inside the abdomen for several hours while it pulls out waste, excess water, sodium, potassium, and other chemicals from the blood vessels that line the abdominal cavity. The fluid and waste are then drained from the abdomen through the catheter and back into the bag. The procedure is repeated four or five times per day. This method is called continuous ambulatory peritoneal dialysis and can be performed at home. Peritoneal dialysis also can be performed using a machine that fills and drains the abdominal cavity throughout the night while the person sleeps. This method is called continuous cycling peritoneal dialysis.

In chronic renal failure, the kidneys lose the same amount of function as in acute renal failure, but the loss occurs slowly over many years. The loss of kidney function is continuous and progressive and may eventually lead to end-stage renal disease (see next page). In the early stages of chronic renal failure, there are no symptoms because of the excess capacity of the kidneys to do their job. When symptoms finally appear, the damage already done is irreversible, so treatment focuses on preventing additional damage to the kidneys and slowing the progression of the disease.

Diabetes and high blood pressure are major causes of chronic renal failure. Polycystic kidney disease (see "Other Urinary Tract Disorders," page 296), sickle-cell disease (see page 239), glomerular diseases (see page 290), obstructive disorders, kidney stones (see page 289), the urinary tract infection pyelonephritis (see page 286), and analgesic nephropathy (see "Other Urinary Tract Disorders," page 296) all can lead to chronic renal failure.

In addition to treating the underlying cause of chronic renal failure, the doctor will take steps to prevent or treat complications that may result from limited kidney function. You may be given erythropoietin (epoetin alfa), a hormone that stimulates bone marrow to produce more red blood cells. You will be placed on a diet that is low in protein, phosphorus, potassium, sodium, and fluids to reduce the strain on your kidneys. If you continue to lose kidney function and progress to end-stage renal disease, you and your doctor will discuss your treatment options so you can make an informed decision.

End-Stage Renal Disease

People in end-stage renal disease (ESRD) have limited options. Because their kidneys have stopped working, they must have their blood cleansed by some means or they will die. They can undergo either hemodialysis or peritoneal dialysis (see previous page), or they can have a kidney transplant. Many people who have the choice will opt for transplantation because it offers a better quality of life over the long term.

Kidney transplantation succeeds in most cases. Unless they are causing high blood pressure or are frequently infected, your own kidneys usually are left in place and the new kidney is placed between them and your bladder. The surgeon connects the artery and vein of the transplanted kidney to one of your arteries and one of your veins and connects the new kidney's ureter to your bladder. The transplanted kidney may start working right away, or it may take up to a few weeks to produce urine.

The donated kidney must match your blood type and be very similar to your kidneys' tissue type. Often a blood relative (a parent, sibling, or child) can supply a kidney for transplantation. Sometimes a spouse or a friend can provide a close match. Otherwise you will need to wait for a donation from someone who has recently died but who has healthy kidneys that match yours.

The surgery will take 3 to 6 hours, and you will stay in the hospital for up to 2 weeks afterward. Your doctor will give you immunosuppressant drugs to reduce the chance of your body rejecting the new kidney. You will take these drugs for the rest of your life. If your body does not accept the new kidney, you will need to continue using dialysis until another donor kidney can be found.

Kidney Cancer

Kidney cancer is the eighth most common type of cancer among men. Twice as many men as women develop kidney cancer. The cause of this type of cancer remains unknown. Possible risk factors include smoking (which doubles the risk of kidney cancer), exposure to asbestos or cadmium, a family history of kidney cancer, eating a high-fat diet, being overweight, and undergoing long-term dialysis.

Different types of cancer can occur in the kidneys. The most common form of kidney cancer in adults is called renal cell cancer. As renal cell cancer grows, it may invade nearby organs, such as the liver, colon, or pancreas, or it may spread via the blood or the lymphatic system to other parts of the body, such as the lungs or the bones. A less common type of cancer, transitional cell cancer, can occur in the kidneys, but occurs more often in the bladder (see next page).

Initially renal cell cancer does not cause symptoms. As the tumor grows, however, symptoms may develop, including blood in the urine, a lump near the affected kidney, fatigue, loss of appetite, weight loss, recurrent fevers, pain in the side, and a vague feeling of being ill. If you have any of these symptoms—which could point to many of the urinary tract disorders discussed in this chapter—your doctor will perform tests to identify the cause of the problem (see "Diagnostic Procedures," page 297). The earlier cancer is diagnosed and treated, the better the chances for recovery.

Once cancer is detected, your doctor will want to determine whether it has spread. This will influence your treatment options. Often, all or part of the cancerous kidney is removed surgically, along with the adrenal gland and any nearby lymph nodes. If the tumor cannot be removed, the doctor may try to block blood flow to the tumor by clogging the renal artery that supplies blood to the diseased kidney; this will starve the tumor of the blood it needs. In either case, the remaining healthy kidney will do the work of both kidneys.

Radiation therapy, while not a cure, may be used to shrink large tumors or to treat metastases (cancer that has spread to other parts of the body) in the bones. Immunotherapy (treatment in which the body's immune system is stimulated to destroy cancer cells), chemotherapy (treatment with powerful anticancer drugs), and hormone therapy (treatment involving hormones that affect the growth of cancer cells) all attack the cancer at the systemic level. This means that the entire body is treated at the same time. Treating cancer at the systemic level may cause more unpleasant side effects (including nausea, vomiting, and hair loss) than other forms of treatment.

Disorders of the Bladder and Urethra

The lower urinary tract consists of the bladder and urethra. If left untreated, disorders of the bladder or urethra can interfere with normal functioning of the urinary tract and lead to kidney damage.

Urethral Stricture

The urethra can become narrowed by scar tissue following catheter placement, surgery, injury, or repeated episodes of urethritis (see page 286). This condition, called urethral stricture, is a common problem following long-term catheter placement. Urethral stricture can interfere with urination and ejaculation. It also can damage the kidneys by causing back pressure (buildup of fluid) in the urinary tract. Urethral stricture also may be a factor in the development of urinary tract infections.

Urethral stricture can be treated in the doctor's office by widening the urethra from within with a thin, flexible instrument called a dilator. Sometimes the scar tissue must be removed surgically using a cystoscope, or a portion of the urethra must be removed surgically. Laser therapy also may be used to remove the scar tissue. Depending on where the stricture is located, a urethral stent (a tiny springlike device that holds the urethra open) can be inserted to keep the passageway open. However, if the stricture is too close to the sphincter muscle (which prevents leakage of urine from the bladder), a stent cannot be used. In some cases the affected segment of the urethra may be surgically reconstructed using tissue taken from another part of the body.

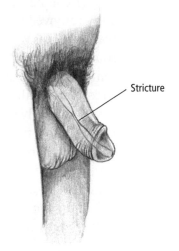

Stricture

Urethral Stricture

Urethral stricture is a condition in which the urethra (the tube that carries urine out of the bladder) is narrowed, potentially interfering with the flow of urine and with ejaculation. The urethra can become narrowed when scar tissue forms after some medical procedures (such as placement of a catheter), surgery, injury, or recurring infections.

Bladder Cancer

Bladder cancer is the fourth most common type of cancer in men. Transitional cell carcinoma, which develops from the cells that line the bladder walls, is the most common type of bladder cancer. This type of cancer also can occur in the kidneys, the ureters, and the portion of the urethra nearest the bladder.

Transitional cell carcinoma that remains confined to the surface of the bladder lining is called superficial bladder cancer. Superficial bladder cancer is the most common type of transitional cell carcinoma (75 to 80 percent of new cases) and is easy to treat, but it tends to recur. In some cases the cancer spreads beyond the bladder lining and invades the muscular wall of the bladder. This is called invasive bladder cancer. The tumor may continue to grow through the bladder wall and spread to nearby organs. Bladder cancer cells also can spread to surrounding lymph nodes and to distant organs such as the lungs or the bones.

Symptoms of bladder cancer can be the same as those for a bladder infection or other urinary tract disorder. Therefore you should talk to your doctor as soon as possible if you experience any symptoms. The most common symptoms of bladder cancer include blood in the urine, painful urination, frequent urination (without an increase in fluid intake), and an urge to urinate with little urine output. If your doctor thinks you may have bladder cancer, he or she will examine the inside of the bladder with a viewing tube called a cystoscope (see "Diagnostic

Procedures," Cystoscopy, page 298) and use other imaging techniques to determine whether the cancer has spread.

Surgery is the most common treatment for bladder cancer. Superficial bladder cancer can be treated with transurethral resection, in which the tumor is surgically removed through a cystoscope. With invasive bladder cancer, all or part of the bladder is removed using a surgical procedure called cystectomy. Often, surrounding lymph nodes, the prostate gland, and the seminal vesicles also are removed. Additional treatment may include radiation therapy, chemotherapy (treatment with powerful anticancer drugs), or immunotherapy (treatment in which the body's immune system is stimulated to destroy cancer cells), depending on where the cancer has spread and how advanced it is.

When the bladder must be removed, the doctor creates an alternative method for storing and passing urine. The doctor often will use an isolated piece of the person's small intestine to create a new channel between the ureters and an opening in the wall of the abdomen (called a stoma) through which urine can pass. A flat bag is attached to the stoma to collect urine, and the person empties the bag as needed. A portion of small intestine also can be used to create a storage pouch inside the body (instead of an external bag), which the person drains by inserting a catheter through the stoma. The storage pouch also can be attached to the remaining portion of the urethra to allow the person to urinate through the urethra.

Until recently, nearly all men experienced erectile dysfunction after bladder removal surgery, but surgical improvements have reduced the likelihood of this side effect. However, men who have had their prostate gland and seminal vesicles removed no longer produce semen, so they do not ejaculate when they have an orgasm, and they are infertile.

Other Urinary Tract Disorders

Other possible disorders of the urinary tract include the following:

- *Polycystic kidney disease.* Polycystic kidney disease (PKD) is a genetic disorder in which numerous fluid-filled cysts (abnormal lumps or swellings) grow in the kidneys. These cysts can slowly displace much of the functional tissue of the kidneys, reducing kidney function and leading to kidney failure. People with PKD can have the disease for decades without developing symptoms. The most common symptoms are pain in the back and the sides (between the ribs and the hips) and headaches. People with PKD also may develop urinary tract infections (see page 286), hematuria (see page 291), cysts in other organs, high blood pressure (see page 217), and kidney stones (see page 289). Doctors use ultrasound scanning (see " Diagnostic Procedures," page 297) to look for cysts in the kidneys, especially in people who have a family history of

PKD. Although there is no cure for PKD, treatment can ease the symptoms and prolong life.

- *Acquired cystic kidney disease.* People who have a long history of kidney disease (especially if they require dialysis) are likely to develop cystic kidney disease similar to PKD (above). The cysts may bleed. People with acquired cystic kidney disease are twice as likely to develop renal cell cancer (see "Kidney Cancer," page 293).

- *IgA nephropathy.* This kidney disorder is caused by deposits of the protein immunoglobulin A (IgA) inside the filtering mechanisms (glomeruli) within the kidney. The IgA protein blocks the normal filtering process, which causes blood and protein to remain in the urine and also causes swelling in the hands and feet. IgA nephropathy is a chronic glomerular disease (see page 290) that may progress over a period of 10 to 20 years.

- *Analgesic nephropathy.* This kidney disease results from long-term use of analgesics (painkillers) and gradually leads to end-stage renal disease (see page 293). Single analgesics such as aspirin have not been found to cause kidney damage. However, medications that combine two or more painkillers (such as aspirin and acetaminophen) with caffeine or codeine are most likely to damage the kidneys. People who already have kidney disease must use caution when taking any painkiller.

Diagnostic Procedures

Urinary tract disorders often can be diagnosed through blood and urine tests. Blood tests can show when the kidneys are failing to adequately remove waste products. Urine tests (urinalysis) can show whether there is bleeding in the urinary tract, whether bacteria have infected the urinary tract, or whether the kidneys are functioning properly. A small sample of urine can be quickly tested for the presence of protein, sugar, blood, and other substances using a dipstick (a strip of paper coated with test chemicals that can be dipped into the urine and checked immediately for results). The relative amount of acid in the urine (pH) can be determined in the same way. Other urine tests require a person to collect all the urine he or she produces over a 24-hour period. Special imaging procedures also may be needed to examine the structure of the kidneys, ureters, bladder, and urethra. The following are the most common tests for diagnosing urinary tract disorders:

- *Serum creatinine.* This blood test measures the amount of creatinine, a waste product that results from eating meat and from muscle repair. High levels of creatinine in the blood indicate that the kidneys are not working properly.

- *Blood urea nitrogen (BUN).* Urea nitrogen is another by-product of protein digestion. As with serum creatinine, high BUN levels on a blood test indicate reduced kidney function.

- *Creatinine clearance.* A creatinine clearance test compares the amount of creatinine present in a 24-hour urine sample with creatinine levels in blood to determine how much blood the kidneys have filtered over a 24-hour period.
- *Specific gravity.* This urine test measures the extent to which the kidneys can concentrate the urine they produce. If the specific gravity is lower than normal, it suggests that the kidneys are not functioning efficiently.
- *Urinary sediment.* Normal urine contains a small number of cells and other materials shed during passage through the urinary tract. Examining the number and type of these substances can help identify specific disorders. For example, the presence of white blood cells and bacteria indicates infection. The presence of white blood cells also may indicate a tumor. Crystals appear when the urine is not acidic enough to dissolve them or when the concentration of crystals in the urine is abnormally high. Casts (cylindrical clumps of material that form in and come from the tubules in the kidney) distinguish kidney problems from disorders of the ureter, bladder, and urethra and help identify the diseased area of the kidney.
- *Intravenous urography.* This series of contrast medium-enhanced X rays allows doctors to view the interior structures of the urinary tract. This test sometimes is called an intravenous pyelogram, or IVP. The contrast medium is injected into a vein, and X rays are taken as it reaches the kidneys and is filtered out. When the contrast medium has filled your bladder, you will be asked to urinate, and X rays will be taken to see if any of the contrast medium remains in your bladder. This procedure is most often performed to look for stones in the kidney or the bladder, cysts in the kidney, tumors, an enlarged prostate, or other possible sources of blockage.
- *Cystoscopy.* For this test, a thin, rigid or flexible tube (with or without a video camera attached) is passed through the urethra into the bladder. This procedure is required to rule out a possible bladder tumor.
- *Retrograde pyelogram.* This procedure usually is performed during a cystoscopy and is used when poor kidney function limits the value of intravenous urography. For this test, contrast medium is injected directly from the bladder into the ureters through the cystoscope. The contrast medium allows the doctor to check for blockages or tumors.
- *Ultrasound scanning.* Ultrasound scanning (also called ultrasonography or a "sonogram") is an imaging technique that allows doctors to see the outline and the interior of the kidneys and, to a lesser extent, the bladder. This procedure offers a noninvasive method of distinguishing between cysts and tumors of the kidney, checking for urinary tract obstruction, detecting inflammation and fluid collection around the kidneys, and identifying the best location for a planned biopsy.
- *Computed tomography (CT) scanning.* CT scanning is a diagnostic technique that uses a computer and low-dose X rays to produce detailed cross-sectional

images of body tissues that are displayed on a video monitor. This technique is performed with or without a contrast medium (a dye) to detect stones and tumors in the urinary tract.

- *Magnetic resonance imaging (MRI)*. MRI is a diagnostic technique that uses a computer, a powerful magnetic field, and radio waves to produce detailed two- and three-dimensional images of body tissues that are displayed on a video monitor. This technique is used to detect tumors in the kidneys and bladder.

CHAPTER 15
Bones and Joints

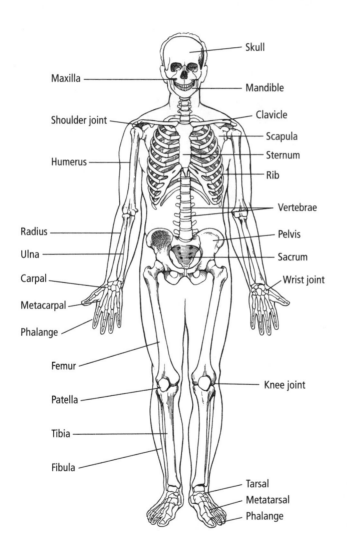

Skull

Maxilla

Mandible

Shoulder joint

Clavicle

Scapula

Sternum

Humerus

Rib

Vertebrae

Radius

Pelvis

Ulna

Sacrum

Carpal

Wrist joint

Metacarpal

Phalange

Femur

Knee joint

Patella

Tibia

Fibula

Tarsal

Metatarsal

Phalange

Your skeleton consists of about 206 separate bones, which range in size from the femur (the long bone in your leg) to the malleus, incus, and stapes (the three tiny bones in your inner ear). The skeleton matures and stops growing at about age 20, although the bone tissue itself remains alive and active, producing blood cells in the bone marrow and storing minerals such as calcium and phosphorus. Tendons attach your muscles to your bones to permit movement of the skeleton. Ligaments connect bone to bone and provide stability to joints. Any point where bone meets bone is a joint. Most, but not all, joints are capable of motion. Your skeleton also supports your body and protects your internal organs.

Disorders of the Bones

Bone is living connective tissue that constantly changes. The bone marrow, where blood cells are produced, is surrounded by cancellous (spongy) bone that fills the medullary canal. Cortical bone, which is made up of the protein collagen infused with minerals, encircles the medullary canal and contains the cells that maintain bone tissue. The thin outer covering of bone is a membrane called the periosteum, which contains nerves and blood vessels and is essential for the formation and growth of new bone. Bone tissue produces its own cartilage to absorb shock and provide a tough, elastic surface between adjoining bones.

Osteoporosis

Osteoporosis is a disease in which the bones become thin, porous, weak, and more susceptible to fractures. Although osteoporosis is generally regarded as a women's health concern, the disease also can develop in men. Because men have larger, denser skeletons, they usually experience bone loss later in life than women. However, older men are at increased risk for hip fracture and other joint fractures as a result of osteoporosis. Men and women lose bone mass at an increased rate after age 65, and calcium absorption decreases with age in both sexes. About a third of men over age 75 have been diagnosed with osteoporosis, and one of every eight men over age 50 will experience a bone fracture as a result of osteoporosis. Therefore all men need to take steps to prevent osteoporosis (see following page).

Bone mass increases throughout childhood and young adulthood, reaching its peak at about age 20. After age 35, bone tissue breaks down faster than new bone is formed. Bone becomes more porous and structurally weaker. Dense, cortical bone tissue is replaced by spongy, cancellous bone. In many cases, osteoporosis is detected only after a fracture occurs. Men who are older, small-framed, or white or Asian are at increased risk for osteoporosis. The following factors can increase your risk of developing osteoporosis:

- long-term use of certain medications (including corticosteroids, heparin, anticonvulsants, aluminum-containing antacids, and some cancer drugs)
- low testosterone level
- excess thyroid hormone
- smoking
- chronic or heavy alcohol consumption
- high intake of caffeine, protein, or sodium (salt)
- insufficient intake of calcium
- vitamin D deficiency
- sedentary lifestyle
- family history of osteoporosis
- disorders that affect absorption of calcium, such as lactose intolerance, peptic ulcers, or celiac disease

To detect bone loss, your doctor will perform urine and blood tests. He or she also will recommend that you undergo a bone density test, which is an imaging technique used to assess bone density and structure. In some cases a bone biopsy (removal of a small piece of bone tissue for microscopic examination) may be required to rule out other possible bone disorders, such as osteomalacia (see page 318).

You can take steps to reduce your risk of developing osteoporosis. Lifestyle changes that focus on your risk factors will help prevent osteoporosis. If some bone loss has already occurred, lifestyle changes and treatment with medications such as calcitonin or alendronate can reduce the risk of fractures.

Here are some steps you can take to help prevent osteoporosis:

- Take in plenty of calcium every day (see "How Much Calcium Do I Need?" on next page).
- Get an adequate supply of vitamin D. Fat-free milk fortified with vitamin D is an excellent source of this essential nutrient.
- Exercise regularly (especially weight-bearing exercise such as brisk walking, jogging, and stair climbing).
- Stop smoking (see page 107).
- Drink alcohol only in moderation.
- Cut back on caffeine.
- Limit your intake of sodium.

Bone Cancer

Primary bone cancer—that is, cancer that begins in the bone versus cancer that spreads to the bone from another part of the body—is rare but occurs most frequently in children and young men. Osteosarcoma is the most common form of primary bone cancer. Osteosarcoma and Ewing's sarcoma (another type of primary bone cancer) usually occur between ages 10 and 25. Other primary bone cancers include chondrosarcoma, fibrosarcoma, malignant giant cell tumor, and chordoma. These cancers occur mainly in adults over age 30.

Symptoms of bone cancer tend to develop slowly. Pain is the most frequent symptom, although in most cases, a firm lump or swelling on the bone can be felt through the skin. Bone cancer is often detected when a bone breaks without obvious cause or fails to repair itself after a fracture.

Tests for bone cancer include blood tests, bone scans, and X rays. If a tumor is detected, additional examinations will be performed to determine whether it is benign (noncancerous) or malignant (cancerous). These procedures include radionuclide scanning (a radioactive substance is injected into the bloodstream to produce images that show where the cancer is growing), computed tomography (CT) scanning (see page 90) or magnetic resonance imaging (MRI; see page 90), and angiography (X rays of the blood vessels taken after a special dye is injected into the bloodstream). A bone biopsy (removal of a small piece of bone tissue for microscopic examination) is performed to identify the type of tumor and to help plan a course of treatment.

Bone cancer is treated with surgery, chemotherapy (treatment with powerful anticancer drugs), and radiation therapy. Most bone tumors are removed surgically, even if they are benign. In many cases, primary bone cancer is successfully treated with a bone graft (replacement of the diseased section of the bone with healthy human bone from a bone bank) and chemotherapy. In some cases, if a tumor is large or has begun to spread throughout the bone, amputation may be performed, followed by chemotherapy. Radiation therapy often is used if the cancer has spread to other tissues.

How Much Calcium Do I Need?

According to nutritional guidelines from the National Institutes of Health, adolescents and young adults should take in 1,200 to 1,500 milligrams of calcium per day; men ages 25 through 65 should take in 1,000 milligrams of calcium per day; and men over age 65 should take in 1,500 milligrams of calcium per day. Good sources of calcium include low-fat and nonfat dairy products; green, leafy vegetables; dried peas and beans; and calcium-fortified foods. The following table lists some good sources of calcium and the approximate amount of calcium they contain:

Good Sources of Calcium

Food	Serving Size	Calcium (in milligrams)
Low-fat or nonfat plain yogurt	1 cup	468
2 percent milk	1 cup	350
Sardines with bones, canned	3 ounces	324
Calcium-fortified orange juice	1 cup	320
1 percent milk or fat-free milk	1 cup	300
Mozzarella cheese, part skim	1 ounce	207
Salmon with bones, canned	3 ounces	181
Tofu (firm)	3 ounces	177
Figs, dried	5 medium	135
Tortilla, corn	2	120
Tortilla, flour	2	106
Great northern beans	½ cup	105
Turnip greens, cooked	½ cup	99
English muffin, plain	1	99
Low-fat cottage cheese	½ cup	69
Orange	1 medium	58
Mustard greens, boiled	½ cup	52
Broccoli, raw	1 cup	42

Fractures

A fracture—a break in bone or cartilage—usually results from injury or an underlying bone disease, such as osteoporosis (see page 301). Fractures are categorized as either simple (closed), in which the broken bone does not break the skin, or compound (open), in which the broken bone punctures the skin. When the two ends of a fractured bone have not separated, it is called a nondisplaced fracture. When the two ends have separated, it is a displaced fracture. Within the categories of simple and compound are other types of fractures (see box), including transverse fracture, spiral fracture, comminuted fracture, and greenstick fracture. The type of fracture determines the choice of treatment.

In general, fractured bones are painful and limit use of the injured limb or body part. Often the injured area appears misshapen. Bruising may occur, and the limb below the fracture may tingle or become numb, cold, or pale. However, sometimes it is possible to walk on a fractured leg or continue to use a fractured arm without realizing it is broken.

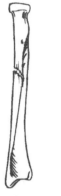 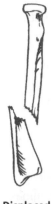

Nondisplaced   **Displaced**
Fracture   **Fracture**

Fractures

Bones can break or crack in various patterns, depending on the direction and force of impact. Here are some of the most common types of fractures and how they are treated:

Transverse fracture. Transverse fractures are breaks straight across a bone that usually arise from a direct blow or an angled force. Doctors treat this type of fracture by immobilizing the bone in a cast.

Spiral fracture. Spiral fractures, which usually affect arm bones or leg bones, often occur when someone violently twists a limb. The bone can break through the skin and damage surrounding nerves and blood vessels. Doctors treat this type of fracture with immobilization in a cast or, sometimes, with traction (the application of tension to a bone to align and immobilize it) or surgery.

Comminuted fracture. Comminuted fractures, in which a bone splinters into three or more pieces, are usually caused by a high-impact injury or a direct blow. This type of fracture is sometimes

difficult to treat because the pieces of bone need to be carefully repositioned.

Greenstick fracture. In greenstick fractures, a long arm bone or leg bone snaps or buckles on only one side, usually from a severe blow or a jarring force. Greenstick fractures are more common in children than in adults. Doctors treat this type of fracture by immobilizing the bone in a cast.

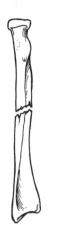 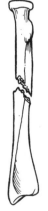 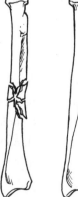

Transverse   **Spiral**   **Comminuted**   **Greenstick**
Fracture   **Fracture**   **Fracture**   **Fracture**

After any serious injury, you should seek medical attention to rule out fractures or detect them before they become worse. If you think you may have a fracture, take immediate steps to immobilize the injured bone to prevent further damage to the bone and surrounding blood vessels and nerves, and elevate the affected body part to reduce swelling. With an open fracture, be sure to place a clean cloth or a bandage gently over the wound to reduce the risk of infection.

Fractured bones must first be restored to their normal position and alignment. This process is referred to as "reduction." A cast or a splint may be sufficient to hold a broken bone in place for healing. If you fracture a large bone or experience a complicated break, you may need surgery. Sometimes bones must be screwed together or rejoined using metal plates or rods. Pins or screws also may be inserted to hold an external frame in place that immobilizes the bone while it heals. You will need to rest the affected limb and avoid overuse until the bone heals.

A stress fracture refers to a condition in which a tiny crack (or cracks) occurs in a bone that has been exposed to repeated injury or overuse. Your lower leg and foot are especially prone to stress fractures. Early symptoms include sharp pain and swelling in the affected area. If the cracks are too small to see on an X ray, the doctor may perform a computed tomography (CT) scan (see page 90) to determine the location and extent of the fracture. Treatment consists of resting the affected area long enough to allow healing to take place.

Disorders of the Soft Tissues

Your muscles, tendons, ligaments, and bursa are all susceptible to damage from daily stress and sports activities. These tissues can be stressed by an imbalance in muscle strength (when one muscle is much stronger than its opposing muscle), lack of flexibility, or weakness caused by a previous injury. A fall, a sudden twisting motion, or a blow to the body is sufficient to cause any of the following problems. Using the injured part before it has healed completely often leads to reinjury.

Bursitis

A bursa is a fluid-filled sac between a bone and a tendon or muscle that allows the tendon to slide smoothly over the bone. Bursitis occurs when repeated stress and overuse cause the bursa to become inflamed and swollen with excess fluid. Bursitis also can result from injury, rheumatoid arthritis, gout, or infection. Bursitis most often occurs in the shoulder but also can affect the hip, knee, elbow, Achilles tendon, or ankle. Often the nearby tendon also becomes swollen. Bursitis usually can be treated with rest, ice, and nonsteroidal anti-inflammatory medication. Occasionally it is necessary for a doctor to withdraw excess fluid from the bursa using a needle and syringe. If an infection is present, the doctor will prescribe antibiotics. If there is no infection, the doctor may inject a corticosteroid drug to relieve symptoms. Even with successful treatment, however, the condition may recur. If bursitis recurs frequently, the affected bursa may be removed in a minor surgical procedure called bursectomy.

Contusion

A contusion refers to a bruised muscle, tendon, or ligament. Following injury, blood pools (collects) in the injured area and discolors the skin. Most contusions respond well to RICE: rest, ice, compression, and elevation (see page 65). However, if you do not see improvement or if the pain worsens, contact your doctor as soon as possible so he or she can take steps to prevent permanent damage to the soft tissues.

Sprain versus Strain

Many people use the terms "sprain" and "strain" interchangeably. However, a sprain refers to stretching or tearing of ligaments (which connect bone to bone), while a strain refers to stretching or tearing of tendons (which connect muscle to bone) and their attached muscles. Sprains most often occur as a result of excessive twisting motion in the ankle, knee, or wrist. Strains often occur in the foot or leg. Mild sprains and strains are treated with RICE (see page 65) followed by gentle exercises to relieve the pain and restore mobility.

Tendinitis

Tendons are cordlike tissues that connect muscle to bone. Inflammation of a tendon is called tendinitis. The condition usually results from excess friction between a tendon and a bone. Tendinitis usually occurs after long-term stress that aggravates a specific tendon. Professional athletes and workers engaged in repetitive job activities are at high risk for tendinitis. Although any tendon can become inflamed, the tendons of the shoulder, wrist, heel (Achilles tendon), and elbow are most susceptible to overuse injuries.

Symptoms of tendinitis include pain, tenderness, and, in some cases, restricted movement of the attached muscle.

Treatment of tendinitis may include making changes in your activities or routine, receiving corticosteroid injections, taking nonsteroidal anti-inflammatory medications such as aspirin or ibuprofen, splinting (immobilizing the tendon), and performing exercises to correct muscle strength imbalance and improve flexibility. Persistent inflammation that does not respond to other forms of treatment may require surgery.

Back Pain

Only the common cold causes more missed days of work than low back pain. The lower (or lumbar) region of the spine connects your upper body (chest and abdomen) to your lower body (hips and legs) and provides tremendous mobility and strength. Twisting, turning, bending, standing, lifting, and walking all rely on the lower back.

Back pain may range from a mild ache or stiffness to severe pain that prevents movement of any sort. Stress on or injury to the muscles and ligaments that support the spine are a common source of back pain. A sedentary lifestyle and being overweight increase the back's vulnerability to stress and injury. Strenuous sports activities and physically demanding jobs can also cause stress and injury to the back. In addition, aging increases the risk of back injury due to age-related changes, osteoporosis, and arthritis. A prolapsed disk (when one of the pads of cartilage between the vertebrae of the spine protrudes and presses on a ligament or a nerve, causing back pain) also is more likely to occur in older adults.

When back pain is chronic or severe or affects a person's ability to function normally, it requires treatment. Contact your doctor if the pain is not relieved within a few days, is severe and constant, recurs, or is accompanied by other symptoms, such as radiating pain, numbness, tingling, weakness, bowel or bladder incontinence, fever, or vomiting. Your doctor can assess the extent and seriousness of a back injury through a thorough physical examination (especially of the back and the legs). Depending on your symptoms and the results of the examination, you may need to undergo X rays, computed tomography (CT) scanning (see page 90), or magnetic resonance imaging (MRI; see page 90).

Most low back pain results from sprains or strains and will respond to self-treatment measures such as limited rest, anti-inflammatory drugs such as aspirin or ibuprofen, back stretching and strengthening exercises, and prevention (see box). In some cases the doctor may prescribe muscle relaxants to relieve symptoms. Your doctor may recommend that you wear a lightweight brace to support your back. He or she also may recommend heat treatments and massage, or traction (a treatment that stretches your spine with weights while you lie on your back). It is important to note that prolonged bed rest weakens the back muscles and is not recommended as a treatment for back pain.

Protecting Your Back

It is easier to prevent back injury than it is to treat it. If you injured your back in the past, you must be especially careful to avoid reinjury. You can protect your back by doing the following:

- Exercise regularly.
- Stretch (especially before exercising).
- Strengthen your abdominal muscles (to support your back).
- Do not smoke.
- Maintain a healthy weight.
- Maintain correct posture (don't slouch).

- Use straight-backed chairs and a firm mattress that support your back.
- Lift objects by bending at your knees rather than at your waist.
- Do not lift heavy objects.
- Avoid standing or sitting in one position for long periods.
- Support one leg on a small stool when standing, to flatten and relax your lower back.
- Sleep on your back with a pillow supporting your bent knees.
- Manage your stress.

Disorders of the Joints

A joint is the point at which two or more bones meet. It is made up of the bones and muscles brought together at the joint, the ligaments (which connect bone to bone), the tendons (which connect muscle to bone), the bursae (which cushion the joint), and cartilage. The cartilage permits smooth movement of the joint and acts as a shock absorber between the bones. The entire joint is enclosed in a fibrous capsule with a special lining (the synovium) that produces fluid to reduce friction within the joint. Inflammation of or damage to any of these components affects the entire joint. This section describes some common problems that can affect the joints.

Osteoarthritis

Arthritis is a general term that refers to inflammation of one or more joints. There are more than 100 arthritic disorders. Osteoarthritis, which most people refer to as simply arthritis, is a chronic joint disease that affects many middle-aged and older Americans. Osteoarthritis that has no obvious cause is called primary arthritis. Osteoarthritis that results from damage to the cartilage that covers the ends of the bones in a joint is called secondary arthritis. Injury and obesity are two factors that may be involved in the development of osteoarthritis. Heredity may also be a factor.

The symptoms of osteoarthritis include pain, tenderness, swelling, redness, and loss of motion or strength in the affected joint or joints. The pain tends to worsen toward the end of the day. In some people the joint may make cracking sounds when it is in motion. In osteoarthritis, joint cartilage gradually wears away, allowing adjoining bones to rub against each other. Painful outgrowths of bone (spurs) also may develop. Although symptoms usually do not appear until middle age, they can begin as early as between ages 20 and 30. Among adults under age 55, men and women are affected equally; after age 55, the incidence of osteoarthritis is higher in women. Joints in the hips, knees, spine, big toe, and fingers are most commonly affected.

Osteoarthritis is diagnosed based on your symptoms and the results of a physical examination. X rays usually are taken to confirm the diagnosis. There is no cure for osteoarthritis. Your doctor probably will prescribe a nonsteroidal anti-inflammatory drug to relieve symptoms. Severe episodes of inflammation may be treated by injecting a corticosteroid drug directly into the affected joint. Massage, heat treatments, and warm baths may help relieve symptoms. Regular, gentle exercise (such as walking or swimming) will help your joints stay flexible. Maintaining a healthy weight (see page 67) will reduce the strain on your joints. For some people doctors may recommend joint replacement (see page 310).

Rheumatoid Arthritis

Rheumatoid arthritis is a chronic autoimmune disease in which the immune system attacks the synovial tissue, the membrane that lines the joints. It is the second most common form of arthritis and usually appears between ages 20 and 40. Although the cause of rheumatoid arthritis is unknown, there is a genetic component: if a close relative is affected, you are more likely to develop the disease. There is no known cure.

In rheumatoid arthritis, the fluid that lubricates the joints contains irritating chemicals that attack and damage the surfaces of the joints. The inflamed membrane swells and thickens, causing a wearing away of the joint cartilage, which leads to erosion of the bone and weakening of supporting tendons, ligaments, and muscles. The small joints in the hands, wrists, feet, ankles, and neck are most frequently affected, but the hips and the knees also can be affected. In most cases, more than one joint is affected and usually the same joints are affected on both sides, such as both hands.

Rheumatoid arthritis alternates between periods during which symptoms are present and periods with no symptoms. These periods can vary in length. When the disease is active, it causes redness, warmth, swelling, tenderness, pain, and stiffness in the affected joints. The severity of symptoms can vary from person to person. The joint damage resulting from the disease is not reversible; in advanced cases, the joints can become deformed.

A diagnosis of rheumatoid arthritis is based on the symptoms and an examination of the joints. The doctor also can use X rays to detect damage— such as erosion of cartilage and bone—in the affected joints. A blood test also may be performed to check for a specific protein (an antibody called rheumatoid factor) that is present in most people who have rheumatoid arthritis.

Treatment of rheumatoid arthritis is similar to the treatment of osteoarthritis (see previous page). If treatment with nonsteroidal anti-inflammatory drugs is not effective, the doctor may prescribe other medications, including gold compounds such as auranofin and aurothioglucose, and oral corticosteroids such as prednisolone and triamcinolone. The doctor also may prescribe antirheumatic drugs such as hydroxychloroquine and penicillamine. In severe cases, medications such as azathioprine, cyclophosphamide, cyclosporine, and methotrexate sometimes are prescribed to suppress the inappropriate immune response.

For most people with rheumatoid arthritis, regular exercise can help maintain flexibility and strength in the joints. Your doctor can recommend suitable exercises and also may recommend that you work with a physical therapist to maintain or restore movement in your joints. For some people, surgery to remove the affected joint lining (a procedure called synovectomy) may provide relief. For severely damaged joints, a total joint replacement (see following page) can reduce pain and restore movement, allowing a person to return to an active life.

Joint Replacement   Because of engineering and medical advances, surgeons can now replace certain joints and restore their normal function. Joint replacement (called arthroplasty) has been used on the ankles, hands, wrists, and toes, but it is most often performed on the knee and the hip. With total joint replacement, the bone ends and cartilage are replaced with metal and plastic joint components. The metal component is inserted into the canal inside each long bone involved, while the plastic part covers or receives the metal "bone ends" as a cartilagelike cushion, where bone meets bone. The joint components are usually attached to the bone tissue with an acrylic cement.

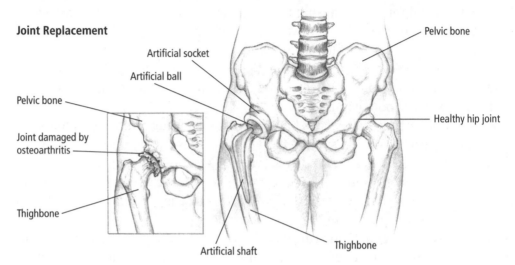

Joint Replacement

Artificial socket

Artificial ball

Pelvic bone

Joint damaged by osteoarthritis

Thighbone

Artificial shaft

Pelvic bone

Healthy hip joint

Thighbone

In hip replacement surgery, the end of the femur is replaced with a metal ball, and a plastic cup is cemented into the pelvis where the acetabulum (pelvic socket) would normally receive the end of the femur. In many patients, particularly younger ones, the plastic cup is not cemented into place to give time (with limited activity) for the natural bone to grow and attach to it. In the knee, damaged bone ends are replaced with metal ends covered with plastic that can permit the same range of motion as a normal knee joint.

Joint replacement surgery lasts approximately 2 to 4 hours and requires a lengthy, structured recuperation period. The amount of recovery time required in the hospital depends on the nature of the surgery, your overall health, and whether you have any complications (such as infection, joint dislocation, or blood clots). You may be walking with support within a day of surgery, and you will start physical therapy immediately. You will probably be hospitalized for about a week, although full recovery can take up to 6 months. It is vital to maintain an appropriate exercise and stretching program after the surgery to keep your new joint in good working order. Although replacement joints usually last at least 20 years, younger and more active patients may need to undergo revision surgery (surgery to repair or replace the artificial joint). Joint replacement surgery has an excellent success rate.

Gout is a metabolic disorder that results from high levels of uric acid (a waste product of cell metabolism) in the blood. The condition can lead to joint inflammation, deposits of uric acid in and around the joints, reduced kidney function, and sometimes the development of kidney stones (see page 289).

Gout is nine times more common in men than in women. Risk factors for gout include obesity, moderate to heavy alcohol consumption, high blood pressure, and kidney disorders. Certain drugs (such as aspirin) can worsen gout, and certain diseases that affect kidney function (such as diabetes and sickle-cell disease) can be a factor. Acute attacks of gout can be brought on by dehydration, joint injury, fever, large meals, high alcohol intake, stress, or recent surgery. Certain foods, such as shellfish, sardines, and organ meats, also may trigger attacks.

The small joint at the base of the big toe is the most common location for an acute gout attack. Other joints affected may include the ankles, knees, wrists, fingers, and elbows. An acute gout attack often begins at night, with severe pain and sometimes a fever. The attack may subside in several hours or several days but usually recurs at irregular intervals.

The symptoms alone usually are sufficient to diagnose gout, but your doctor can confirm the diagnosis by examining your blood for elevated uric acid levels and your joint fluid for signs of uric acid crystals.

Future attacks can be prevented by increasing fluid consumption (at least eight 8-ounce glasses every day), losing weight (see page 73), reducing alcohol intake, modifying your diet, and taking nonsteroidal anti-inflammatory drugs (such as ibuprofen) to relieve the pain and inflammation and medications (such as allopurinol or probenecid) to lower blood levels of uric acid.

Disorders of the Wrist and the Hand

The hand consists of the wrist, palm, and fingers. The wrist has eight bones (carpals); four are connected to the forearm bones (radius and ulna), and four are connected to the five bones of the palm (metacarpals). Each of the bones of the palm is connected to one of the finger bones (phalanges). Each finger has three phalanges; the thumb has two phalanges. Hand movements are controlled by a complex network of ligaments, tendons, and muscles. The hand has a wide range of motion that allows you to perform a wide variety of manual tasks. The complexity and versatility of the hand make it particularly vulnerable to injury.

Carpal Tunnel Syndrome

Carpal tunnel syndrome is a common repetitive-stress injury that can affect one or both hands. Repeating the same hand motions over a prolonged period may lead to swelling of the tendons that bend the fingers and the thumb, which in turn puts pressure on the median nerve where it enters the hand (the carpal tunnel). Repetitive motions such as keyboard work (including operating a computer, adding machine, or cash register), assembly line work, painting, driving, and some sports (such as handball and racquetball) can cause this injury.

Common symptoms of carpal tunnel syndrome include numbness, tingling, and pain in the hand and forearm (especially at night), pain or weakness when gripping objects, and clumsiness in handling objects.

Diagnosis of carpal tunnel syndrome is based on your symptoms and the results of a doctor's examination of your hand and wrist. If pain shoots down into your hand and fingers or up into your forearm when the doctor taps lightly on the front of your wrist, you probably have carpal tunnel syndrome. Nerve conduction tests such as electromyography (EMG) may be performed to determine whether there is any nerve damage.

Your doctor probably will recommend that you rest the affected hand and avoid the repetitive activity that is causing the problem. You also may need to wear a splint or a brace to immobilize your wrist while allowing you to continue using your hand. Nonsteroidal anti-inflammatory drugs such as aspirin or ibuprofen can relieve pain and inflammation. Injections with corticosteroids may be prescribed if pain persists. Surgery to relieve the pressure on the median nerve (a procedure called carpal tunnel release) is performed in severe cases that do not respond to other forms of treatment.

Baseball Finger

Baseball finger (also known as a jammed finger or mallet finger) refers to a tear in the tendons at the outermost joint in the finger. The condition results from a sudden blow to the fingertip, such as when the finger is hit by a ball. Symptoms include pain, swelling, and bruising. If the injury is severe, you will not be able to straighten the affected finger.

To reduce pain and swelling, place an ice pack on the finger immediately after the injury occurs. See your doctor as soon as possible. He or she may X ray the finger to make sure it is not broken. The doctor probably will immobilize your finger with a splint for 2 to 3 months to help the joint heal properly. In some cases the doctor may insert a wire through the joint to hold the finger straight while the tendons are healing. Nonsteroidal anti-inflammatory medications such as aspirin or ibuprofen will help relieve pain and reduce swelling.

You should avoid athletic activities until after the injury has healed. Your doctor may recommend that you work with a physical therapist or an athletic trainer on exercises that will strengthen the tendons and help restore normal function to the joint. Apply ice packs to the finger if swelling occurs. If the injury is severe, you may never be able to fully straighten the affected finger.

Trigger Finger

Trigger finger (tenosynovitis of the hand) is inflammation of the tendons and surrounding tendon sheaths in a finger. This condition prevents the finger joints from moving smoothly. Trigger finger is a repetitive-stress injury caused by repetitive motions such as keyboarding or assembly line work.

You may have difficulty straightening the affected finger. You also may feel a slight clicking sensation when you straighten or bend the finger. Once the affected finger is bent, the tendon may catch for a few seconds and then suddenly release with a jerking motion (like a trigger). Symptoms include pain, tenderness, and swelling in the hand and wrist.

Nonsteroidal anti-inflammatory medications such as aspirin or ibuprofen will help relieve pain and reduce swelling. Your doctor probably will recommend that you rest your hand and change your work habits or avoid the activity that is causing the problem. You also may need to wear a splint or brace to immobilize your wrist while allowing you to continue using your hand. If the pain persists, your doctor may prescribe injections of a corticosteroid drug such as cortisone. In severe cases, surgery may be performed to relieve pressure on the tendons.

Disorders of the Elbow

The elbow is a hinge joint between the humerus (upper arm bone) and the ulna and radius. The elbow allows you to bend and straighten your arm and to rotate your forearm without moving your upper arm. Your biceps muscle bends the forearm, while your triceps muscle straightens the forearm. The bony projection that forms the point of the elbow is the olecranon. Popularly known as the "funny bone," because bumping the nerve (the ulnar nerve) that passes over it produces a familiar tingling sensation, the olecranon prevents overextension of the elbow.

Epicondylitis

Tendons attach the forearm muscles to the elbow at bony outgrowths called epicondyles. These tendons can become inflamed and painful, especially with repetitive motions of the forearm (such as using a manual screwdriver, washing windows, or swinging a baseball bat). This inflammation is called epicondylitis. The two types of epicondylitis are called tennis elbow (the outer tendons are inflamed) and golfer's elbow (the inner tendons are inflamed).

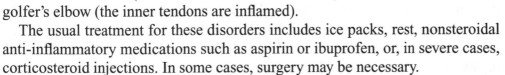

Elbow

The usual treatment for these disorders includes ice packs, rest, nonsteroidal anti-inflammatory medications such as aspirin or ibuprofen, or, in severe cases, corticosteroid injections. In some cases, surgery may be necessary.

Trapped Nerve

A trapped ulnar nerve is another common injury that occurs when the nerve that crosses the point of the elbow is compressed or pinched. This causes numbness, tingling, weakness, and pain in the forearm and hand. Rest, ice, and avoiding reinjury can relieve symptoms and help the damaged nerve heal. Surgery to reposition the ulnar nerve may help prevent repeated compression.

Other possible elbow disorders include bursitis (see page 305), fractures (see page 304), and osteoarthritis (see page 308).

Disorders of the Shoulder

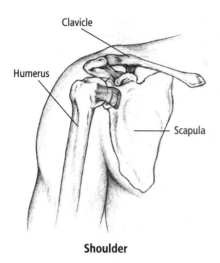

Shoulder

You may think of your shoulder as a single unit, but this joint is actually made up of three bones—the clavicle (collarbone), the scapula (shoulder blade), and the humerus (upper arm bone)—and three joints. The acromioclavicular joint is between the tip of the shoulder blade (acromion) and the collarbone. The scapulothoracic joint is between the shoulder blade and the thorax (rib cage), and the glenohumeral joint, commonly called the shoulder joint, is between the glenoid cavity (shoulder socket) and the head of the humerus. The shoulder is a ball-and-socket–type joint that permits a wide range of motion. In fact, the shoulder is the most movable—and, because of this, the most unstable—joint in the body.

Shoulder Dislocation

Shoulder dislocation occurs when the humerus (upper arm bone) comes out of the shoulder joint. The bone is usually displaced in front of and below the shoulder. Ligaments and other connective tissues are stretched or torn. In severe cases, nerves and blood vessels also may be damaged. The injury is caused by falling onto an outstretched hand or arm or onto the shoulder itself. It also may be caused by a powerful direct blow to the shoulder. Shoulder dislocation is sometimes accompanied by a fracture (see page 304).

Symptoms of shoulder dislocation include severe pain in the shoulder accompanied by swelling and bruising. The shoulder also may look misshapen.

To reduce pain and swelling, place an ice pack on the injured area immediately after the injury occurs. Then see your doctor or go to a hospital emergency department without delay. (With a recurring dislocation, you may be able to "pop" the shoulder back into place.) To immobilize the shoulder and to aid healing, the doctor may place your arm in a sling or strap your arm to your chest. He or she may prescribe an analgesic (pain-relieving) medication such as codeine with aspirin or acetaminophen. The doctor also may prescribe a nonsteroidal anti-inflammatory drug such as aspirin or ibuprofen to relieve pain and reduce swelling. (**Warning:** Do not take these medications at the same time unless your doctor tells you to do so.)

You should avoid athletic activities until after the injury has healed. Your doctor will probably recommend that you apply an ice pack to the injured area for 20 to 30 minutes three or four times per day for 2 to 4 days to reduce swelling and inflammation. After the swelling has gone down, apply a heating pad to your shoulder to increase circulation to the injured area and speed healing. (**Warning:** Apply heat only after swelling has subsided, or swelling in the injured area may increase. Be careful when using a heating pad; too much heat can cause tissue damage or burns.)

Once you have had a shoulder dislocation, you are at risk for a recurrence of the injury. Raising your arm over your head or sleeping with your arm above your shoulder could cause another dislocation. Your doctor may recommend that you work with a physical therapist or an athletic trainer on exercises that will stabilize the ligaments and tendons, strengthen the shoulder muscles, and help prevent another dislocation. A shoulder dislocation is usually a more serious injury than a shoulder separation (see below).

Shoulder Separation

Shoulder separation occurs when the ligaments that attach the clavicle (collarbone) to the scapula (shoulder blade) are torn. The injury is caused by falling onto an outstretched hand or arm or onto the shoulder itself. It also may be caused by a direct blow to the shoulder. Symptoms include severe pain, swelling, and bruising. There may be limited movement in the shoulder. In some cases the collarbone is pushed out of its normal position and sticks up under the skin. Also, the shoulder may look misshapen.

To reduce pain and swelling, place an ice pack on the injured area immediately after the injury occurs. If symptoms persist, see your doctor as soon as possible, or go to a hospital emergency department. To immobilize the shoulder and to speed healing, the doctor may place your arm in a sling or strap your arm to your chest. A nonsteroidal anti-inflammatory drug such as aspirin or ibuprofen will help reduce pain and inflammation. In severe cases, surgery to repair the damaged ligaments may be required.

You should avoid athletic activities until after the injury has healed. Your doctor probably will recommend that you apply an ice pack to the injured area for 20 to 30 minutes three or four times per day for 2 to 4 days to reduce swelling and inflammation. Use a heating pad on the injured area once the swelling has gone down, to increase circulation and speed healing. (**Warning:** Apply heat only after swelling has subsided, or swelling in the injured area may increase. Be careful when using a heating pad; too much heat can cause tissue damage or burns.) Ask your doctor if he or she has a list of recommended exercises or if you should work with a physical therapist or an athletic trainer on exercises that will stabilize the ligaments and tendons and strengthen the shoulder muscles. Shoulder separation usually does not cause any lasting adverse effects.

Disorders of the Hip

The hip is the joint between the upper end of the femur (thighbone) and the acetabulum, the cuplike structure in your pelvic bone. This ball-and-socket joint allows your leg to move forward and backward, to move from side to side, and to rotate to the left and the right. The femur and the pelvis are attached by ligaments. The hip supports the pelvis, the abdomen, and the chest and allows you to stand and move.

Wear and tear on the hip can result in bursitis (the most common cause of hip pain; see page 305) or osteoarthritis (see page 308). Bursitis can cause pain on the outer side of the hip that worsens after lying on that side, walking, or climbing stairs. Bursitis in the area of the upper buttocks is most noticeable while walking uphill or after sitting for a long period on a hard surface.

Osteoarthritis in the hip can progress to the point where joint replacement is required (see page 310). The bones in the hip also can be weakened by osteoporosis (see page 301), which can result in a hip fracture after a fall or an injury.

Disorders of the Knee

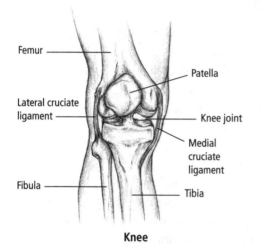

Knee

The knee is a modified hinge joint between the femur (thighbone) and the tibia (shin bone). The knee allows you to bend and straighten your leg. It also allows slight rotation of the lower leg when the knee is bent. Your hamstring muscles bend the knee, while your quadriceps muscles straighten the knee. Strong ligaments join your femur to your lower leg bones (tibia and fibula) and limit side-to-side movement, overextension, and overbending of the knee. The ligaments also limit sliding movement between the bones. Your knee also has two menisci (crescent-shaped disks of cartilage) to reduce friction and distribute the weight-bearing load evenly during walking or running. The knee joint is vulnerable to injury from the front or either side, as well as from overextension. Injury can affect the menisci or any of the ligaments, bursae, cartilage, bones, or tendons that form the knee. The knee is prone to a number of disorders and injuries because of its special design and because it bears weight and provides movement.

Torn Ligament

A torn ligament usually results from a severe twist or a forceful blow to the knee when the knee is bent and then straightened. It also can occur when the foot is placed firmly on the ground and the leg is straightened while the knee is twisted. Each ligament in the knee is subjected to tremendous stress and strain. Injuries to ligaments usually cause immediate pain that is present even at rest. The pain increases when the knee is bent or when weight is put on the knee. The joint also may be swollen and warm. There may be stiffness, and movement may be limited. You may hear or feel a "pop," and your knee may give out when the ligament tears. Injury to a ligament on the side of the joint causes pain in that side of the knee. Injury to a ligament within the joint causes pain deep inside the knee.

Ligament injuries are first treated with RICE (see page 65). You also must use some form of support (such as crutches or a cane) to avoid putting weight on the injured knee joint. In some cases a splint or a brace is needed for long-term immobilization of the joint. Nonsteroidal anti-inflammatory drugs such as aspirin or ibuprofen will help relieve pain and reduce inflammation. Arthroscopy (see box) often is needed to repair the ligament. Your knee joint may be unstable after this injury and may be more susceptible to recurring ligament or cartilage tears. Your doctor may recommend working with a physical therapist or an athletic trainer on exercises that will stabilize the ligaments and tendons and strengthen the leg muscles.

Arthroscopy

Arthroscopy is a procedure that uses an arthroscope (a viewing tube with a tiny video-camera at its tip) to examine, diagnose, and treat joint problems. The procedure is usually done on the knee joint, but it can be performed on other joints, such as the shoulder, elbow, ankle, hip, and wrist. For arthroscopic surgery, the surgeon makes a small incision and inserts the arthroscope directly into the joint. The procedure can be observed on a video monitor and videotaped. Surgical instruments are inserted into the joint through other small incisions. Any loose bone, cartilage, or other material in the joint also can be removed. A biopsy (removal of a small piece of tissue from the joint for examination under a microscope) can be easily performed during arthroscopy.

Arthroscopic surgery is performed to examine and repair the following:

- torn rotator cuff (the muscles and tendons surrounding the shoulder joint)
- torn meniscus (a crescent-shaped disk of cartilage found in the knee joint)
- torn or damaged ligaments

- torn cartilage
- inflamed tendon sheaths

General, local, or spinal anesthesia is used, depending on the joint. Most people do not require strong pain medication afterward and can usually resume light normal activities within a few days. However, after arthroscopic knee surgery, a person must wear a knee brace and have physical therapy on the joint for several weeks or months to promote healing and prevent further injury.

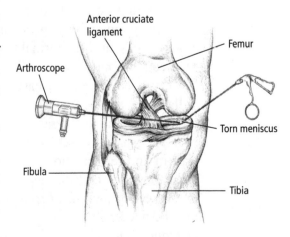

Arthroscopic Knee Surgery

Torn Cartilage

Either meniscus in the knee can be torn during sharp, rapid, twisting motions. The incidence of this type of injury rises with age and participation in sports that require quick, reactive movements, such as basketball, downhill skiing, and soccer. Certain knee motions cause a popping sensation, sometimes accompanied by swelling, warmth, and instability in the joint. Treatment for torn cartilage is similar to treatment for a torn ligament (see page 316). A torn meniscus is often repaired using arthroscopy (see box on previous page).

Other Knee Disorders

Tendinitis (see page 306) can occur in the front of your knee below the patella (kneecap) or in the back of the knee at the popliteal tendon. As with ligament injury, tendinitis is treated with RICE (see page 65) and nonsteroidal anti-inflammatory medication such as aspirin or ibuprofen. Rehabilitative exercise programs can begin when the swelling is gone. Because corticosteroid injections can rupture knee tendons, they are rarely, and very carefully, given. Surgical repair of a severely ruptured tendon may be necessary.

Bursitis (see page 305) of the knee commonly occurs on the inside of the knee and on the front of the kneecap. Treatment is similar to that for the ligament and tendon injuries described above. Osteoarthritis (see page 308) is a common cause of pain and inflammation in the knees. In severe cases, surgery to replace the damaged knee joints (see Joint Replacement, page 310) may be necessary.

Other Bone and Joint Disorders

Here are some less common diseases and disorders that can affect the bones and joints:

- *Paget's disease.* Also called osteitis deformans, this chronic disorder disturbs the normal process of bone formation. The disease is more common among men and among adults age 40 and older. The cause of the disease is unknown. With Paget's disease, normal bone breaks down more rapidly than usual and is replaced by abnormal bone. The new, abnormal bone is larger but weaker than healthy bone. Paget's disease usually affects the leg bones, upper arm bone, collarbone, and pelvis. Bone pain, deformity, and fractures are the most common symptoms. A diagnosis of Paget's disease is confirmed with X rays and blood tests. Most cases do not require treatment other than painkillers such as aspirin and regular monitoring of the affected bones. In severe cases, treatment may include calcitonin or etidronate to relieve pain and to promote natural bone formation. In some cases, surgery to correct the bone deformities may be necessary.
- *Osteomalacia.* This condition weakens the bones of adults through demineralization (excessive loss of calcium and phosphorus). Osteomalacia is caused

by vitamin D deficiency, which usually results from insufficient vitamin D intake, limited exposure to sunlight, or inadequate absorption of vitamin D by the intestines. Kidney disease, certain metabolic disorders, and some medications also can increase the risk of developing osteomalacia. Symptoms include bone pain, usually in the neck, ribs, hips, and legs; restricted mobility; and difficulty walking. Diagnosis is based on symptoms, X rays, and the results of blood tests. Treatment focuses on increasing vitamin D levels in the body. The doctor also may recommend calcium supplements. Any underlying cause of the disease also must be treated.

- *Ankylosing spondylitis.* Ankylosing spondylitis is a form of arthritis that primarily affects the spine, shoulders, hips, and knees. Ankylosing spondylitis frequently begins between ages 20 and 40 and is more likely to occur in men than in women. It appears to run in families. Symptoms include pain and stiffness (in the lower back, especially after resting), chest pain, loss of appetite, and redness and pain in the eye (due to inflammation of the iris). As the disease progresses, it can be extremely painful and crippling. In severe cases, the vertebrae in the spine may fuse. Diagnosis is based on symptoms, blood tests, and X rays. There is no cure for ankylosing spondylitis. However, symptoms may be relieved with heat treatments, massage, and a supervised exercise program to strengthen the back muscles. The doctor also may prescribe nonsteroidal anti-inflammatory drugs to reduce pain and stiffness.

CHAPTER 16
Brain and Nervous System

Your brain is the most complex and least understood organ in your body. It interprets information gathered through the senses, initiates all body movement, stores information for later use, and controls thought and behavior. The cerebellum helps maintain posture and balance and the coordination of movements. The brain stem controls vital functions such as breathing. The uppermost part of the brain stem, known as the midbrain, controls some reflex actions and is involved in voluntary eye movements.

Your forebrain—the cerebrum and the structures inside it—manages abstract reasoning, learning, communication, sensation, emotion, and all other higher functions. The cerebrum is coated with a thin layer of gray tissue, called the cerebral cortex, where information processing occurs. Voluntary responses, such as movement and speech, are initiated inside the cerebrum, influenced by structures that control emotional state and modify perceptions. The hypothalamus is an important center of emotion and controls body temperature and sleep. The thalamus serves as a clearinghouse for information moving between the cerebrum and the brain stem and spinal cord. The hippocampus indexes memories. The basal ganglia (clusters of nerve cells adjacent to the thalamus) integrate movements.

Although your nervous system has many types of cells, the neuron serves as the main functional unit and is often referred to by the terms nerve cell or brain cell. Neurons have a central cell body, threadlike extensions called dendrites that spread out like short branches of a tree to receive messages from other nerve cells, and axons, which transmit messages between nerve cells. Other cells wrap around the axon, providing insulation and helping signals travel faster. At the end of each axon is a synapse, where signals pass from one nerve cell to another.

Chemicals called neurotransmitters enable brain cells to communicate with each other. Some neurotransmitters, such as acetylcholine or norepinephrine, make neurons react quickly. A neurotransmitter called gamma-aminobutyric acid (GABA) makes cells less excitable. Other neurotransmitters are serotonin, dopamine, and glutamate. Some medications used to treat neurological disorders adjust the level of specific neurotransmitters to restore normal function.

Your spinal cord, a complex bundle of nerves, carries messages between your brain and your body. Your brain and spinal cord together make up the central nervous system. Nerves that branch off from your spinal cord form the peripheral nervous system. Eight sets of nerves branch off from the cervical spine (neck), 12 sets from the thoracic spine (chest), five sets from the lumbar spine (lower back), and six sets from the sacrum (base of the backbone and tailbone). These nerves transmit instructions to all parts of the body and carry sensory information to the brain.

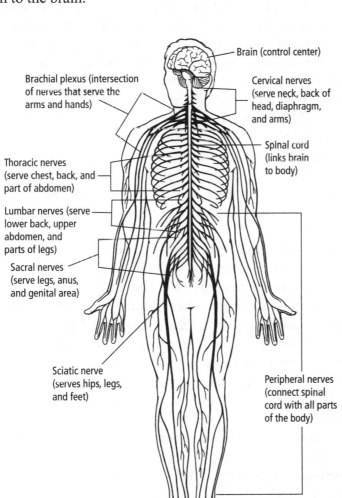

Brain (control center)

Brachial plexus (intersection of nerves that serve the arms and hands)

Cervical nerves (serve neck, back of head, diaphragm, and arms)

Spinal cord (links brain to body)

Thoracic nerves (serve chest, back, and part of abdomen)

Lumbar nerves (serve lower back, upper abdomen, and parts of legs)

Sacral nerves (serve legs, anus, and genital area)

Sciatic nerve (serves hips, legs, and feet)

Peripheral nerves (connect spinal cord with all parts of the body)

The Nervous System

The central nervous system is made up of the brain and spinal cord. The nerves that emanate from the spinal cord to the rest of the body make up the peripheral nervous system.

With spinal injuries, the exact location of nerve damage determines the function lost. For example, nerves in the arms or legs may be injured by compression. This occurs in carpal tunnel syndrome (see page 311), which affects peripheral nerves that pass through the wrist. Some disorders such as diabetes can affect many nerves at the same time, resulting in a condition called polyneuropathy.

Common Neurological Symptoms

The following are common symptoms of neurological disorders. Familiarity with these symptoms will help you to recognize the onset of a disorder or a new characteristic of an existing disorder.

- *Seizure.* A seizure is excessive electrical activity in the brain that can result in temporary loss of consciousness, memory, or motor control. The most common type of seizure, called a generalized seizure, begins with a loss of consciousness and motor control followed by violent, repetitive jerking of the limbs. During a partial seizure, a person usually remains conscious, although he or she may have hallucinations involving smell or vision, experience repetitive involuntary movements, or exhibit unusual behavior.
- *Tics.* Tics are involuntary and repetitive movements or actions that can be simple or complex. Simple tics are sudden, brief movements such as eye blinking, shoulder shrugging, facial grimacing, head jerking, yelping, and sniffing. Complex tics are coordinated patterns of movement involving several muscle groups such as jumping, smelling objects, touching the nose, touching other people, biting the lips, banging the head, and shouting obscenities or repeating the words of others.
- *Aphasia.* Aphasia refers to a disturbance or loss of language skills (comprehension, expression, or both) caused by injury to tissues in the language centers (called Broca's area and Wernicke's area) of the brain. Injury to Broca's area causes problems with language expression. Damage to Wernicke's area affects language comprehension. Global aphasia describes a loss of both language comprehension and expression caused by widespread damage to that side of the brain. Nominal aphasia refers to difficulty naming objects or thinking of a particular word. This may be caused by injury to a specific language center of the brain or by widespread brain dysfunction.
- *Apraxia.* Apraxia refers to the inability to perform certain tasks, such as tying one's shoes or dressing, because of loss of the ability to recall the sequence of steps that are necessary to perform such tasks. The person understands the task and sometimes can perform individual components of the task but cannot complete the entire task.
- *Amnesia.* Amnesia refers to loss of the ability to store information in memory or to recall information stored in memory. Amnesia can be classified broadly as immediate (lasts for a few seconds), intermediate (lasts for a few days), or

long term (lasts indefinitely). Sudden amnesia can be a sign of a serious neurological disorder.

- *Delirium and dementia.* Delirium refers to a temporary condition in which a person is disoriented and also may be irritable, fearful, delusional, or confused. Dementia refers to a permanent and progressive decline in intellectual function, insight, judgment, memory, and personality. In dementia, aphasia and apraxia (see above) may occur, along with depression, anxiety, paranoia, or an inability to recognize familiar faces, locations, or objects (agnosia).
- *Tremor.* Tremors are involuntary, rhythmic, back-and-forth movements caused by alternating contraction and relaxation of muscles. The most common type is a slight rapid tremor in the hands when the arms are stretched out in front of the body. Anxiety, fatigue, stress, and certain drugs can also cause tremors. Tremors that occur during intentional movements may result from injury to the cerebellum, the area of the brain that controls balance and coordination. Tremors that occur when a person is at rest may be due to Parkinson's disease.

Stroke

A stroke (also called a cerebrovascular accident) occurs when brain tissue is deprived of its blood supply. A stroke is the equivalent of a heart attack, but in the brain. Strokes can result from a blockage of blood flow to the brain (called an ischemic stroke) or from a ruptured blood vessel that bleeds into the brain (called a hemorrhagic stroke). Damage to the brain from a stroke begins within seconds of the interruption in blood flow.

About 80 percent of all strokes are ischemic strokes that result from a blockage in a blood vessel in the neck or the brain. Ischemic strokes can cause severe disability. There are three ways that blood flow can be blocked in an artery leading to the brain: when a clot forms inside the blood vessel (called cerebral thrombosis), when a clot travels from another part of the body and becomes lodged in a blood vessel (called cerebral embolism), or when an artery becomes severely narrowed (called stenosis).

Hemorrhagic strokes can result from rupture of an aneurysm (a weak, thin blood vessel wall); from changes in small arteries resulting from high blood pressure or diabetes; or, less commonly, from an arteriovenous malformation (see "Other Neurological Disorders," page 341). When the bleeding occurs within the brain itself, the stroke is classified as an intracerebral hemorrhage. If the bleeding occurs within the membranes between the brain and the skull, it is called a subarachnoid hemorrhage.

Sometimes blood flow to the brain is diminished or blocked for just a few minutes. This temporary cutoff of blood is called a transient ischemic attack (TIA). The symptoms of a TIA clear up quickly. Just as angina indicates an increased risk for heart attack, a TIA is a warning sign for a future stroke. Familiarize yourself with the following warning signs of stroke.

Warning Signs of a Stroke

Symptoms of a stroke often appear suddenly, without warning. If you have one or more of the following symptoms, call your doctor, 911, or your local emergency number immediately. The sooner you get treatment for a stroke, the more likely you are to recover. These symptoms may be accompanied by drowsiness, nausea, or vomiting.

* sudden numbness or weakness in your face, an arm or a leg, or on one side of your body
* sudden confusion or difficulty speaking or understanding speech
* sudden difficulty with vision (such as dimness or double vision) in one or both eyes
* sudden difficulty walking, dizziness, or loss of balance or coordination
* sudden severe headache with no obvious cause

A stroke can occur in anyone at any age. However, the following factors can increase your risk of having a stroke:

* *High blood pressure* is the leading risk factor for stroke. If your blood pressure is high (more than 140/90), work with your doctor to lower it (see page 217). High blood pressure in blood vessels in the brain can cause them to rupture. It also can cause blood vessels to narrow by thickening their walls. Obstructions such as blood clots and tiny pieces of fatty plaque may lodge in blood vessels that supply blood to the brain.
* *Smoking* has been linked to the buildup of fatty deposits in the walls of the carotid arteries, the main arteries in the neck that supply blood to the brain. Blockage of these arteries is a leading cause of stroke in white Americans. In addition, smoking raises blood pressure, reduces the amount of oxygen in the blood, and makes blood thicker and more likely to clot. (For information on quitting smoking, see page 107.)
* *Heart disease* can produce blood clots that may break loose and block blood vessels in or leading to the brain. Preventing or treating heart disease can reduce the risk of developing blood clots.
* *Prior TIAs or strokes* indicate that a problem exists in the blood vessels supplying the brain. Contact your doctor as soon as possible if you think you have had a TIA. Carefully following your doctor's advice will reduce your risk for stroke.
* *Diabetes* (see page 365) increases fatty deposits inside blood vessels throughout the body, including the brain. If blood glucose levels are high at the time of a stroke, the damage to the brain can be severe. Keeping diabetes under control will help reduce the risk of stroke.

If you have one or more of the above disorders or conditions, work closely with your doctor to reduce your risk for stroke. If you smoke, the sooner you quit, the sooner your risk for stroke will begin to decline. Most people at risk for stroke are advised by their doctors to take anticoagulants (blood thinners) such as warfarin, or platelet inhibitors (drugs that discourage formation of blood clots) such as aspirin, clopidogrel, or ticlopidine.

If the arteries that supply blood to your brain—the carotid arteries—are narrowed, your doctor may recommend a carotid endarterectomy (a surgical procedure to remove fatty deposits from the walls of the carotid arteries). Before surgery, your carotid arteries will be examined for blockages using a procedure called cerebral angiography (see "Diagnostic Procedures," page 342). In people who have significant narrowing of the carotid arteries that has caused a stroke or TIAs and who are at low risk for complications, carotid endarterectomy can significantly reduce the risk of stroke.

The severity of a stroke may range from mild to disabling to life-threatening, depending on the type of stroke and its location in the brain, the amount of tissue affected, and the amount of time that passes before treatment begins. Because each side of the brain controls the opposite side of the body, a stroke in the left side of the brain affects the right side of the body, and a stroke in the right side of the brain affects the left side of the body. Strokes in areas of the brain that carry out specific functions (such as speech, sight, or memory) will interfere with or possibly eliminate that ability. Strokes in vital brain structures can result in coma or even death. In a hemorrhagic stroke, bleeding from a ruptured artery can irritate other blood vessels in the brain, causing them to go into spasm and damage adjacent brain tissue.

The amount of damage caused by a stroke is directly related to promptness of treatment. Ideally, treatment should begin during the stroke. If injected within 3 hours of the onset of symptoms, a thrombolytic (clot-dissolving) drug such as tissue plasminogen activator (tPA) can greatly reduce long-term damage from an ischemic stroke. When contacting emergency medical personnel, be sure to tell them that you (or a family member or friend) have symptoms of a stroke.

For hemorrhagic strokes, doctors bring blood pressure under control, if necessary. In some cases blood may be drained to reduce pressure on surviving brain tissue and prevent further damage. The person may need to undergo surgery to repair a bleeding artery or to remove blood clots.

When blockages or other types of damage occur in small blood vessels in the brain, they may gradually destroy brain tissue in many areas. Over time, symptoms of dementia may develop, including confusion, loss of short-term memory, getting lost in familiar places, bladder or bowel incontinence, emotional disturbances, difficulty following instructions, or difficulty handling money. Symptoms usually begin after age 60.

Recovery after a Stroke

Loss of function after a stroke may be temporary or limited; some people recover most of the functions they have lost and continue to live independent lives. However, some people who have strokes need assistance with daily tasks (such as bathing or dressing). Others may become permanently dependent on family members, friends, or healthcare providers for all their daily care. Many people who do not immediately or fully recover from a stroke work with professional therapists who help them adapt to their limitations and function as independently as possible.

A physical therapist can help the person recover physical strength and mobility and prevent immobility by providing treatments such as exercise, massage, and manipulation. A physical therapist also can help the person learn to use equipment such as a walker or a cane properly. An occupational therapist can help the person regain muscle control and coordination and learn to compensate for his or her limitations. A speech therapist can work with the person to recover as much of his or her speech as possible and can teach the person (and his or her family) other methods of effective communication. A speech therapist also can help the person deal with breathing and swallowing problems.

After a stroke, many people experience feelings of depression (see page 345). They may feel frustrated or isolated, especially if they have not been able to return to their usual routine or if they are having problems communicating with others. Symptoms of depression include sleeplessness, indifference, and withdrawal. For most of these people, the depression is temporary. It may be helpful for the person to join a support group to share experiences and information with others who are in a similar situation. Talking with a psychiatrist or another mental health professional may help the person cope with and overcome his or her depression. To treat prolonged depression, a doctor may prescribe antidepressant medications such as tricyclic antidepressants, serotonin reuptake inhibitors, monoamine oxidase inhibitors, or bupropion.

Some people who have had a stroke may experience inconsistent and unpredictable mood changes. For example, they may laugh or cry inappropriately or may become irritable without apparent cause. In such cases it is important for family members and friends to understand that the person cannot control this behavior and that he or she will benefit from their patience and ongoing support.

Tumors of the Central Nervous System

In the brain and spinal cord, even benign (noncancerous) tumors can be debilitating or life-threatening. Because the brain and the spinal cord are enclosed within bony structures, there is no room for tissue expansion. Any abnormal growth or swelling puts pressure on delicate tissues and can cause damage and impair function. Benign tumors growing next to critical nerves, brain structures, or blood vessels can compress them and cause problems. Tumors deep in the brain or surrounding tissue can be difficult or even impossible to remove surgically. Cancerous tumors can damage tissue and impair function. They may spread to the brain from other parts of the body or originate in the brain or spinal cord.

Except for tumors that have spread from other parts of the body, the cause of brain and spinal cord tumors is unknown. Brain tumors can develop at any age. Spinal cord tumors are less common and are most likely to develop in young and middle-aged adults. Some genetic disorders, such as neurofibromatosis (in which many soft tumors grow from nerves in the skin) and tuberous sclerosis (a disorder causing an acnelike skin condition, mental retardation, and epilepsy), also can cause benign tumors to grow throughout the central nervous system.

Tumors of the central nervous system are named for the type of cell or tissue from which they grow. The most common types of tumors in adults include the following:

- *Chordoma.* This slow-growing tumor, which usually appears between ages 20 and 40, develops from tissue in the upper spinal cord.
- *Glioma.* This type of tumor grows from the glial cells in the brain. Gliomas account for about half of all brain tumors and about a fifth of all spinal cord tumors. Gliomas are categorized according to the type of glial cells from which they arise: astrocytoma (from astrocytes), oligodendroglioma (from oligodendroglia cells), ganglioneuroma (from glial cells and immature neurons), and mixed glioma (usually from astrocytes and other glial cells).
- *Meningioma.* Meningiomas develop from the meninges (the thin membranes that cover the brain and spinal cord). Meningiomas affect people of all ages but are most common among those in their 40s. Meningiomas grow slowly and rarely spread. Most are noncancerous. Small meningiomas may not cause any symptoms and may be detected by chance during a brain scan performed for another reason.
- *Pineal tumor.* Pineal tumors grow in the pineal gland, a small structure deep within the brain, and account for about 1 percent of brain tumors.
- *Pituitary adenoma.* The pituitary gland is an endocrine gland in the brain that releases hormones that help control the function of other endocrine glands and influence growth, metabolism, and maturation. Pituitary adenomas are noncancerous tumors that account for about 10 percent of brain tumors. If a pituitary adenoma grows, it can press on the optic nerves and impair side vision.
- *Schwannoma.* This type of noncancerous tumor arises from Schwann cells (cells that form a protective sheath around each neuron). One of the more common forms of schwannoma (an acoustic neuroma) affects the major nerve in the brain that is responsible for balance and hearing.

Tumors in the spinal cord are also named according to their location. For example, extradural tumors develop between the vertebrae and the dura (the tough membrane that protects the spinal cord). Tumors within the dura are either extramedullary (outside the spinal cord) or intramedullary (inside the spinal cord).

Brain tumors often do not cause symptoms until they have grown large enough to press on tissue, nerves, and blood vessels and affect brain function. When this occurs, a brain tumor can interfere with a specific sense, learned skill, or bodily function.

Warning Signs of a Brain Tumor

The symptoms described below may indicate a brain tumor or another neurological disorder. If you experience any of these symptoms, see your doctor as soon as possible.

- *Seizure.* Talk to your doctor immediately if you experience a seizure for the first time.
- *Loss of movement or sensation.* Gradual loss of movement or sensation in part of your body can indicate a growing brain tumor.
- *Unsteadiness.* Problems with balance, especially if accompanied by a headache, may be caused by certain brain tumors. Loss of balance should always be checked by your doctor.
- *Visual changes.* Partial, temporary, or gradual loss of vision—or double vision that occurs along with a headache—should never be ignored. Tell your doctor as soon as possible if you experience any changes in your vision.
- *Hearing loss.* Loss of hearing, especially in young to middle-aged adults, can result from certain brain tumors. Hearing loss due to a brain tumor is sometimes (but not always) accompanied by dizziness.
- *Difficulty speaking.* Gradual changes in your ability to speak or to use speech correctly (such as a persistent inability to recall words) should never be ignored. Tell your doctor about even minor changes in your ability to communicate.
- *Behavior changes.* Gradual—sometimes barely noticeable at first—changes in behavior and emotional stability can indicate a brain tumor. Memory loss, inability to concentrate, confusion, depression, apathy, and mood swings are sometimes symptoms of a brain tumor.
- *Headache.* Certain types of headaches are more likely to be caused by a brain tumor: a constant headache that is worse in the morning and eases slightly as the day goes on; a persistent headache that is accompanied by nausea or vomiting; or a headache that is accompanied by double vision, weakness, or numbness. If you experience any of these types of headaches, see your doctor as soon as possible.

Common symptoms of brain tumors include headaches and numbness or weakness in the arms and legs. The headaches tend to become more severe and last longer as the tumor grows, and they may be accompanied by nausea and vomiting. If the tumor disturbs the normal flow of electrical signals through the brain, seizures can occur. Pressure on certain nerves can lead to vision or hearing problems. Tumors that arise in the cerebrum, especially toward the front of the brain, can alter normal behavior, personality, memory, language, and learning skills. Tumors located toward the base of the brain can lead to weakness or paralysis (partial or complete loss of movement), lack of coordination, or difficulty walking.

A tumor on or near the spinal cord can disrupt the flow of sensory information (including pain) to the brain, or movement commands from the brain to the body. Pain caused by a spinal cord tumor may feel like it is coming from elsewhere in the body. Such pain is usually constant, sometimes severe, and often described as burning or aching. Tumor-related changes in sensation include numbness and decreased sensitivity to temperature. Because all muscles are controlled by nerves, tumors in the spinal cord can cause weakness, spasticity (stiffness and restriction of movement), paralysis, difficulty walking, or loss of bladder or bowel control.

Tests to diagnose a tumor in the brain or spinal cord include computed tomography (CT) scanning and magnetic resonance imaging (MRI; see "Diagnostic Procedures," page 342). You may also have cerebral angiography (see "Diagnostic Procedures," page 342)—an examination of the arteries deep inside the brain to assess the tumor's type and determine its exact position. Another possible test is an electroencephalogram (EEG), in which electrodes are attached to your scalp to monitor the electrical activity in your brain and help determine if the tumor is causing seizures or otherwise affecting brain function.

Specialized surgical techniques may be used to remove the tumor. Microsurgery uses a high-power microscope that allows the surgeon to view and access delicate brain tissue. Laser surgery uses powerful, concentrated beams of light to destroy the tumor. Ultrasonic aspiration uses high-frequency sound waves to break up the tumor and an aspirator to vacuum up the pieces. If a tumor cannot be removed and the flow of cerebrospinal fluid inside the brain or skull is blocked, a flexible tube called a shunt will be inserted to reroute and drain the fluid, relieving pressure on the brain.

If a tumor is malignant (cancerous) and cannot be removed completely, radiation therapy probably will be used to destroy tumor cells and shrink the tumor. Because radiation therapy destroys only dividing cells, it is particularly useful for treating brain tumors. Doctors use CT scanning and MRI to help focus treatment on the tumor and prevent radiation damage to healthy brain tissue.

Chemotherapy (treatment with powerful anticancer drugs) is used to shrink or destroy tumors. Other medications may also be used to relieve problems associated with the tumor. For example, corticosteroids are often prescribed to control the swelling in the brain or spinal cord that can result from a tumor.

Disorders of Brain Function

The underlying causes of certain neurological disorders such as Alzheimer's disease are not yet known. However, much is known about other neurological disorders—such as Parkinson's disease, multiple sclerosis, and migraines—although they are not yet fully understood. Research is ongoing to understand these disorders better and to develop effective treatments.

Alzheimer's Disease

Alzheimer's disease is a progressive disease in which brain cells degenerate and die, causing memory loss, confusion, loss of intellectual abilities (including thinking, reasoning, judgment, and memory), physical deterioration, and eventually death. It can also cause significant changes in mood, personality, and behavior. Alzheimer's disease is the most common form of irreversible dementia (progressive deterioration of mental functioning). The disease usually occurs after age 65, and progresses over a course of about 8 to 10 years. However, it can take as few as 2 or as many as 20 years.

The cause of Alzheimer's disease is unknown. Most people who develop Alzheimer's disease have no family history of it. Women are affected more often than men, but this may be related to the fact that women generally live longer and the disease occurs later in life. Alzheimer's disease is not a normal part of aging.

Symptoms of Alzheimer's disease, which vary from person to person, appear gradually and worsen over time. Initial symptoms—such as inability to concentrate, forgetfulness, anxiety, and depression—often go unnoticed or may be mistakenly attributed to normal aging. Memory problems eventually worsen, and the person also experiences impaired intellectual skills. He or she becomes apathetic and withdrawn. In later stages of the disease the person becomes severely confused and disoriented and also may become irritable, fearful, suspicious, delusional, agitated, and even violent. Eventually the person will be unable to perform daily activities (such as bathing, dressing, eating, and using the toilet) and will need total care.

Diagnosis of Alzheimer's disease is based on symptoms (as described by the person or his or her family members) and tests that evaluate various aspects of mental functioning (such as short-term memory). To make a diagnosis of Alzheimer's disease, the doctor

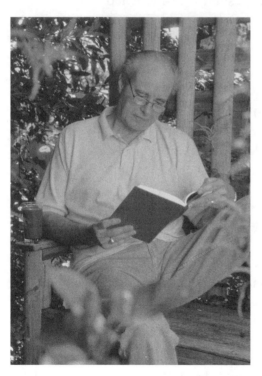

Stimulate Your Mind

Just as exercise strengthens your muscles, neurological research shows that "exercising" your brain may help keep it strong as you age. Engaging in intellectually stimulating activities such as reading, doing crossword puzzles, and learning new things increases the number of connections between the cells in your brain. Doctors now think that these extra connections may provide a buffer against the destructive effects of Alzheimer's disease and, in some cases, postpone the onset of symptoms.

needs to rule out other possible causes of the person's symptoms, such as depression (see page 345), kidney failure (see page 291), liver disease, thyroid disorders, excessive alcohol intake, side effects of medication, drug interactions, fatigue, poor diet, vision problems, and hearing problems. Parkinson's disease (see page 337), stroke (see page 323), and other neurological disorders, such as meningitis (see page 341) or encephalitis (see page 341), also can cause similar symptoms. Computed tomography (CT) scanning and magnetic resonance imaging (MRI; see "Diagnostic Procedures," page 342) are not performed to diagnose Alzheimer's disease but often are used to rule out other possible causes of dementia, such as a brain tumor (see page 326) or a stroke.

Although there is no cure for Alzheimer's disease, some people in the early to middle stages of the disease may benefit from medications (such as donepezil or tacrine) that help improve memory and manage some of the behavior problems caused by the disease. Other medications to treat or cure Alzheimer's disease are currently under investigation.

Caring for a Person Who Has Alzheimer's Disease   Caregiving can be demanding, stressful, and exhausting. If you are caring for a loved one who has Alzheimer's disease, learn all you can about the disease so you can be adequately prepared to deal with this challenging situation. Here are some useful recommendations for caregivers:

- Watch for warning signs of Alzheimer's disease (see next page) such as forgetfulness, confusion, or withdrawal. Some symptoms may be due to another underlying disease or condition—such as depression (see page 345)—that can be treated and cured.
- Gather useful information (such as educational materials and referrals to support groups) from reliable sources such as your doctor, your local library, your local hospital, and your local chapter of the Alzheimer's Association.
- Make all necessary legal and financial arrangements (including advance directives, durable power of attorney, and payment of healthcare costs) as soon as possible. This will help prevent potential legal and financial problems in the future. Contact a lawyer for additional information and assistance.
- Take all necessary precautions to protect your loved one from potential dangers such as falls, burns, poisoning, and wandering away from home. Taking steps such as locking away hazardous objects and materials (including medications, cleaning fluids, matches, lighters, and firearms), installing special locks on doors and windows, and placing night-lights along the route from the bedroom to the bathroom and in the bathroom itself can help prevent serious injuries. The Alzheimer's Association offers a nationwide program called Safe Return that registers people with memory problems and provides them

with special identification. The program maintains a 24-hour, toll-free number to call when a registered person is either lost or found. Contact your doctor or the Alzheimer's Association for additional information.

The Warning Signs of Alzheimer's Disease

The Alzheimer's Association has developed the following checklist of common symptoms to help you recognize the warning signs of Alzheimer's disease. (Some of these symptoms also may apply to other forms of dementia.) If you know someone who has several of these symptoms, he or she should see a physician for a complete examination.

- *Recent memory loss that affects job skills.* It is normal to occasionally forget assignments, colleagues' names, or business associates' telephone numbers, then remember them later. People who have dementia, such as Alzheimer's disease, may forget things more often and not remember them later.
- *Difficulty performing familiar tasks.* Busy people can be so distracted from time to time that they may leave the carrots on the stove and only remember to serve them at the end of the meal. People with Alzheimer's disease could prepare a meal and not only forget to serve it, but also forget they prepared it.
- *Problems with language.* Everyone has trouble finding the right word sometimes, but a person with Alzheimer's disease may forget simple words or substitute inappropriate words, making what he or she says incomprehensible.
- *Disorientation of time and place.* It is normal to forget the day of the week or your destination for a moment. But people with Alzheimer's disease can become lost on their own street, not knowing where they are, how they got there, or how to get back home.
- *Poor or decreased judgment.* People can become so immersed in an activity that they for-

get for a moment about the child they are watching. People with Alzheimer's disease could forget entirely about the child under their care. They may also dress inappropriately—for example, wearing an overcoat on a hot day or wearing several shirts or blouses at once.

- *Problems with abstract thinking.* Balancing a checkbook may be difficult for anyone when the task is more complicated than usual. A person with Alzheimer's disease could forget completely what the numbers are and what needs to be done with them.
- *Misplacing things.* Anyone can temporarily misplace a wallet or keys. A person with Alzheimer's disease may put things in inappropriate places—for example, an iron in the freezer or a wristwatch in the sugar bowl.
- *Changes in mood or behavior.* Everyone becomes sad or moody from time to time. A person with Alzheimer's disease can exhibit rapid mood swings—from calm to tears to anger—for no apparent reason.
- *Changes in personality.* People's personalities ordinarily change somewhat with age. But a person with Alzheimer's disease can change drastically, becoming extremely confused, suspicious, or fearful.
- *Loss of initiative.* It is normal to get bored with housework, a job, or social obligations from time to time but most people soon regain their initiative. A person with Alzheimer's disease, however, may become very passive for long periods of time and require cues and prompting to become involved.

- Seek help and support from others. Do not try to do everything yourself. Keep an updated list of things that need to be done, and ask reliable family members or friends for help whenever you need it. Contact your doctor, local hospitals, and volunteer, community, and health organizations for information and referrals. Join a support group to share information and experiences with others in a similar situation. Consider hiring a professional caregiver through a licensed home health agency.

- Be realistic about the inevitable outcome of the disease. Prepare yourself to deal with the loss of your loved one. Talking things over with a close friend or relative or with members of a support group will help you come to terms with your grief.

- Be prepared to make informed decisions about long-term care. A person with late-stage Alzheimer's disease needs total care. As soon as you learn that your loved one has Alzheimer's disease, begin gathering information about long-term-care facilities in your area so you will be able to make an informed decision when necessary.

- Take care of yourself. Take regularly scheduled breaks; eat a nutritious, well-balanced diet (see page 4); exercise regularly (see page 11); do not smoke (see page 107); and get plenty of sleep. Limit your intake of caffeine and alcohol, and use relaxation techniques (see page 119) such as meditation and deep-breathing exercises to help relieve stress.

Contact the Alzheimer's Association (800-272-3900) for additional information and advice on caring for a person who has Alzheimer's disease.

Amyotrophic Lateral Sclerosis

Amyotrophic lateral sclerosis (ALS), also called Lou Gehrig's disease, is a progressive motor neuron disease that has no known cause. In ALS, the motor neurons (nerve cells in the brain and spinal cord that control muscular activity) gradually degenerate, causing the muscles to weaken and waste away, eventually leading to paralysis. ALS occurs during middle age, and men are more likely to develop the disease than women.

Symptoms of ALS include tripping and falling, weakness in the hands and arms, and twitching and cramping of the muscles. As the disease progresses, it can cause difficulty speaking, swallowing, and breathing. In the final stages, although the person is aware and his or her intellect is unimpaired, he or she is unable to speak or move.

Diagnosis of ALS is based on the symptoms and on the results of various diagnostic procedures, including electromyography (an examination that measures the electrical activity of the muscles), blood tests, muscle biopsies (removal of small samples of muscle tissue for microscopic examination), and computed tomography (CT) scanning and magnetic resonance imaging (MRI; see "Diagnostic Procedures," page 342).

There is no way to prevent the disease or to reverse or slow its progression. Most people with ALS die within 5 years of diagnosis. Treatment focuses on relieving discomfort and helping the person stay independent for as long as possible. The person's life may be prolonged through the use of a ventilator (a machine that takes over breathing when a person can no longer breathe on his or her own) and feeding through a tube when a person has difficulty swallowing.

Epilepsy

In a person who has epilepsy, abnormal electrical activity in the brain causes seizures (temporary loss of consciousness or memory, or uncontrolled movements or behaviors). Epilepsy refers to a pattern of repeated seizures. The disorder can result from a brain tumor, stroke, head injury, lead poisoning, alcohol or other drug withdrawal, metabolic imbalances, or brain infections (such as encephalitis or meningitis).

There are two basic categories of seizures: generalized seizures, which affect the entire brain, and partial seizures, which affect only one area of the brain. The two most common types of generalized seizures are grand mal seizures and petit mal (or absence) seizures. During a grand mal seizure, the person experiences loss of balance and coordination, loss of consciousness, and uncontrollable jerking movements. In some cases the person may also experience loss of bladder or bowel control. A grand mal seizure can last for several minutes and leave the person disoriented and exhausted. The person usually does not remember the seizure.

Petit mal seizures occur most often in children. During a petit mal seizure, the person experiences loss of awareness that may last from a few seconds to about half a minute. Some people also experience brief confusion, muscle twitching, or rapid eye movements. The person is not aware of the seizure, and the symptoms are often subtle and may go unnoticed; the person may appear to be inattentive or daydreaming. This type of seizure may occur hundreds of times per day, seriously impairing the ability to concentrate or complete even simple tasks.

During a simple partial seizure, a person may experience sudden muscle twitches, tingling sensations, or hallucinations that affect smell, taste, or vision. This type of seizure lasts for several minutes. The person is aware of the seizure as it occurs and can recall what happened afterward.

During a complex partial seizure, a person appears dazed and may perform involuntary actions such as walking in circles, laughing, speaking nonsensically, or smacking his or her lips. The person is not aware of his or her actions. Afterward the person is confused and does not remember the seizure.

A diagnosis of epilepsy is based on the results of a thorough neurological examination (see "Diagnostic Procedures," page 342) and an evaluation of the type and pattern of the person's seizures. Because most people do not remember their seizures, information about the seizures is usually obtained from witnesses. The person will probably undergo an electroencephalogram (see "Diagnostic Procedures," page 342) to examine the electrical activity of the brain. Computed tomography (CT) scanning or magnetic resonance imaging (MRI; see "Diagnostic Procedures," page 342) will probably be performed to rule out other possible causes of the seizures, such as a brain tumor (see page 326) or a stroke (see page 323).

The risk of having a seizure increases with stress, sleep deprivation, fatigue, inadequate food intake, or failure to take prescribed medications. Seizures often occur spontaneously, but they can also be triggered by certain stimuli such as flickering or flashing lights, loud noises, or monotonous sounds. If you have grand mal seizures, you may be able to sense an oncoming seizure through feelings of unease or a recognizable sensory change (such as a specific sound, smell, or visual disturbance) called an aura.

Epilepsy is usually treated with anticonvulsant medications (such as primidone or diazepam) that prevent or control seizures. In rare cases, if medication does not control the seizures, surgery may be performed to remove the affected brain tissue. A special diet helps some people. Biofeedback (see page 118) also may be helpful. Most people with epilepsy live normal, productive lives with the help of medication.

How to Help During a Seizure

A person who is having a seizure may lose consciousness, fall to the ground, and move about violently. Here are some things you can do to help ensure that a person is not injured during a seizure.

- Do not panic.
- Do not try to restrain the person.
- Do not place your fingers or any object in the person's mouth during the seizure.
- Move away any large or sharp objects.
- After the seizure, make sure nothing is blocking the person's mouth or airway (such as food, gum, or dental devices).
- Place the person on his or her side.
- After the person regains consciousness, call a physician or take him or her to the nearest hospital emergency department.
- Call 911 or your local emergency number if the seizure lasts longer than 5 minutes or if the person has not had a seizure before.
- Call 911 if a second seizure begins shortly after the first seizure ends.

Multiple Sclerosis

Multiple sclerosis (MS) is a progressive, disabling disease of the central nervous system (the brain and spinal cord). MS is an autoimmune disease, in which the body's immune system mistakenly attacks and destroys its own tissue (in this case, the myelin that surrounds and protects nerve cells). Early in the disease, inflammation occurs at random sites in the brain or spinal cord, damaging myelin and causing scarring (sclerosis) that interferes with the transmission of messages between the brain and the body.

The initial symptoms of MS may include blurred or double vision, red color distortion, or blindness in one eye. Muscle weakness, lack of coordination and balance, fatigue, partial or complete paralysis, and spasticity (stiffness) can occur in the early stages of the disease. Other symptoms include numbness, tingling, tremors, dizziness, and slurred speech. About half of all people with MS also experience problems with concentration, attention, memory, and judgment, although intellectual and language skills remain unchanged. Depression and paranoia can occur, as can inappropriate mood swings. Sexual dysfunction and loss of bowel and bladder control also can occur. The symptoms may worsen when the body heats up from high environmental temperature, exercise, taking a hot bath, or having a fever. Early in the disease, symptoms often come and go. Later they may gradually worsen.

The symptoms of MS usually appear between ages 20 and 40, although a diagnosis may not be made immediately. A diagnosis is based on eliminating other possible causes of the symptoms, such as stroke (see page 323) or a brain tumor (see page 326), and detecting characteristic features of MS. For example, certain changes in the brain can be observed with magnetic resonance imaging (MRI; see "Diagnostic Procedures," page 342) after sufficient damage has occurred, and sometimes increased inflammatory proteins (antibodies) can be found in cerebrospinal fluid (obtained during a lumbar puncture; see "Diagnostic Procedures," page 342). These antibodies, which are produced for no known reason, are strongly associated with MS. In some cases the doctor may perform an evoked response test, in which electrodes are placed on the person's head, and electrical activity in the brain is recorded as he or she is exposed to various sensory stimuli such as sound or light.

The cause of MS is unknown. Evidence suggests that the disease may result from a combination of a person's genetic susceptibility (the disease tends to run in families) and a viral infection early in life. Environment also appears to have a role in susceptibility to MS. People who spend the first 15 years of their lives in a temperate climate have a higher risk of developing the disease later in life than those who spend their first 15 years in a tropical climate. This is thought to be the period when the viral infection occurs in susceptible people.

Whites are twice as likely as blacks to develop MS, and women are twice as likely to be affected as men (although, when the disease starts later in life, men are as likely as women to be affected). Most people with MS live a normal life span.

There is no cure for MS, although new treatments, such as interferon beta and glatiramer acetate, can reduce the likelihood of episodes and can slow progression of symptoms. Treatment will depend on symptoms. Corticosteroids (such as dexamethasone, methylprednisolone, or prednisone) or adrenocorticotropic hormone are prescribed to control inflammation in the nervous system during acute episodes, especially when the symptoms affect movement rather than sensation. To relieve fatigue, your doctor may prescribe amantadine or modafinil. He or she also will advise you to help prevent fatigue by staying cool (such as with air conditioning).

The doctor may prescribe muscle relaxants to relieve muscle spasms and also may recommend that you swim or participate in a water therapy program. Physical therapy can help maintain muscle strength and improve your balance and coordination. Occupational therapy can help you learn easier ways to perform daily tasks. For urinary incontinence, your doctor may prescribe an antispasmodic medication (such as dicyclomine or hyoscyamine) to relax the bladder and control muscle contractions.

Parkinson's Disease

Parkinson's disease is a progressive degenerative disease like amyotrophic lateral sclerosis (see page 333), though it has a much slower course. Researchers believe that a combination of factors—including environmental toxins, genetic predisposition, accelerated aging, or damage to cells from free radicals—may bring about the disease. The average age of onset is 60, but many younger adults have early symptoms. Men and women are affected equally by Parkinson's disease.

In Parkinson's disease, the neurons in the basal ganglia (clusters of paired nerve cells deep inside the brain) that control muscular activity become damaged or die. These nerve cells produce an important neurotransmitter (chemical messenger) called dopamine, which has an essential role in controlling muscle actions. Without sufficient dopamine, the nerve impulses are disrupted, causing the primary symptoms of the disease: tremor (trembling) in the hands, feet, arms, legs, and head; stiffness and weakness; slow movement; and impaired balance and coordination.

The early symptoms of Parkinson's disease are subtle and appear gradually. The hands and feet may tremble slightly. Eventually the person's speech may become slow and halting, and his or her handwriting will become very small. Some people may have a flat facial expression and become stiff and unsteady. As the disease progresses, they may experience problems with memory and thought processes. The skin may become oily (especially on the forehead, nose, and scalp) or very dry, or excessive sweating may occur. People with Parkinson's disease often have difficulty sleeping. Depression also is common.

A diagnosis of Parkinson's disease is based on the symptoms. There is no cure for the disease, but medication can relieve the symptoms for most people in less severe stages of the disease. The most common medication is levodopa (also called L-dopa), which the body converts to dopamine. Not all symptoms respond well to levodopa, and those that do will return if the medication is stopped. Anticholinergic drugs such as benztropine may be prescribed to relieve tremor. Brain surgery to reduce tremor and rigidity may be performed on some people for whom medication has not been effective. Although the progression of Parkinson's disease cannot be slowed, treatment to relieve symptoms can help people continue to lead active lives.

Tourette's Syndrome

Tourette's syndrome is a rare inherited disorder characterized by involuntary movements and nasal and vocal sounds. Researchers believe that the abnormality in the gene or genes responsible for the disease affects the way the brain controls neurotransmitters (chemical messengers such as serotonin and dopamine). Symptoms usually begin before age 18, and men are up to four times more likely to have the disease than women. In some cases the symptoms are not noticeable or do not continue into adulthood.

Early symptoms of the disease include facial tics such as eye blinking, nose twitching, or grimaces. (Note that most such tics are not due to Tourette's syndrome.) Over time the tics may become more noticeable and may include head jerking, neck stretching, foot stamping, and body twisting or bending. The person also may make strange noises, such as coughing, sniffing, grunting, yelping, barking, or shouting. More disturbing symptoms, such as involuntary shouting of obscenities, constantly echoing words of others, touching others excessively, or repeating actions obsessively, also may occur. In severe cases people with Tourette's syndrome may harm themselves by biting their lips and cheeks and banging their heads against hard objects.

Tics periodically change in number, frequency, type, and location. They also may disappear for a time and then reappear. If a person tries to suppress a tic, tension will build until the tic occurs, often in a more dramatic manner. Tics tend to worsen in stressful situations and improve during periods of relaxation or when the person concentrates on another activity.

Tourette's syndrome is diagnosed through monitoring of symptoms (the tics must be present for at least 1 year) and confirmation of a family history of the disease. In some cases neurological tests may reveal another cause of the symptoms.

There is no cure for Tourette's syndrome, although symptoms tend to decrease with age. The disorder does not affect the intellect. The person may not require any treatment, but the doctor may prescribe medications to reduce specific symptoms that interfere with daily routine. Relaxation techniques (see page 119) and biofeedback (see page 118) can help prevent tics.

Headaches

A headache is a very common type of pain. The pain of a headache may extend over the entire head, or it may be limited to a specific area. Headache pain may range from mild to severe. Unusual or sudden changes in posture or prolonged coughing, sneezing, or exposure to sunlight can lead to a headache. In some cases, however, a headache may be a symptom of a serious underlying condition, such as a stroke or a brain tumor.

Call your doctor immediately if your headache is severe or persistent, if it occurs after a blow to the head, or if it is accompanied by any of the following:

- fever
- nausea
- stiff neck
- pain in your eye or ear
- dizziness, confusion, or loss of consciousness
- weakness or paralysis
- seizures

Tension headaches (also called muscle contraction headaches) are the most common type of headache. These headaches produce mild to moderate pain that feels as though pressure is being applied to the head or neck. The pain may be accompanied by muscle tenderness. Tension headaches can be brought on by head or neck injury, anxiety, stress, eyestrain, or poor posture. If the headaches occur almost every day, they are referred to as chronic daily headaches, and they may cause fatigue, depression, and difficulty sleeping.

A *migraine* is a severe, persistent headache accompanied by certain recognizable symptoms. Migraine headaches produce intense throbbing pain that occurs on one side of the head and may spread to the other side. Evidence suggests that susceptibility to migraines is inherited.

Symptoms may include nausea, vomiting, diarrhea, sensitivity to light and noise, fever, chills, aches, and sweating. Some people experience a specific warning sign called an aura, such as a visual disturbance, just before the onset of a migraine. Migraine attacks usually last for a few hours, but more severe episodes may last for a few days. Attacks can occur several times per week or once every few years. A migraine can be completely disabling; following an attack, the person is often exhausted, irritable, or unable to concentrate.

People who have migraines may be able to identify triggers (specific substances, conditions, or circumstances that can bring on a headache), such as alcohol, monosodium glutamate (MSG; found in processed foods), tyramine (found in aged cheese and red wine), or nitrates and nitrites (found in processed meat products). Other potential triggers include fluorescent lights, glaring light (such as from computer screens), high altitudes, strong smells, and sudden changes in temperature or barometric pressure.

A *cluster headache* is a series of headaches that affects one side of the head. Cluster headaches come on suddenly and produce intense symptoms, which may include a runny nose; drooping eyelid; and an irritated, watery eye on the affected side. The pain often centers just behind the eye. Cluster headaches often occur early in the morning and can be as brief as 15 minutes or as long as 3 hours. With episodic cluster headaches, attacks occur daily or several times per day for many weeks or months and then disappear for an extended period (months or years). With chronic cluster headaches, attacks occur at least once per week.

Over-the-counter pain relievers such as aspirin, acetaminophen, and ibuprofen will relieve most headaches. Some antidepressants are useful for treating chronic pain and may help reduce the occurrence of most types of headaches. Muscle relaxants may reduce the pain of muscle contraction headaches. People with migraine headaches can take ergot alkaloids or serotonin agonists at the onset of symptoms to help reduce the severity and duration of their headaches. Migraines

Headache Diary

Keeping a headache diary is a good way to help you identify the factors that trigger your headaches so that you can take steps to prevent future headaches. Whenever you have a headache, carefully mark down the following information:

- date
- time headache began
- time headache ended
- intensity of pain (such as mild, moderate, or severe)
- type of pain (such as aching, throbbing, or stabbing)
- location of pain
- other symptoms (such as nausea, vomiting, or sensitivity to light)
- medication taken for headache (type and amount) and results
- self-treatment for headache (such as sleep, cold compresses, or relaxation techniques) and results

- activity you were engaged in (such as sleeping or exercising) when headache began
- your location when headache began (such as indoors or outdoors)
- potential allergens nearby when headache began (such as pollen, tobacco smoke, dust, or pets)
- other environmental factors (such as noises, odors, or weather)
- food or drink consumed before headache began
- your emotional state before headache began (such as angry, stressed, or tired)
- medication you are taking for other reasons (both prescription and over the counter)

Take your headache diary with you when you visit your doctor. The information it contains will reveal any patterns related to your headaches, which is helpful for determining the triggers of your headaches and recommending appropriate treatment.

often can be reduced or prevented in people who experience frequent episodes by daily use of medication. If you have frequent headaches you will benefit from keeping a headache diary (see previous page) to track your headache triggers, symptoms, and sources of relief.

Other Neurological Disorders

This section describes several less common disorders of the central nervous system.

- *Meningitis.* Meningitis is inflammation of the meninges (the membranes that surround the brain and spinal cord), usually caused by a viral or bacterial infection. Symptoms often appear suddenly and include high fever, severe and persistent headache, sensitivity to light, stiff neck, nausea, and vomiting. In viral meningitis the symptoms are less severe. Symptoms of bacterial meningitis develop more rapidly and are followed by drowsiness and, in some cases, loss of consciousness. Viral meningitis usually clears up within a week or two and requires no treatment other than medication to relieve pain. Bacterial meningitis is a medical emergency and requires immediate treatment with large doses of antibiotics given intravenously. Contact your doctor immediately if you have symptoms of meningitis.
- *Encephalitis.* Encephalitis is inflammation of the brain, usually caused by a viral infection. Symptoms include sudden fever, headache, vomiting, sensitivity to light, stiff neck and back, confusion, drowsiness, clumsiness, unsteady gait, and irritability. More serious symptoms include muscle weakness, changes in behavior, memory loss, impaired judgment, seizures, and loss of consciousness. Some types of encephalitis may be treated with drugs such as acyclovir. In most cases, however, treatment focuses on relieving symptoms, keeping the person comfortable, and allowing the body's immune system to fight the infection. The doctor may prescribe anticonvulsant medication to prevent seizures and corticosteroid drugs to reduce swelling in the brain. Some cases of encephalitis are short and relatively mild. Other cases can be severe, causing long-term disability or even death. Symptoms of encephalitis require immediate evaluation by a physician because early diagnosis and treatment may prevent serious, perhaps fatal, complications.
- *Arteriovenous malformation.* An arteriovenous malformation (AVM) is a congenital (present from birth) disorder in which there is a tangled web of arteries and veins in the brain or spinal cord. Symptoms include bleeding (at the site of the malformed blood vessels), seizures, headaches, paralysis, loss of speech or vision, or other neurological symptoms. Once detected, the AVM can be removed surgically, closed off by injecting a special medicinal glue (in a procedure called embolization), or shrunk with radiation. If an AVM is untreated it can bleed into the brain or spinal cord, causing severe disability or death.

- *Bell's palsy.* Bell's palsy is a temporary paralysis of facial muscles due to inflammation of one of the facial nerves. Usually only one side of the face is affected. Symptoms include weakness, twitching, or paralysis (which may prevent the eye from closing completely), drooling, and impairment of taste. Other symptoms may include pain, watery eye, and hypersensitivity to sound. Bell's palsy can occur in anyone at any age but is more common among pregnant women and people who have diabetes or a viral infection such as the flu, a cold, or cold sores. There is no specific treatment, and symptoms often clear up on their own in people who do not have other related illnesses. Sometimes facial weakness is caused by a more serious disease. If you have other symptoms, or if the condition does not improve quickly, see your doctor.

Diagnostic Procedures

If you have symptoms of a neurological disorder, your doctor will use one or more of the following diagnostic procedures to determine the cause of your symptoms. He or she may refer you to a neurologist (a physician who specializes in treating disorders of the brain and spinal cord) for further evaluation and treatment.

- *Neurological examination.* During a neurological examination, a physician performs a variety of physical tests to check the functioning of a person's nervous system. He or she will test vision (by examining eye movement, pupil reaction, and other eye reflexes); reflexes (by tapping the knee with a rubber hammer, for example); hearing; sensation (by gently sticking the foot with a pin); movement (by asking the person to perform simple tasks); and balance and coordination (by asking the person, for example, to balance on one foot, touch the nose with the eyes closed, or walk heel-to-toe).
- *Lumbar puncture.* For a lumbar puncture (also called a spinal tap), a hollow needle is inserted into the spinal column in your lower back to obtain a sample of cerebrospinal fluid, which circulates around the brain and spinal cord. The fluid is examined for signs of infection, cancer, bleeding, or inflammation. A lumbar puncture also is performed as part of myelography (see next page).
- *Electroencephalography.* This is a painless examination in which electrodes are placed on the scalp to record the electrical activity of the brain. Electroencephalography helps identify signs of a tumor, epilepsy, or other neurological disorders.
- *Computed tomography (CT) scanning.* CT scanning uses computer and low-dose X rays to produce detailed cross-sectional images of body tissues such as the brain and spinal cord. The images, which are clearer than conventional X-ray images, are displayed on a video monitor. During the procedure, you lie on a table inside a circular opening in the scanner. A contrast medium (a dye) may be injected before the scan to highlight blood vessels, organs, or any abnormalities. The procedure is painless.

- *Magnetic resonance imaging (MRI).* MRI uses a computer, a powerful magnet, and radio waves to create detailed two- or three-dimensional images of body tissues. The images are displayed on a video monitor. MRI often produces better images than CT scanning, especially when the tissue being examined is located near bone. The procedure is painless and has no known side effects. During the procedure, you lie in a tunnel inside the magnet. Some people feel claustrophobic during an MRI. You are given a signal button to hold so that you can signal the technician to stop the procedure if you become anxious. If you think that you might feel claustrophobic during the MRI, ask the doctor for a tranquilizer before the procedure. Because the magnet makes loud knocking noises, you may be offered headphones to wear during the procedure, to help block the noise. Also, because of the powerful magnetic field that is created during the procedure, you cannot carry or wear any metal objects (such as jewelry or a watch) or electronic devices (such as a hearing aid or a pager). You cannot have an MRI if you have a pacemaker or any magnetic metal (including plates, screws, or artificial joints) implanted in your body.

- *Cerebral angiography.* This diagnostic procedure is used to examine the arteries in the brain and the carotid arteries in the neck and to help diagnose problems such as narrowed or blocked arteries, aneurysms (see page 323), and arteriovenous malformations (see page 341). In cerebral angiography, a catheter (a thin, flexible tube) is inserted into the femoral artery, a large blood vessel in the groin area, and threaded up through the main blood vessels of the abdomen and chest and into the main arteries in the neck (carotid arteries). Contrast medium (a dye) is injected through the catheter into the arteries, and a series of rapid-sequence X rays (similar to a movie) is taken. The images are displayed on a video monitor. Cerebral angiography produces better images than carotid ultrasound (see below) and allows the doctor to look deeper inside the brain.

- *Myelography.* Before CT scanning and MRI (see above) became available, doctors relied on myelography to look inside the spinal canal. In this procedure, contrast medium is injected into the spinal canal after a lumbar puncture, and a series of X rays is taken. Because the procedure is lengthy and may be painful, myelography is generally used only when CT scanning or MRI cannot be performed or do not provide enough information.

- *Carotid ultrasound.* If you are at risk for stroke (see page 323) or have experienced a transient ischemic attack (see page 323), you will likely undergo a carotid ultrasound. In this procedure, sound waves are used to produce images that help the doctor detect changes in the rate of blood flow through the carotid arteries (the major arteries in the neck that supply blood to the brain). The images, which are displayed on a video monitor, reveal blockages or potential blockages in the carotid arteries.

CHAPTER 17

Mental Disorders

A mental disorder is a condition that affects a person's thinking and shows in his or her feelings and behavior. The term "mental disorder" is misleading because it implies that a mental disorder is distinct from a physical disorder. In reality, many forms of mental illness arise from a physical cause, such as an imbalance in brain chemistry. In addition, the experience of a person with a mental disorder is no less real than the experience of a person with a physical disease, and it can be just as devastating.

Common mental disorders include mood disorders, anxiety disorders, sleep disorders, and psychotic disorders. They can cause a wide variety of symptoms, such as inappropriate anxiety, disturbances of thought and perception, and mood disturbances. These disorders are legitimate medical problems. They do not go away just by trying to shake off the symptoms, and they do not come about because the affected person has a character flaw or weakness. Mental disorders can be triggered by stressful negative or positive life events, such as the loss of a job, a promotion, the birth of a child, or a divorce. Sometimes, however, they occur with no obvious cause, changing the person's personality and affecting his or her work and relationships.

Many mental disorders go untreated in men because some men may not recognize the symptoms of a mental disorder. Other men may feel ashamed or fear the social stigma of having a mental disorder and may be reluctant to seek help. Many men do not even know that help is available. In fact, only about 20 percent of people with mental disorders seek treatment. In addition, health insurance coverage for mental problems is often inadequate. This is unfortunate because medical science has made great advances in determining the causes of and appropriate treatment for many mental disorders. A wide range of effective treatments for mental disorders is now readily available. If you think you may have a mental disorder, talk about the problem with your doctor. He or she can refer you to the proper mental health specialist so you can get the help you need.

Mood Disorders

Mood disorders, sometimes referred to as affective disorders, are a type of mental illness that affects a person's mood. Everyone experiences occasional periods of sadness or euphoria (a strong sense of well-being), but people with a mood disorder feel these emotions more strongly than other people and for longer periods. About one in seven people is affected by a mood disorder each year. Possible causes include an inherited predisposition, an imbalance in brain chemicals that regulate mood, and environmental factors—or a combination of all three. The most common mood disorders include depression, bipolar disorder (formerly known as manic depression), and seasonal affective disorder (SAD). In general, mood disorders are among the most treatable of all mental disorders.

Depression

It is normal to feel unhappy in response to a personal loss or stressful situation, but such feelings usually go away with the passage of time. Depression, on the other hand, can cause deep feelings of sadness or despair that can last for months or even years. Depressed men often feel overwhelmed by life and become emotionally and physically withdrawn.

Depression is a serious condition that can have profound effects on a man's quality of life. Long-term bouts of depression can negatively affect your ability to function at work and in social situations. It can also severely limit your capacity to enjoy the basic pleasures of life—your family, your friends, your favorite activities, and your sex life. More than 18 million people experience depression in the United States every year. It can occur at any age but usually seems to first appear between ages 25 and 45. Although men are only half as likely to have severe depression as are women, depressed men are four times as likely to commit suicide than depressed women (although women attempt suicide more frequently). In fact, men over age 55 have the highest risk of suicide among Americans. Untreated depression is the leading cause of suicide in the United States.

Symptoms of depression include persistent sadness or despair, insomnia, decreased appetite, irritability, apathy, withdrawal from social situations, loss of energy, poor self-esteem, feelings of hopelessness or helplessness, an inability to enjoy former interests, a decreased interest in sex, and suicidal thoughts. Depression also can cause you to lose interest in your appearance. The tone of your voice may be dull and flat and your pattern of speech monotonous. Frequent bouts of crying, often with no apparent cause, are common.

The Warning Signs of Suicide

Depression is the number one risk factor for suicide. In fact, 70 percent of all people who commit suicide are depressed. Although men attempt suicide only a third as often as do women, men are more likely to be successful in the attempt. The highest suicide rates are for men over age 85, but suicide also is the third leading cause of death among younger men aged 15 to 24 years. Married men are less likely to attempt or commit suicide than are separated, divorced, or widowed men. Facing adverse life events, such as financial loss, can alter the chemistry in the brain, increasing the risk for suicide, especially if the person already has an emotional disorder or is abusing drugs or alcohol. Risk factors for suicide include a family history of an emotional disorder, substance abuse, suicide, or physical or sexual abuse; a prior suicide attempt; having a gun in the home; imprisonment; impulsive behavior; and exposure to the suicidal behavior of others (especially for teens or young men).

A suicide attempt—or even talking about suicide—should never be dismissed as a mere attention-getting ploy. Attempted suicide is always a cry for help from a person who is usually battling some type of emotional disorder, such as depression, or a substance abuse problem. Most people with depression or substance abuse can be treated successfully and go on to lead healthy lives. If someone you know begins talking about or threatening to commit suicide, take the person seriously and try to get him or her to see a doctor, or call a suicide hot line. A suicide attempt is often preceded by certain telltale warning signs, such as:

- talking about suicide or death, even jokingly
- difficulty dealing with the loss of a loved one or some other adverse life event
- withdrawal from friends and activities
- hoarding of pills or purchase of a gun
- abuse of drugs or alcohol
- giving away prized possessions
- a previous suicide attempt
- writing notes or poems about death
- changes in eating or sleeping habits
- neglect of personal appearance

The best way to prevent a suicide attempt is to get professional help for an emotional disorder or substance-abuse problem. Recognition of depression in older men can go a long way toward preventing suicide, especially if they are living alone. Limiting access to guns, especially in combination with treatment of an emotional disorder, also is an effective way to prevent suicide attempts in high-risk men. If someone you know is in immediate danger, call 911 or your local emergency number.

Some people have a recurrent but less severe form of depression, called dysthymia. Dysthymia is diagnosed when a depressed mood persists for at least 2 years and is accompanied by at least two other symptoms of depression. People with this milder form of depression are susceptible to periodic episodes of major depression.

Doctors think that a number of factors may combine to cause depression. A deficit in certain brain chemicals—particularly serotonin and norepinephrine—seems to cause the anxiety, irritability, and fatigue often experienced in the disorder. A family history of depression also can increase your chances of having the disorder. Certain environmental factors—such as exposure to violence or emotional or physical abuse—also seem to have a role. People who have low self-esteem or a pessimistic outlook seem to be more susceptible to depression than those who are more self-confident and optimistic.

The good news is that depression responds very well to treatment, even in people who have had the disorder for many years. Up to 90 percent of depressed people who receive treatment experience a reversal of their symptoms. If you have symptoms of depression, your primary care doctor probably will refer you to a psychiatrist (a doctor who specializes in treating mental disorders) for treatment. Before he or she prescribes any form of treatment, the psychiatrist will request that your primary care doctor perform a complete physical examination. If these evaluations reveal no physical cause for your symptoms, your psychiatrist will then conduct a psychological evaluation.

Doctors usually treat depression with antidepressant medication, often combined with psychotherapy or psychological counseling. The purpose of drug treatment is to correct any imbalance in brain chemistry. The most common drugs prescribed to treat depression are selective serotonin reuptake inhibitors (such as fluoxetine, fluvoxamine, and paroxetine) and tricyclic antidepressants (such as amitriptyline, desipramine, and nortriptyline). These drugs are not tranquilizers or sedatives and are not addictive. Antidepressant medications can improve the symptoms of depression in 4 to 6 weeks, although the person needs to continue taking them for at least 5 months (usually longer) after symptoms improve.

Psychotherapy may be recommended for an individual or a family, or in a group setting with other people who are experiencing depression. Individual psychotherapy takes place in the office of a psychiatrist or psychologist, in regularly scheduled 30- to 45-minute sessions. The goal of psychotherapy is to relieve the person's distressing symptoms so that he or she can resume a normal routine. There are different types of psychotherapy. One type involves helping the person understand unconscious and unresolved conflicts. Another emphasizes changing negative patterns of thinking. A third attempts to replace ineffective behaviors with more positive constructive behaviors. Ask your therapist which type he or she recommends and why. Treatment can last several weeks, months, or years, depending on the severity of the depression.

In extreme cases of severe depression, a psychiatrist may admit the person to the psychiatric unit of a hospital for full, 24-hour care. The doctor will develop a treatment plan, which will be carried out by a team of mental health professionals that includes the psychiatrist, psychiatric nurses, a clinical psychologist, a social worker, rehabilitation therapists, and an addiction counselor, if needed. The treatment plan usually includes individual, group, or family therapy, along with medication. The person usually remains hospitalized for about 6 to 12 days.

Bipolar Disorder

Bipolar disorder, in which periods of deep depression alternate with episodes of euphoria or mania, affects about 1 percent of Americans. The disorder's wide mood swings continue indefinitely, interrupted by periods of remission or normal mood. The depressed phase produces typical symptoms of depression, such as sadness or despair, loss of interest in favorite activities, fatigue, and thoughts of suicide (see page 346). During the manic phase, affected people experience persistently elevated mood and energy, delusions of grandeur, feelings of invincibility, unrealistically high self-esteem, agitated movement, talkativeness, abrasive and rapid speech, racing thoughts and distractibility, poor judgment, poor impulse control, and a decreased need for sleep. Some people in the manic phase also go on unrestrained buying sprees or have impulsive, indiscreet sexual encounters. Extreme mania can lead to delirium (mental confusion) or paranoia (excessive or irrational suspiciousness). Manic states can last for days, weeks, or months and may begin gradually or suddenly. They are followed by a period of normal mood or by an episode of depression. Initial episodes of mania frequently occur between ages 15 and 25.

Bipolar disorder affects an equal number of men and women. It tends to run in families; up to 90 percent of those affected have a relative with either bipolar disorder or depression. The illness also has been linked to both an imbalance in brain chemistry and a deficiency in the production of certain hormones (substances produced by the body that control key bodily functions). The severe mood swings characteristic of the disorder can seriously affect a person's life, upsetting personal relationships and disrupting routines at work. Although everyday occurrences can trigger a manic episode, dates that have significant meaning for the person, such as the anniversary of a parent's death, are especially likely to trigger one.

Like depression (see page 345), bipolar disorder is readily treatable, but because the affected person feels so elated and invincible, he or she may dismiss the need for treatment or refuse to comply with prescribed treatment. Medications that are most commonly used to treat bipolar disorder include mood stabilizers (such as lithium), antidepressants (such as fluoxetine or bupropion), and antipsychotic drugs (such as haloperidol), often in combination. The hallmark mood stabilizer for bipolar disorder is lithium carbonate, a naturally occurring mineral salt. Lithium controls the manic phase of bipolar disorder by affecting the central nervous system's control over emotion. Its effectiveness depends on the amount of the drug in the bloodstream, so lithium must be taken exactly as prescribed. A blood test can be performed to ensure a therapeutic level. For people who do not respond well to lithium, doctors may use other mood stabilizers, such as divalproex sodium or carbamazepine. Most mood stabilizers produce side effects, including weight gain, thirst, hand tremors, and muscle weakness.

Doctors may prescribe antidepressants during the depressive phase of bipolar disorder, but they usually instruct the person to resume taking a mood stabilizer once the depressive phase has ended. Antipsychotic drugs are used predominantly for people whose manic phase has escalated into a psychotic episode (loss of awareness of reality).

Psychotherapy, also called talk therapy, can boost the effectiveness of the drugs used to treat bipolar disorder by helping those with the illness learn how to become more aware of their symptoms, deal with stressful life events, and comply with drug treatment. This kind of therapy works best when the therapist is experienced in treating bipolar disorder. Because families also are affected by the disorder, family members may be offered counseling to help strengthen relationships that have been strained by the illness. People with very severe cases of bipolar disorder may need hospitalization or, in extreme cases, electroconvulsive therapy, in which a current of electricity is passed through the brain to induce seizures. This treatment may be highly effective within a few weeks (usually three treatments per week). Memory loss may occur, but the memory returns within a few months.

Seasonal Affective Disorder

Seasonal affective disorder (SAD) is a type of mood disorder that brings on depression when the seasons change. The most common type of SAD is known as winter depression, which usually starts in the late fall or early winter and ends in spring. Many people without SAD feel "blue" and more fatigued when the days get shorter. However, people with winter depression experience true depression, along with symptoms that are not typical of a depressive disorder, including excessive sleeping, increased appetite, a craving for high-carbohydrate foods, irritability, and weight gain. A smaller number of people experience another form of the disorder known as summer depression, which usually begins in late spring or early summer. Signs of summer depression include the more typical depressive symptoms of decreased appetite, weight loss, and sleeplessness. The cause of summer depression is not known. Both forms of SAD seem to recur at the same time each year. SAD can occur along with a bipolar disorder (see previous page) or depression (see page 345). Women are affected by SAD four times as often as men.

Doctors think that winter depression may be brought on by the reduction in the amount of sunlight that occurs during the winter months. A good argument for this theory is that SAD is more common in people living in the northern latitudes than in those living farther south. In addition, artificial, bright-light therapy, also known as phototherapy, is very effective in treating winter depression. In a typical phototherapy session, people with the disorder sit in front of a desktop light box or wear a light visor, initially for 10 to 15 minutes per day, increasing to 30 to 45 minutes per day. Benefits may not be seen for several days to several weeks. It is important to continue phototherapy until spring, when the person can obtain increased natural light from the sun. Phototherapy appears to have few side effects, although some people may experience headaches, fatigue, irritability, and insomnia if they take light therapy too late in the day. These side effects can be reduced by sitting farther from the light source or by decreasing the length of the phototherapy sessions.

Tanning beds are not recommended for the treatment of winter depression because they emit high levels of ultraviolet rays, which are harmful to the eyes and the skin. Phototherapy is often combined with drug therapy or psychotherapy to treat winter depression. The drug of choice for this type of SAD is called a monoamine oxidase inhibitor (such as isocarboxazid or phenelzine).

Doctors treat summer depression differently than the winter form of SAD. Summer depression responds better to the antidepressants usually prescribed for nonseasonal depression (see page 345).

Anxiety Disorders

Fear is the driving force behind anxiety disorders. Each of us experiences fear throughout the course of our lives. But instead of feeling the reasonable fear that helps us recognize and respond to immediate danger, such as narrowly avoiding a traffic accident, people with an anxiety disorder experience fear that occurs in response to dangers that are either imagined or not immediately threatening. Such people experience almost constant feelings of worry or dread that interfere with their daily activities, along with symptoms of anxiety such as rapid heartbeat and increased perspiration.

Anxiety disorders are the most prevalent mental disorders in adults. About 30 million people in the United States have some type of anxiety disorder, and twice as many women as men are affected. Anxiety disorders appear to arise from a combination of stressful life experiences, psychological traits, and genetic inheritance, although certain disorders—such as panic disorder (see page 352)—appear to have a stronger genetic component than others. The most common anxiety disorders include generalized anxiety disorder, phobias, panic disorder, obsessive-compulsive disorder, and posttraumatic stress disorder.

Generalized Anxiety Disorder

People who have generalized anxiety disorder experience ongoing but unrealistic worry or dread about the circumstances of daily life. The excessive worries often pertain to many areas of the affected person's life, including work, relationships, finances, personal health, the well-being of one's family, perceived misfortunes, and impending deadlines. Affected people can experience a variety of symptoms, including feelings of fear and dread, restlessness, muscle tension, a rapid heart rate, light-headedness, poor concentration, insomnia, increased perspiration, cold hands and feet, and shortness of breath. Symptoms typically worsen during stressful periods.

Generalized anxiety disorder affects only half as many men as women. It begins in childhood or adolescence in about 50 percent of affected people but does not seem to run in families.

Phobias

There are three major types of phobias: specific phobias, social phobias, and agoraphobia. Specific phobias are those triggered by fear of a specific object, such as snakes or spiders. Claustrophobia (fear of enclosed spaces), acrophobia (fear of heights), and fear of flying or driving also fall into this category. About 8 percent of American adults experience one or more specific phobias in any given year. Typically developing in childhood, many specific phobias disappear by adulthood. Those that last into adulthood usually require treatment.

Social phobia describes persistent anxiety in social situations, based on fear of embarrassment or ridicule. People with a social phobia become preoccupied with concern that other people will notice their anxious symptoms—such as blushing, sweating, or trembling—or that their mind will go blank when speaking to someone else. Like stage fright, social phobia causes intense fear when the person is aware that other people can observe him or her doing even simple things, such as eating a meal in a restaurant or putting on a coat. A more general form of the disorder provokes fear during most interactions with other people. People with a social phobia often avoid socializing and even can have difficulty attending school or keeping a job. Performance anxiety and fear of public speaking also fall into this category of phobias. Social phobia affects men and women in equal numbers and usually develops in childhood or adolescence. It has been linked to shyness and tends to run in families.

Agoraphobia, a term that literally means "fear of the open marketplace," refers to fear of being in public places, such as streets, shopping malls, theaters, airplanes, and other places where people gather. People with agoraphobia fear that they will not be able to escape from a given place or that no one will be available to help them in such circumstances. People with agoraphobia often do not venture out of their homes unless accompanied by someone else. Agoraphobia is the most serious type of phobia because in the most extreme cases, affected people refuse to leave their homes at all. The disorder most often develops from the constant worry, preoccupation, and avoidance that occurs following a series of panic attacks (see below). Agoraphobia occurs twice as often in women as in men.

Many doctors use desensitization techniques to treat phobias. Desensitization involves gradually exposing a person to the trigger (object or situation that he or she fears) in an attempt to teach the person to react without fear. Medication and psychotherapy also are typically used to treat phobias.

Panic Disorder

Panic attacks are brief and very intense episodes of a high level of anxiety that often occur with no apparent cause. A panic attack can produce sweating, shortness of breath, rapid heart rate, chest pain, numbness or tingling, trembling, and nausea or stomach pains. Most affected people also report feeling that they are losing control, "going crazy," or dying. An attack typically starts suddenly and builds to its maximum intensity in 10 to 15 minutes, rarely lasting more than 30 minutes. The experience provokes a strong urge to flee and often causes the person to seek help at a hospital emergency department. After the person experiences one or more panic attacks, he or she begins to anticipate more of them and may begin to avoid activities or situations, such as riding in an elevator, that seem to trigger them. Anxiety caused by merely thinking of the possibility of another attack can cause the person to become reclusive. Extreme cases of panic disorder can lead to agoraphobia (fear of being in public places).

Panic disorder is about twice as common in women as in men. Typically the disorder first appears between late adolescence and middle age. Panic attacks do not always indicate an underlying mental illness; up to 10 percent of people experience an isolated panic attack each year. A panic disorder can occur when other mental disorders, such as social phobia (see previous page), generalized anxiety disorder (see previous page), or depression (see page 345), also are present. Doctors can confirm a diagnosis of panic disorder when the person has experienced at least two panic attacks and develops persistent concern about having additional attacks.

Obsessive-Compulsive Disorder

Obsessions are recurrent, intrusive thoughts, impulses, or images that the affected person perceives as being inappropriate, grotesque, or forbidden. These thoughts seem unlike the person's usual thoughts and can cause anxiety and distress. The obsessions also seem uncontrollable, and the person becomes afraid that he or she will lose control and act upon them. Common themes of obsessions include contamination with germs, worry that the person has unknowingly inflicted harm upon someone else, or loss of control over violent or sexual impulses.

Compulsions, on the other hand, are repetitive behaviors or patterns of thought that reduce the anxiety that accompanies an obsession or that "prevent" some dreaded event from occurring. Compulsions can take the form of repeated, ritualistic patterns of hand washing, checking, counting, or praying. For example, the person may count to ten 30 times or may count backward. He or she may recite a certain prayer or passages from the Bible in a specific sequence. Compulsive rituals can consume long periods of time. The presence of both obsessions and compulsions constitutes obsessive-compulsive disorder.

Obsessive-compulsive disorder affects about $2\frac{1}{2}$ percent of Americans and is equally common among men and women. It typically begins in adolescence or young adulthood in males. As with generalized anxiety disorder (see page 351), symptoms tend to worsen during stressful periods. There is strong evidence that the disorder runs in families.

Posttraumatic Stress Disorder

Posttraumatic stress disorder refers to the anxiety and disturbances in behavior that develop after experiencing an extreme trauma, such as witnessing a murder, experiencing torture, being in a serious accident, or participating in military combat. A critical feature of posttraumatic stress disorder is the psychological symptom of dissociation, a perceived detachment of the mind from the person's emotional state or even from the body. Dissociation is also characterized by a dreamlike or unreal perception of the world and may be accompanied by poor memory of the traumatic event. Other symptoms of posttraumatic stress disorder include general anxiety, a heightened sense of arousal, avoidance of situations that elicit memories of the trauma, and intrusive recollections of the event in flashbacks, dreams, or recurrent thoughts. Symptoms of the disorder may be immediate or delayed, beginning 6 months or more after the traumatic event.

A person with posttraumatic stress disorder experiences decreased self-esteem and a loss of long-held beliefs about people or society. He or she begins to feel hopeless and permanently damaged by the traumatic experience and begins to have difficulty with personal relationships. Substance abuse often develops as the person attempts to relieve such feelings by using alcohol, marijuana, or sedatives.

Posttraumatic stress disorder is most common among women who are rape victims. Women are twice as likely to have the disorder as men. The disorder is also common in concentration-camp survivors and Vietnam War veterans. About half of all people with posttraumatic stress disorder recover within 6 months. For the others, the disorder typically persists for years and may dominate their lives.

Treatment of Anxiety Disorders   Anxiety disorders are usually treated with some form of counseling or psychotherapy (see page 347), often combined with drug treatment. Doctors now use more focused, time-limited forms of therapy that teach the affected person how to cope with the symptoms of anxiety rather than exploring unconscious conflicts. A critical element of such therapy is gradual but increasing exposure to the object or situation that causes the anxiety in order to stop the affected person from avoiding anxiety-inducing situations.

Medications that doctors typically prescribe to treat anxiety disorders are those that readjust imbalances in neurotransmitters (chemicals that carry messages between brain cells). Such medications include benzodiazepines, antidepressants (such as paroxetine or fluoxetine), and an antianxiety medication called buspirone. Benzodiazepines such as clonazepam, diazepam, and lorazepam have antianxiety and sedative effects but can be habit-forming. Buspirone is useful for treating generalized anxiety disorder and, unlike the benzodiazepines, is not addictive.

Sleep Disorders

The amount of sleep needed each night varies from person to person, but most healthy men need 8 to 8½ hours of sleep per night to be fully alert during the day. If a man does not get enough sleep—even for one night—he may experience drowsiness that disrupts his daily routine.

Certain medical conditions and drugs also can interrupt sleep and cause daytime drowsiness. Problems such as asthma (see page 245), congestive heart failure (see page 233), and rheumatoid arthritis (see page 309) or any other painful condition can keep you from getting a good night's sleep. Medication used to treat high blood pressure or heart disease, and asthma medications such as theophylline, also can interfere with sleep. Alcohol can help you to fall asleep but causes sleep disruption later in the night and can produce early morning headaches. The sedative effects of alcohol also can put you at increased risk for motor vehicle collisions if you drink and drive. Caffeine, which stays in the body for 3 to 7 hours after ingestion, makes it harder to fall asleep and stay asleep. The nicotine in cigarettes and nicotine patches is a stimulant that also can disrupt sleep.

Many men who work the night shift have difficulty sleeping. Most night-shift workers get less sleep overall than day workers. The human sleep-wake cycle is designed to prepare the body for sleep at night and wakefulness during the day. These natural rhythms make it harder for a person to sleep during the day and to work at night. In addition, lights, noise (such as from telephones), and family members can be annoying distractions that disrupt daytime sleep.

If you have problem with sleepiness, monitor your sleep-wake patterns. If you are consistently getting fewer than 8 hours of sleep per night, try to get more sleep by gradually moving to an earlier bedtime. If your schedule does not permit you to go to bed earlier, try to squeeze in a 30- to 60-minute daily nap. If you are sleepy, do not drive; sleepiness will increase your risk of having a collision.

If you think you are getting enough sleep but still feel sleepy during the day, you may have a sleep disorder. Talk to your doctor, who can evaluate your symptoms and prescribe appropriate treatment.

Some men have medically recognized sleep disorders. The most common sleep disorders are insomnia, sleep apnea, narcolepsy, and restless legs syndrome.

Insomnia

Most people need a full 8 hours of sleep, while some can function well with less. Many people, however, are unsatisfied with the amount of sleep they get. Insomnia refers to inadequate or poor-quality sleep, usually the result of difficulty falling asleep, frequent waking during the night, or rising too early in the morning. Once the person wakes during the night or early in the morning, he or she has difficulty going back to sleep. Insomnia can cause fatigue, lack of energy, difficulty concentrating, and irritability.

Insomnia that lasts only a few weeks or less is called transient insomnia. If episodes of insomnia occur from time to time, the problem is called intermittent insomnia. Insomnia that occurs on most nights and lasts a month or longer is called chronic insomnia.

Factors that may contribute to insomnia include being older and having a history of depression (see page 345). Although insomnia occurs in men and women of all ages, it seems to be more common in women and older people. Transient insomnia and intermittent insomnia often occur in people who are experiencing temporary problems such as stress, noisy sleeping conditions, extreme heat or cold, jet lag, or side effects of medications.

The causes of chronic insomnia are more complex, often involving a number of underlying disorders. One of the most common causes of chronic insomnia is depression (see page 345). Other causes include arthritis (see page 308), kidney disease (see page 288), heart failure (see page 233), asthma (see page 245), sleep apnea (see next page), narcolepsy (see page 357), restless legs syndrome (see page 358), Parkinson's disease (see page 337), and hyperthyroidism (see page 374).

Lifestyle factors such as overuse of caffeine, alcohol, or other drugs; shift work; smoking cigarettes before bedtime; excessive daytime napping; or chronic stress also have a role in the development of insomnia. Stopping these behaviors may help eliminate insomnia.

If you have insomnia, your doctor will take a complete health history (see page 82) and a sleep history. To obtain a sleep history, the doctor will ask you to keep a sleep diary or interview your sleep partner to find out how much sound sleep you typically get each night. Transient and intermittent insomnia may require no treatment because it often clears up when the underlying problem, such as jet lag, is resolved. If your daytime performance is adversely affected by transient insomnia, your doctor may prescribe a short-acting sleeping pill for a brief period.

To treat chronic insomnia, your doctor will first diagnose and treat any underlying medical or psychological problems you may have. He or she may prescribe a sleeping pill, but only for a brief period to minimize unwanted side effects or dependence on the pills for sleep. Certain behavioral techniques also are often used to improve sleep. One such technique is relaxation therapy, which is used to eliminate anxiety and muscle tension. Some people with insomnia benefit from sleep restriction, which at first allows only a few hours of sleep each night, and gradually increases sleep time to a more normal span of time. Another helpful treatment is called reconditioning, which teaches the affected person to associate the bed and bedtime with sleep by avoiding use of the bed for any activity other than sleep or sex.

Sleep Apnea

Sleep apnea is a serious, potentially life-threatening breathing disorder that is characterized by brief, involuntary interruptions of breathing during sleep. There are two types of sleep apnea: obstructive and central. Obstructive sleep apnea, the most common type, occurs when air cannot flow into or out of the person's nose or mouth because of an obstruction caused by a relaxed and sagging tongue or a sagging uvula (the small piece of tissue that hangs from the center of the back of the throat) during sleep. Central sleep apnea, which is less common, occurs when the brain fails to send the proper signals to the muscles used in breathing to continue regular inhalation and exhalation during sleep.

During any given night, a person with sleep apnea may involuntarily stop breathing 20 to 30 times per hour. These pauses in breathing are usually accompanied by snoring, although not everyone who snores has sleep apnea. The snoring occurs because, although the person continues to try to breathe, air cannot flow easily in and out of the mouth. Choking also can occur.

During the pause in breathing, the person is unable to inhale oxygen and exhale carbon dioxide, resulting in increased levels of carbon dioxide in the blood. This increase in carbon dioxide alerts the brain to wake the person. Breathing often resumes with a loud snort or a gasp. The frequent arousal prevents the person from getting enough sleep and often causes early morning headaches and daytime drowsiness. Daytime concentration and performance suffer due to sleep deprivation.

Sleep apnea occurs in all age groups but is more common in men than in women. More than 12 million people in the United States are estimated to have the disorder. People most likely to have sleep apnea are those who snore loudly and also are overweight, have high blood pressure, or have a physical abnormality inside the nose or upper airway. The problem appears to run in families, suggesting a possible genetic cause.

To diagnose sleep apnea, doctors use two tests, performed either at a sleep center or at home. One test is polysomnography, which records various body functions—such as the electrical activity of the brain, eye movement, muscle activity, heart rate, and blood oxygen levels—during sleep. A test called the multiple sleep latency test measures how fast a person falls asleep. (It takes most people 10 to 20 minutes to fall asleep; people who habitually fall asleep in fewer than 5 minutes are likely to require treatment for a sleep disorder.)

Treatment for sleep apnea depends on the underlying cause. Lifestyle changes are enough to reverse the disorder in some people. Such changes may include avoiding the use of alcohol, tobacco (see page 107), and sleeping pills, all of which can make the airway more likely to collapse during sleep. Overweight people can benefit from losing weight (see page 73). People in whom sleep apnea occurs only when they sleep on their backs are advised to sleep on their sides. The most common treatment for the disorder is called continuous positive airway pressure, in which the person wears a mask over the nose during sleep so that pressure from an air blower can force air through the nasal passages. The process also helps prevent the airway from collapsing during sleep. Side effects may include nasal irritation and drying, facial skin irritation, sore eyes, headaches, and abdominal bloating. Dental appliances can reposition the lower jaw and tongue during sleep to reduce the risk of airway obstruction. Medications are generally not effective for treating sleep apnea.

Some people with sleep apnea undergo surgery to increase the size of their airways. Common surgical procedures include removal of the adenoids (tissue at the back of the nasal cavity that helps the body fight infection), tonsils, nasal polyps, or uvula and part of the soft palate. People with life-threatening sleep apnea may need a tracheostomy, in which a small hole is made in the windpipe and a tube is inserted through which air can flow directly into the lungs while the person sleeps.

Narcolepsy

People who have narcolepsy experience such overwhelming daytime sleepiness—even after adequate sleep at night—that they become drowsy or fall asleep at inappropriate times and places during the day. Such "sleep attacks" can occur repeatedly during a given day and may come on without warning. Another classic symptom of narcolepsy is cataplexy (sudden episodes of loss of muscle function that cause the person to collapse suddenly or his or her neck to go limp). Sleep paralysis often occurs, preventing the affected person from moving while falling asleep or waking up. Some people also have vivid hallucinations while falling asleep. Such symptoms can seriously disrupt the person's life and limit his or her activities.

Narcolepsy occurs in both men and women and can begin at any age. As many as 200,000 people are affected, although the problem is often underdiagnosed or misdiagnosed as depression, epilepsy, or side effects of medication. Doctors think that a disturbance in the normal order of sleep stages causes narcolepsy. Most people first go through a stage of nonrapid eye movement (NREM) when falling asleep, followed by a stage of rapid eye movement (REM), when dreaming and muscle relaxation occur. In people with narcolepsy, these stages are reversed.

To diagnose narcolepsy, doctors perform two tests—polysomnography and the multiple sleep latency test (see page 356)—at a sleep center or at the person's home.

There is no cure for narcolepsy, but certain treatments can relieve symptoms. Drugs called central nervous system stimulants (such as methylphenidate, dextroamphetamine, or modafinil) can help manage the excessive daytime sleepiness caused by narcolepsy. Antidepressants (such as amitriptyline or fluoxetine) also are prescribed. An important part of treatment is scheduling short naps two to three times per day to help relieve daytime sleepiness. Some people with narcolepsy and their families find it helpful to join a support group where they can learn to deal with the emotional effects of the disorder, talk about occupational limitations, and find out how to avoid situations that could cause injury.

Restless Legs Syndrome

Restless legs syndrome is a sleep disorder in which a person experiences unpleasant sensations in the legs. People who have this disorder often describe the sensations as creeping, crawling, tingling, pulling, or painful feelings in the calves, although the entire leg can be affected. These sensations can occur when the person lies down or sits for long periods, such as in bed, at a desk, or riding in a car. Moving, rubbing, or massaging the legs brings relief, at least briefly. People with restless legs syndrome find it difficult to relax and fall asleep, often sleeping best during the morning hours. A lack of sufficient sleep at night causes daytime drowsiness and affects performance at home and at work. Many people with restless legs syndrome have periodic limb movement, which is characterized by involuntary jerking or bending leg movements that occur every 10 to 60 seconds during sleep.

The cause of restless legs syndrome remains unknown, but certain factors have been linked to the disorder. They include a family history of the disorder; pregnancy; low levels of iron in the blood; diseases such as kidney failure (see page 291), diabetes (see page 365), and rheumatoid arthritis (see page 309); and a high caffeine intake.

Both men and women can develop restless legs syndrome, which is more common and more severe among older people. An accurate diagnosis often depends on how well the person can describe his or her symptoms because there is no visible abnormality in the legs and there is no diagnostic test to detect the disorder. Mild cases of restless legs syndrome respond well to self-treatments such as taking a hot bath, massaging the legs, using a heating pad or an ice pack, exercising, and eliminating caffeine. More serious cases are treated with benzodiazepines (such as clonazepam or diazepam) and opioids (such as codeine or propoxyphene). These drugs do not cure restless legs syndrome but only treat the symptoms. Some people respond well to a nondrug treatment called transcutaneous electric nerve stimulation (TENS), in which electrical stimulation is applied to the legs or feet for 15 to 30 minutes before bed to reduce leg jerking during sleep.

Psychotic Disorders

A psychosis is a serious mental disorder in which a person loses touch with reality and cannot tell whether he or she is having a real-life experience or an unreal one. The two most common types of psychosis are schizophrenia and delusional disorder.

Schizophrenia

Schizophrenia is a devastating brain disorder that can be extremely disabling. The first signs of the disorder are often confusing and shocking to family and friends. Schizophrenia is characterized by profound disruptions in thought and emotion that can affect language, perception, and a person's sense of self. It can produce a wide array of symptoms. Some symptoms, called positive symptoms, show an excess of or distortion in normal functioning. They include hearing voices or other hallucinations, delusions (such as the belief that radio or television programs are sending special messages directly to the affected person), disorganized or incoherent speech, unpredictable agitation, purposeless and bizarre behavior, and catatonia (unawareness and rigid or unusual postures). So called negative symptoms reflect a loss of normal functioning. They include a flat facial expression and tone of voice, a lack of speech fluency, apathy, and the inability to begin or maintain any type of goal-oriented behavior. No single symptom defines the disorder, but rather a pattern of symptoms that is accompanied by difficulty holding a job or functioning in society. Several subtypes of schizophrenia, defined by their predominant symptom, have been identified. For example, a person with paranoid schizophrenia is preoccupied by delusions or "hearing voices."

Schizophrenia is often misunderstood. Many people mistakenly think that the disorder causes multiple personalities. Some people may fear that a person with schizophrenia is violent and dangerous, although most people affected with schizophrenia are not violent. The best way to think of schizophrenia is to compare a normal brain to a functioning telephone switching system in which the calls (in the form of perceptions) come in and are routed to the proper destination. But in the brain of a person with schizophrenia, the switching system malfunctions. Incoming calls can be sent along the wrong pathway, leave the pathway, or arrive at the wrong destination. Incoming perceptions and outgoing messages become disorganized or blocked.

More than 2 million people in the United States have schizophrenia. It usually appears during young adulthood. Onset can be either sudden or gradual. Researchers have found that susceptibility to schizophrenia may be inherited, but there is also some evidence that impairment in fetal brain development may also have a role in the disorder. Many people with schizophrenia are severely disabled and stigmatized by the disorder, which affects their careers and relationships.

Antipsychotic medications (such as haloperidol, thioridazine, or fluphenazine) are prescribed to treat the hallucinations and delusions that frequently occur and may also help improve emotional expression. Most of these medications are taken by mouth, but seriously affected people may have to take them by injection. Antipsychotic medications can produce side effects such as muscle spasms, drowsiness, faintness, dry mouth, blurred vision, sensitivity to sunlight, and constipation. Some men who take these medications have difficulty with sexual function.

Only one person in five fully recovers from schizophrenia, and about 10 percent of affected people remain severely ill over long periods, even with treatment. In another 50 percent, symptoms improve, sometimes significantly. Most people with schizophrenia will need treatment for the rest of their lives. Some people with schizophrenia may deny that they need medications and refuse to take them. Others forget to take their medications because of the disorganized thinking that is characteristic of the disease.

This behavior makes it difficult to help a friend or family member who may be showing signs of schizophrenia. If you know someone who may have schizophrenia, you may be more successful in getting him or her to seek treatment by focusing on one symptom, such as depression or difficulty sleeping. Above all, try to maintain a caring, helpful manner when approaching someone who may have this type of psychotic disorder, since they often are anxious and suspicious of others.

Delusional Disorder

Many people with schizophrenia have delusions (tenaciously held false beliefs), but not all people with delusions have schizophrenia. Doctors diagnose a person with a delusional disorder if he or she has a persistent delusion that involves a situation that could occur in daily life, such as being poisoned or followed, but shows no other signs of schizophrenia. Aside from the odd manifestations of the delusion, the person's behavior is not unusual, and his or her functioning at home and work is not impaired.

Delusions fall into a number of distinct categories. The most common type of delusion is that of persecution by others. People with this type of delusional disorder believe that their friends, family, or coworkers are conspiring to drug or spy on them or to ruin their reputations.

Another form of delusional disorder that is frequently encountered is delusional jealousy, in which the person takes everyday occurrences, such as a partner's returning home a bit late from work, as evidence of unfaithfulness. Erotic delusions compel the affected person to believe that he or she is loved by someone with high status, such as the president of the company he or she works for or a famous actor. People who have grandiose delusions believe that they have special powers that could save the world or cure a disease. Delusional disorder also can take the form of somatic delusions, in which the person thinks that there is something seriously wrong with his or her body—that it is misshapen, produces a foul odor, or has insects crawling on it.

The treatment of choice for a delusional disorder is drug therapy, but drugs are not always successful in treating the disorder. Delusions that persist for a long period can be difficult for doctors to treat. If the affected person is unable to function in daily life, or if he or she poses a threat to himself or herself or others, the person will have to be hospitalized.

Living with a Person Who Has a Mental Disorder

About 51 million people in the United States have some form of emotional or mental disorder. Because mental illness is so common, many Americans cope with the day-to-day struggle of sharing a home with a person who is mentally ill. Living with a person who has a mental disorder can be challenging and stressful, and most family members are not adequately prepared for the experience. Many families also fear the stigma that still surrounds many types of mental illness. But effective treatments exist for many mental disorders, and help is readily available. The first step in dealing with a loved one's problems is to recognize the warning signs of a mental disorder:

- confused thinking
- long periods of depression
- extreme mood swings (from elation to sadness)
- high levels of fear, worry, or anxiety
- withdrawal from people and activities
- significant changes in eating or sleeping habits
- rage
- delusions or hallucinations
- thoughts of suicide or homicide
- denying the existence of a problem
- unexplained physical illnesses
- substance abuse

The symptoms of many mental disorders are similar, so many families share the same experiences. The behaviors—including withdrawal, angry outbursts, or disorganized speech—that characterize certain mental disorders can be shocking and embarrassing when performed in public. If you are in such a situation, remember that the person cannot help what he or she is doing. Try to encourage the person to move to a more private place until he or she is calm. Discuss with the person's doctor what to do in such situations so that you can be prepared the next time.

To help fight the stigma of mental illness, you can become an advocate for your loved one. Ask the doctor about the person's specific needs and try to fill them. For example, someone who has delusional disorder (see page 360) may be able to hold a job but may need an understanding boss who is willing to overlook the person's delusional behavior as long as it does not interfere with work. Many people have misconceptions about mental illness; you can work to correct these misconceptions and help them change their attitudes and the way they interact with people who are mentally ill.

Many people who live with someone who has a mental disorder find it helpful to join a support group. These groups offer a protective environment in which you can share your concerns and learn coping strategies from people who face similar challenges. If there is no local support group that deals with your particular situation, consider starting one. Other people in similar situations may be happy to participate.

Family or individual counseling often benefits partners or family members. A therapist or counselor familiar with the type of mental disorder involved can teach you about the disorder and suggest ways to handle typical situations you may encounter. Talk to a number of therapists before beginning counseling to find one who is knowledgeable about the disorder and with whom you feel comfortable.

Having a person with a mental disorder in the family alters the dynamics of family life. The affected person tends to become the focal point around which family life revolves. Caregivers or other family members can often feel slighted and overwhelmed, and may become resentful. Children, especially, can feel ignored. They also may feel embarrassed when an insensitive friend makes fun of the affected person. It is important to try to balance the needs of the person with the needs of the other members of your household. Plan special activities with the other members of your family—especially your children—to make them feel included and to draw you together as a family.

Caregivers can easily become overwhelmed by their responsibilities. Because of this, you should not attempt to handle everything yourself; the full responsibility of caregiving should never fall on one person. A caregiver who is on call 24 hours a day will burn out quickly. Schedule regular breaks from your caregiving duties. When you need an unscheduled break, arrange to have a dependable relative or a friend fill in for you.

Keep an updated list of things that need to be done. Identify as many people as possible who can provide help. Every member of your household can participate or contribute in some way. Ask your friends and relatives, too. Offer them choices from your list, such as doing chores, running errands, preparing meals, making telephone calls, and providing company. Be direct. Do not hesitate to ask for help whenever you need it.

If family members or friends cannot help, contact volunteer and community organizations, as well as your doctor and local hospitals and health organizations. If you belong to a support group, ask the group members for suggestions. You also may want to hire a professional caregiver through a licensed home health agency, such as a visiting nurse association.

Caring for yourself is an essential part of being a caregiver. To succeed as a caregiver, it is vital that you follow a healthy lifestyle. Eat a nutritious, well-balanced diet (see page 4), exercise regularly (see page 11), do not smoke (see page 107), and get plenty of sleep. Try to limit your intake of caffeine and alcohol. And be sure to use relaxation techniques (see page 119), such as meditation and deep-breathing exercises, to relieve stress.

CHAPTER 18
Endocrine System

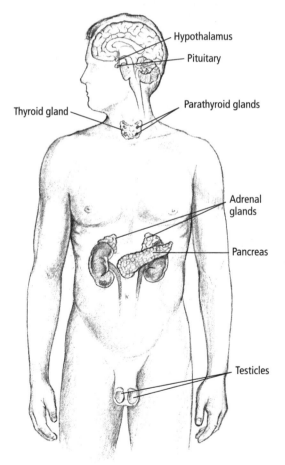

Endocrine System

The endocrine system is a network of glands, organs, and tissues designed to release directly into the bloodstream hormones that control many essential body processes. The glands of the endocrine system include the following:

- *Hypothalamus.* The hypothalamus is the region of the brain that coordinates production and release of hormones by the pituitary gland, the thyroid gland, the adrenal glands, and the testicles.
- *Pituitary gland.* The pituitary gland is the most important endocrine gland. It is often called the master gland because it produces hormones that control other endocrine glands and many essential body processes.
- *Thyroid gland.* The thyroid gland produces the hormones thyroxine and triiodothyronine, which have an important role in metabolism (the chemical processes that take place in your body), and calcitonin, which helps regulate the calcium level in your blood and helps your bones retain calcium.
- *Parathyroid glands.* The parathyroid glands produce parathyroid hormone, which helps regulate the calcium level in your blood.

- *Adrenal glands.* The adrenal glands produce corticosteroid hormones, which have an important role in metabolism; epinephrine, which helps your body respond to stress or danger; aldosterone, which helps regulate your blood pressure and the sodium and potassium levels in your blood; and testosterone, which regulates your reproductive system.
- *Pancreas.* The pancreas produces insulin and glucagon, hormones that regulate the use of sugar (glucose), fats, and proteins in your body.
- *Testicles.* The testicles produce androgens (male sex hormones), the most important of which is testosterone, which regulates your reproductive system.

Disorders of the Pancreas

Located just behind the stomach, your pancreas releases hormones—such as insulin—that control how your body uses the sugar, fats, and protein consumed in your diet. The most common disorders of the pancreas are diabetes and pancreatitis (see page 277). Cancer also can affect the pancreas.

Diabetes

Diabetes is a serious, chronic condition that affects an estimated 16 million Americans. Up to 95 percent of people with diabetes have type 2 diabetes, also referred to as adult-onset or non–insulin-dependent diabetes. One-third of these people do not know they have the disease because type 2 diabetes seldom causes symptoms in the early stages.

When you have diabetes, the amount of glucose (a simple sugar that is the body's main source of fuel) in your blood is too high. Your blood always has some glucose in it, but excessive amounts are not good for your health.

Diabetes affects the way your body uses food for energy and growth. Most of the food you consume is broken down into glucose, which passes into the bloodstream and is transported throughout the body for use by the cells. To get inside the cells, a hormone called insulin must be present. Insulin is produced by the pancreas.

When you eat, the pancreas normally produces the proper amount of insulin to allow glucose to enter your cells. But in people with diabetes, either the pancreas produces insufficient insulin or the cells do not respond to the insulin produced. Glucose builds up in the blood and overflows into the urine. During urination, the body loses its vital source of energy.

Diabetes is widely recognized as one of the leading causes of death and disability in the United States. It can produce serious, long-term complications that affect every major part of the body. Some of these complications are heart disease, stroke, nerve damage, blindness, kidney failure, and amputations.

Type 1 Diabetes   Type 1 diabetes, the less common form of the disorder, occurs when the body's immune system (see page 376) attacks the insulin-producing cells in the pancreas and destroys them. The pancreas then loses its ability to produce an adequate supply of insulin.

Type 1 diabetes is sometimes referred to as insulin-dependent diabetes because people who have it need daily injections of insulin to stay alive. If the person's insulin level is not sufficient, symptoms appear quickly, including increased thirst, feeling hungry, frequent urination, weight loss, blurred vision, irritability, and extreme fatigue. Without insulin these symptoms worsen, and the person can lapse into a life-threatening coma.

At present, the cause of type 1 diabetes is unknown, but both a person's genetic makeup and environmental factors such as viruses may have a role in the development of the disorder. Type 1 diabetes accounts for 5 to 10 percent of all cases of diagnosed diabetes in the United States. It most often develops in children and young adults, but it can appear at any age. This type of diabetes occurs equally among men and women. Type 1 diabetes most frequently occurs in whites.

To diagnose type 1 diabetes, your doctor will give you a thorough physical examination and will ask you questions about your symptoms, your family health history (see page 80), and your personal health history (see page 82). He or she will order blood tests to measure the level of glucose in your blood. Your blood also will be tested for changes in levels of electrolytes such as sodium and potassium. The doctor may also order a urine test that can detect the presence of substances known as ketones that accumulate in your urine if your body does not produce enough insulin.

To treat this type of diabetes, the doctor will teach you how to give yourself daily injections of insulin. He or she may recommend an insulin pump, which is implanted just under the skin on the abdomen and provides insulin continuously 24 hours a day according to a plan programmed just for you. The steady infusion of insulin keeps your blood glucose level in the healthy range between meals and overnight. When you eat, you program the pump to deliver an extra dose of insulin based on the amount of food you eat.

You will also learn how to test your blood glucose level at home using a home glucose meter that measures the amount of glucose present in a small drop of blood taken from your finger. (Newer monitors are available that allow you to measure the blood glucose level without sticking your finger.) Frequent monitoring of your blood glucose level can help you gauge how often to take your insulin injections or how well your insulin pump is working.

Diet is a key component of diabetes management. A dietitian will help you to plan meals that are tailored to your individual needs. The diet plan will tell you not only what types of food to eat—mostly complex carbohydrates and high-fiber foods—but also when to eat, because it is important to balance your insulin injections with your food intake. This balance will ensure that you keep your blood glucose level as close to normal as possible.

Regular exercise actually helps to reduce the level of glucose in your blood by improving your body's ability to convert the food you eat into energy. Exercise also strengthens your heart and blood vessels, which can be adversely affected by uncontrolled diabetes. Work with your doctor to plan an exercise program that fits your schedule and includes activities you like. Be sure to plan your exercise sessions around your mealtimes and insulin injections so you can keep your blood glucose level within the normal range.

Type 2 Diabetes   The more common form of diabetes is type 2 diabetes. Ninety to 95 percent of people with diabetes have this form. In people with type 2 diabetes, the pancreas produces insulin, but the body's cells cannot effectively use it. The end result is the same as that in type 1 diabetes: an unhealthy buildup of the sugar glucose in the blood and the body's inability to make efficient use of its main source of fuel.

The symptoms of type 2 diabetes develop very gradually and are barely noticcable at first. Over time, however, people with type 2 diabetes may feel tired, urinate frequently (cspccially at night), be unusually thirsty, lose weight, and have blurred vision. Eventually, they may develop frequent infections—especially of the skin—and sores that are slow to heal.

Type 2 diabetes usually develops in adults over age 40 and is most common over age 55. About 80 percent of people with this form of diabetes are overweight, and obesity is an important risk factor for type 2 diabetes. It is morc common in older women than in older men. In contrast with type 1, the incidence of type 2 diabetes is about 60 percent higher in African Americans and up to 120 percent higher in Hispanic Americans than it is in whites. Native Americans have the highest incidence of diabetes in the world. People who have family members with type 2 diabetes are at greater risk of developing the disease.

Doctors use a number of tests to diagnose type 2 diabetes. If you have a family history of type 2 diabetes or are otherwise at risk of developing it, you will be given a screening blood test to measure the level of glucose in your blood. A high or a low glucose level in a screening blood test will warrant a fasting blood glucose test, which measures the glucose level in your blood after you have fasted for 10 to 12 hours, usually overnight. Blood glucose levels of 125 mg/dL (milligrams of glucose per deciliter of blood) or more on two or more fasting blood glucose tests show that you have diabetes. If your blood glucose levels fall between 105 and 124 mg/dL, or if your fasting blood glucose levels are normal but you have symptoms of diabetes, the doctor may recommend an oral

---

Warning Signs of Type 1 Diabetes

Symptoms of type 1 diabetes appear suddenly and develop most often in children and young adults. See your doctor right away if you have any of the following symptoms:

- increased thirst
- frequent urination
- constant hunger
- abdominal pain
- nausea
- weight loss
- blurred vision
- fatigue

glucose tolerance test. Before taking this test, the doctor will ask you to eat a carbohydrate-rich diet for a few days and then to fast overnight. You will then receive a glucose-containing liquid to drink, and your blood glucose level will be monitored for 2 hours through blood tests taken every 30 minutes. High levels (over 200 mg/dL) of glucose in the blood indicate that you have type 2 diabetes. Moderately high levels show that you have a condition called impaired glucose tolerance, which places you at an increased risk of developing type 2 diabetes and at an increased risk of developing heart disease.

A test called a glycosylated hemoglobin test measures the percentage in your blood of a particular type of hemoglobin (the substance in red blood cells that carries oxygen). If you have too much glucose in your blood, the extra glucose forms a link with (glycosylates) the hemoglobin. The blood test can determine the average level of glucose in your blood over the past 120 days. In a person who does not have diabetes, about 6 percent of all hemoglobin is glycosylated. In a person whose diabetes has been poorly controlled for a long time, the level of glycosylated hemoglobin can be as high as 25 percent. If you are diagnosed with diabetes, your doctor is likely to recommend that you have a glycosylated hemoglobin test twice a year to monitor the effectiveness of your treatment.

Obesity is the number one cause of type 2 diabetes, so weight reduction is the primary goal of treatment. A balanced weight-loss diet and regular exercise are often all that are needed to reach and maintain a normal blood glucose level. If not, your doctor will prescribe oral medication (including sulfonylureas such as glipizide or glyburide, or other medications such as metformin or acarbose) that reduces the level of glucose in your blood. Although most people with type 2 diabetes take oral medication, some people who have the disorder need to take daily injections of insulin. The doctor will probably recommend that you routinely check your blood glucose level at home using a simple test so that you can determine whether your program of diet, exercise, and medication is working.

Managing Diabetes Before the discovery of insulin in 1921, people with type 1 diabetes died within a few years after getting the disease. Insulin is not considered a cure for the disease, but daily injections of the hormone help the affected person live a normal life. The insulin injections have to be balanced with diet, proper timing of meals, and exercise. Frequent blood glucose testing helps to monitor the level of glucose in the blood. Diet, exercise, and blood glucose testing also are indispensable for the management of type 2 diabetes. Some

Warning Signs of Type 2 Diabetes

Type 2 diabetes is the more common form of the disease. The symptoms of type 2 diabetes develop gradually and are not as noticeable as those of type 1 diabetes. See your doctor right away if you experience any of the following symptoms:

- frequent urination, especially at night
- unusual thirst
- weight loss
- blurred vision
- fatigue
- frequent infections
- slow healing of sores

people with this form of diabetes also take drugs or insulin to lower their blood glucose level.

People who have either type of diabetes must take responsibility for their own day-to-day care to keep their blood glucose level from getting too low or too high. If the blood glucose level drops too low, usually because the person has taken too much insulin or oral medication or has not balanced the insulin or medication with the proper food intake, a condition known as hypoglycemia occurs. Hypoglycemia causes the person to tremble and become weak, confused, hungry, and dizzy. Pale skin, headache, irritability, sweating, rapid heartbeat, and a cold and clammy feeling are additional symptoms of hypoglycemia. In severe cases the person can lose consciousness and even lapse into a coma. The symptoms of low blood glucose can be mistaken for those of other conditions, such as anxiety or overindulgence in alcohol. The best way to correct a low blood glucose level is to eat or drink something—such as hard candy, soda pop, or orange juice—that contains sugar. Many people with diabetes carry glucose tablets for just such an emergency. A person who has diabetes should always wear a medical identification bracelet or necklace and carry a wallet card containing up-to-date personal medical information. This will identify the person's condition and help ensure appropriate medical treatment if he or she ever has a hypoglycemic reaction while in public.

A person also can become very ill if the blood glucose level rises too high, a condition known as hyperglycemia. This usually happens when the person has not taken enough insulin or oral medication or has not properly regulated his or her blood glucose level with diet. Symptoms are the same as those of type 1 diabetes. Hypoglycemia and hyperglycemia can occur in people with both types of diabetes, and both are potentially life-threatening emergencies.

Keeping the blood glucose level as close to normal as possible reduces the risk of developing serious complications. In a person who does not have diabetes, the normal level of glucose in the blood ranges from 60 to 110 mg/dL. The blood glucose level goes up after eating but returns to the normal range within 1 or 2 hours. Most people with diabetes should aim for a blood glucose range of about 90 to 120 mg/dL before a meal and less than 150 mg/dL about 2 hours after their latest meal.

The doctor will monitor how well you control your diabetes and check for any possible complications, such as nerve damage. Doctors who specialize in treating diabetes and other disorders of the endocrine system are called endocrinologists. People with diabetes should also see an ophthalmologist (a doctor who specializes in treating diseases of the eyes) for eye examinations (see page 370) and a podiatrist (a doctor who specializes in care of the feet) for routine foot care (see page 371).

The biggest problem for people with diabetes is heart and blood vessel disease, which can lead to heart attacks, stroke, and high blood pressure. Diabetes also can cause poor circulation (blood flow) in the legs and feet. To check for heart and blood vessel disease, the doctor will order certain tests, including an electrocardiogram (which measures and records the flow of electricity through the heart) and a cholesterol test. The doctor will take your blood pressure at each visit and check the pulse in your feet and legs to make sure you have good circulation. He or she will recommend that you eat foods low in fat and salt, lose weight if you need to, and exercise regularly. Your doctor will also advise you not to smoke and to limit your intake of alcohol.

Having diabetes also is a risk factor for kidney disease. After several years, a high blood glucose level can cause your kidneys to stop functioning. This condition is called kidney (or renal) failure (see page 291). Diabetes is the primary preventable cause of kidney failure in the United States. The doctor will check your urine at least once a year for protein, a sign of kidney damage. A blood pressure medication called an angiotensin-converting enzyme (ACE)

Diabetic Eye Disease

People who have diabetes are at high risk for a number of eye problems that can cause severe vision loss or blindness. The most common diabetic eye disease is diabetic retinopathy, which is damage to the blood vessels in the retina, the light-sensitive membrane at the back of the eyeball. In some people with diabetic retinopathy, blood vessels in the retina may swell and leak fluid. In other people, abnormal new blood vessels grow on the surface of the retina. These changes can produce loss of vision or blindness.

In the early stages of the disease, no pain or other symptoms may be present. This is why, if you have diabetes, you should have your eyes examined at least once a year. During the examination, the doctor will use eyedrops to dilate (enlarge) your pupils so that he or she can see inside your eyes to check for signs of the disease. As diabetic retinopathy progresses, the person may experience blurred vision or vision loss.

Doctors treat diabetic retinopathy by using laser surgery to seal the leaking blood vessels or to shrink abnormal vessels. Diabetic retinopathy cannot be prevented, but you can reduce your risk of developing the disease and slow its onset and progression by keeping your blood glucose level within normal range.

A cataract (see page 390) is a cloudy covering that appears over the normally clear lens of the eye. People with diabetes are twice as likely to develop cataracts as are people without diabetes. Cataracts also develop at an earlier age in people with diabetes. Usually cataracts can be surgically removed.

If you have diabetes, you also have twice the normal risk of developing glaucoma (see page 388). This disease is caused by abnormally high pressure from excess fluid in the eyeball. The increased pressure damages the optic nerve and blood vessels in the eye, resulting in vision loss. Doctors treat glaucoma with medications or laser surgery.

Early detection and treatment, before vision loss occurs, are the best ways to control diabetic eye disease. If you have diabetes, make sure you have a thorough eye examination at least once a year. For more information on diabetic retinopathy, cataracts, and glaucoma, see chapter 20.

inhibitor can sometimes help prevent kidney damage, even if your blood pressure is normal. It is very important to control your blood pressure to prevent kidney damage. Be sure to take your blood pressure medication as prescribed. See your doctor right away if you think you might have a bladder or kidney infection, indicated by cloudy or bloody urine, pain or burning during urination, and frequent urination or an urgent need to urinate. Back pain, chills, and fever also are possible symptoms of a kidney infection.

Over time, a high blood glucose level can damage the nerves in your body. Nerve damage due to diabetes can produce a loss of sensation or cause pain and

Foot Care Tips for People with Diabetes

People with diabetes are prone to developing severe infections that are slow to heal. The feet are especially susceptible to infection, even from something as common as an ingrown toenail. Nerve damage produced by diabetes can cause numbness in the feet that reduces the person's ability to feel pain from an injury or infection. An infection can become so serious that it results in the need for amputation.

Controlling your blood glucose level with diet, exercise, and your daily insulin intake can go a long way toward preventing foot problems. The following tips also can help you take better care of your feet:

- Check your feet every day. Look for cuts, blisters, red spots, and swelling, and use a mirror to check the bottoms of your feet.
- Wash your feet every day. Bathe your feet in warm (not hot) soapy water every day and dry them well, especially between the toes.
- Keep your feet soft and smooth. Apply a moisturizing lotion over the tops and bottoms of your feet but not between your toes.
- Smooth corns and calluses gently. Use a pumice stone to gently rub rough spots away.
- Trim your toenails each week. Cut them straight across and file the edges gently with an emery board or nail file.
- Always wear shoes and socks. Never walk barefoot, because you could injure your feet. Wear shoes that are comfortable and fit well.
- Protect your feet from hot and cold. Wear shoes at the beach or on hot pavement. Wear socks if your feet get cold at night.
- Keep the blood circulating to your feet. Put your feet up when sitting. Wiggle your toes and move your feet up and down for a few minutes two or three times a day. Do not cross your legs for long periods. Do not smoke.
- Be more active. Ask your doctor to help you plan a regular exercise program.
- See your doctor regularly. The doctor will check your feet for any potential problems. Call your doctor right away if a cut, sore, blister, or bruise on your foot does not begin to heal after a day. Follow your doctor's advice about routine foot care.

burning in your feet. Nerve damage happens slowly, and you may not realize that you have a problem. Your doctor will routinely check the sensation and the pulse in your feet to look for signs of nerve damage.

A high level of blood glucose also can damage the small blood vessels and nerves in and around the penis. Therefore diabetes can interfere with both the nerve impulses and the blood flow necessary to produce and maintain an erection. About 60 percent of men with diabetes experience erectile dysfunction (see page 146).

Diabetes can cause infection of the gums and the bones that hold your teeth in place. Like any infection, gum disease (see page 409) can cause your blood glucose level to rise, making the problem worse. Without treatment, your teeth can become loose and begin to fall out. To help prevent gum disease, see your dentist twice a year and tell him or her that you have diabetes. And be sure to brush and floss your teeth twice a day.

Cancer of the Pancreas

Pancreatic cancer is one of the leading cancers in men, with 26,000 new cases diagnosed each year. It is the fifth most common cause of cancer deaths in the United States and around the world. Most pancreatic cancer begins in the ducts that carry pancreatic juices into the first section of the small intestine. A rare type of pancreatic cancer begins in the cells inside the pancreas (known as the islets of Langerhans) that produce insulin. As the cancer grows, the tumor invades organs—such as the stomach and the small intestine—that surround the pancreas. Cancer cells also can break away from the main tumor and spread to other parts of the body—most commonly the lymph nodes or the liver—through the bloodstream.

Cancer of the pancreas has been called a "silent" disease because it usually does not cause symptoms in the early stages. The cancer may grow for some time before it causes symptoms. When symptoms occur, they may be so vague that they go unnoticed. For these reasons, cancer of the pancreas is often not detected until the later stages, when the cancer has already spread outside the pancreas.

Symptoms include pressure in the upper abdomen that sometimes spreads to the back. The pressure may worsen after the person eats or lies down. Other symptoms include nausea, loss of appetite, weight loss, and weakness. If the tumor blocks the duct through which bile (a fluid produced by the liver that helps digest fat) passes into the small intestine, the person develops jaundice (yellowing of the skin and the whites of the eyes), and his or her urine may become dark.

The cause of cancer of the pancreas is unknown, but certain factors can increase your risk of developing the disease. Age is a risk factor; the disease rarely occurs before age 40, and the average age at diagnosis is 70. Smoking and heavy drinking are also risk factors for cancer of the pancreas. Cigarette smokers develop the disease two to three times more often than nonsmokers. Having diabetes also increases your chances of developing cancer of the pancreas. People with diabetes develop the disease about twice as often as the general population. The risk of developing pancreatic cancer is higher in people who consume a diet that is high in fat and low in fruits and vegetables.

To diagnose cancer of the pancreas, the doctor will perform a physical examination and ask about the person's health history (see page 82). He or she will order tests that will produce images of the pancreas. Such tests also will help the doctor determine how far the cancer has progressed. Computed tomography (CT) scanning (which uses a series of X rays and a computer to produce cross-sectional images), magnetic resonance imaging (MRI; which uses a powerful magnetic field and a computer to produce three-dimensional images), and ultrasound scanning (which uses high-frequency sound waves to produce images) are commonly used to diagnose cancer of the pancreas. To view the pancreatic ducts, the doctor probably will order a test called endoscopic retrograde cholangiopancreatography (ERCP). In ERCP, an endoscope (a lighted, flexible viewing tube) is passed down the throat, through the stomach, and into the small intestine. After the endoscope is in place, contrast medium (a type of dye) is injected into the pancreatic ducts, and a series of X-ray images is produced.

Images of the pancreas and nearby organs may not provide adequate information for the doctor to make a firm diagnosis of pancreatic cancer. He or she also may have to perform a biopsy, in which a small sample of tissue is taken from the pancreas for analysis under a microscope. A biopsy can be performed in three ways. In a needle biopsy, the doctor inserts a long needle into the abdomen and then into the pancreas to obtain a tissue sample. A brush biopsy is performed at the same time as the ERCP. The doctor inserts a tiny brush into the endoscope and rubs off some cells for later analysis. Sometimes the doctor performs the biopsy during a surgical procedure known as a laparoscopy. During this procedure, the doctor inserts a laparoscope (a viewing tube equipped with a precision optical system that sends clear images to a video monitor) into the abdomen through a small incision and removes a small tissue sample. The doctor also can use the same tube to see inside the abdomen to determine the location and the extent of the cancer.

Cancer of the pancreas can be cured only in its early stages. However, because of the lack of early symptoms, the disease is not often detected until it is in its later stages, when treatment is difficult. Therefore, treatment often focuses on improving the person's quality of life by controlling the symptoms of the disease. Pain relievers are usually prescribed.

Depending on the type of pancreatic cancer, its location, and whether it has spread, the doctor may attempt to remove the tumor or stop its growth by using surgery, radiation therapy, or chemotherapy (treatment with powerful anticancer drugs). Surgery involves removing all or part of the pancreas and possibly some surrounding tissue. Doctors also use surgery to help relieve symptoms that occur if a duct is blocked. During radiation therapy, the doctor uses a radioactive substance or X rays to damage cancer cells and stop them from growing and spreading. The radiation affects cells only in the treated area. Chemotherapy uses drugs to kill cancer cells. It is given in cycles so the person can have a period of recovery between treatments. Sometimes doctors use surgery, radiation therapy, and chemotherapy in combination to treat cancer of the pancreas. All three forms of treatment have side effects that your doctor will describe for you.

Surgery to treat cancer of the pancreas is major surgery that requires a lengthy recovery period. Pain, fatigue, and weakness are common. Fatigue is also a side effect of radiation therapy, which also can cause hair loss, darkening of the skin, nausea, vomiting, and diarrhea. People undergoing chemotherapy may be more susceptible to infection; may bruise or bleed easily; may have nausea, vomiting, and diarrhea; and may develop sores in the mouth. The side effects vary from person to person.

People living with cancer of the pancreas (and their families) face many problems and an uncertain future. Coping with these problems may be easier when they can share their concerns in a support group and if they have help with home care. Your doctor or a social worker at your local hospital can refer you to appropriate sources of information and assistance.

Other Endocrine System Disorders

Here are two closely related disorders of the endocrine system that are more common in women but also can occur in men:

- *Hyperthyroidism.* This condition occurs when an overactive thyroid gland produces excessive amounts of thyroid hormone, increasing your metabolic rate and your heart rate. Graves' disease (see below) is the most common cause of hyperthyroidism. Early symptoms develop gradually and usually include irritability, anxiety, mood swings, dry skin, weight loss, increased appetite, and increased sweating. In more advanced cases, symptoms can include an enlarged thyroid gland (called a goiter), muscle wasting, tremor, abnormal heart rate and rhythm, and bulging eyeballs. A goiter is visible as a swelling on the neck. A large goiter may press on the esophagus or the trachea, making it difficult or painful to swallow or breathe. Doctors diagnose hyperthyroidism based on the symptoms, a physical examination, and blood levels of thyroid hormone and thyroid-stimulating hormone. Doctors often prescribe beta-blockers (see page 225) to relieve symptoms such as a rapid heart rate. Antithyroid medications (such as methimazole and propylthiouracil) that reduce production of thyroid hormones also are prescribed. If treatment with medication is ineffective, you may be treated with a single dose of radioactive iodine (in liquid or pill form), which collects in the thyroid gland, eventually destroying some thyroid tissue and inhibiting production of thyroid hormones. Some people may require additional radioactive iodine treatments. (In some cases, a doctor may treat a person with radioactive iodine before prescribing medication.) If a goiter is particularly unsightly or if it is causing problems with swallowing or breathing, a doctor may recommend surgery to remove the enlarged portion of the thyroid gland.

- *Graves' disease.* Also called diffuse toxic goiter, Graves' disease is an autoimmune disease (a disturbance in the body's immune system) in which the body produces antibodies that attack the cells of the thyroid gland. Because these antibodies imitate thyroid-stimulating hormone, they cause the thyroid gland to produce excessive amounts of thyroid hormone, resulting in a condition known as hyperthyroidism (see above). Graves' disease tends to run in families. Symptoms, diagnosis, and treatment are the same as for hyperthyroidism.

CHAPTER 19
Immune System

The immune system is an intricate network of specialized cells and organs that defends your body against attacks by infectious microorganisms such as bacteria, viruses, and fungi, and by larger invaders such as worms. The human body provides an ideal habitat for many microorganisms, both beneficial and harmful. When a harmful microorganism tries to enter the body, the immune system will attempt to block its entry. If that fails, the immune system will search out and destroy the invader. The immune system also has a role in allergies, autoimmune diseases, and controlling cancer.

The immune system has several remarkable characteristics. When working properly, it can distinguish between the body's own cells and those that come from outside of the body. It also can remember previous exposures to certain microorganisms. For example, if you have had chickenpox, you usually will not develop it again because your immune system knows that you have already been exposed and will respond even more aggressively to that virus. Not only can the immune system recognize millions of different invading microorganisms, it also can produce specific molecules to fight each one. The success of the immune system depends on an elaborate system of communication and checks and balances that quickly pass information back and forth along pathways.

Bone marrow (the soft tissue in the hollow shafts of the long bones) is a key component of your immune system. It produces white blood cells called lymphocytes, which are essential components of the immune system. Another important part of the immune system is the spleen (a fist-sized organ in your upper left abdomen). The spleen produces lymphocytes and phagocytes (another type of white blood cell). Other organs of the immune system include the thymus gland (a gland in the upper chest), tonsils (masses of lymph tissue at the back of the throat), adenoids (swellings of lymph tissue at the back of the roof of the

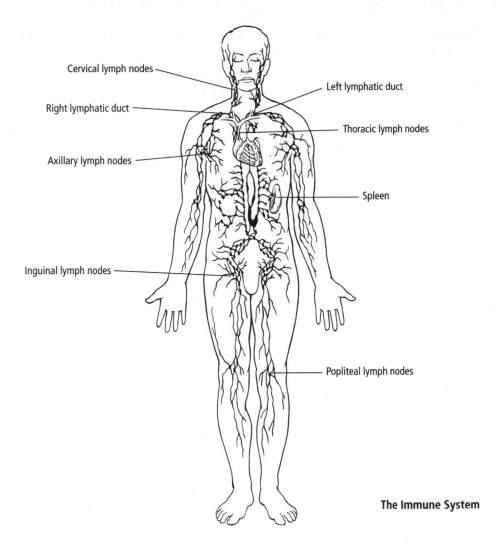

Cervical lymph nodes

Left lymphatic duct

Right lymphatic duct

Thoracic lymph nodes

Axillary lymph nodes

Spleen

Inguinal lymph nodes

Popliteal lymph nodes

The Immune System

mouth), appendix (a small, fingerlike projection from the large intestine), and lymph nodes. The lymph nodes are bean-shaped organs in the head, neck, chest, abdomen, and groin. They filter a watery fluid called lymph, which bathes the body tissues and contains lymphocytes.

Once a foreign cell or infectious microorganism is detected, your body begins an immune response to defend itself. Several different types of white blood cells travel to the site of infection to stop the invader from going any farther. White blood cells called phagocytes surround the invading microorganisms and destroy them, dying in the process. Other white blood cells, called mast cells, release chemicals at the site of the infection to trigger the swelling and redness that are characteristic of inflammation.

If the invading microorganism survives, it is subjected to a second attack. The body sends more sophisticated white blood cells, known as B lymphocytes and T lymphocytes (also called B cells and T cells), to the site of the infection.

B lymphocytes can recognize specific microorganisms and produce proteins called antibodies, which are specially designed to destroy these microorganisms. Some B lymphocytes will become "memory cells," which will recognize the invading microorganism if it tries to enter the body again and will automatically produce antibodies to destroy it.

There are two types of T lymphocytes—killer cells and helper cells. Killer T lymphocytes destroy microorganisms that have infected the cells of the body by attaching to the invading microorganisms and releasing chemicals that destroy them. Killer T lymphocytes also rid the body of cancer cells. Helper T lymphocytes protect the body from both invading microorganisms and cancer cells by enhancing the actions of the killer T lymphocytes and by controlling various aspects of the immune response.

Some people may lack one or more components of the immune system, or a component may not function properly. This is called an immunodeficiency disorder, which means that the person cannot adequately fight off infection. In other people, a specific substance such as ragweed pollen or saliva on cat dander (flakes of dead skin), which is harmless to most people, can provoke an inappropriate immune response. This is commonly called an allergy. In some other people the immune system mistakenly attacks the body's own cells and tissue, resulting in what is known as an autoimmune disease. One such disease is type 1 diabetes (see page 365).

Immunodeficiency Disorders

A weakened immune system can be congenital (present from birth), or it may result from an inherited disorder or an infection. It also may occur as a side effect of drug treatment. People with weakened immune systems have difficulty fighting infections that are easily handled by a healthy immune system. When a person's immune system is ineffective, harmful microorganisms can thrive and multiply rapidly, causing life-threatening infections.

A small number of infants are born with defects in their immune systems. Infants born with defective B lymphocytes are unable to produce antibodies and therefore are vulnerable to a wide variety of infections. Doctors treat this type of disorder with injections of live antibodies. Some infants lack T lymphocytes because they were born without a thymus gland or because the thymus gland is small and abnormal. This disorder requires a thymus gland transplant. In very rare cases, infants are born without an immune system, a condition known as severe combined immunodeficiency disease. Children with this disease gained notoriety by living for years in germ-free rooms or "bubbles." A few of these children have been successfully treated with bone marrow transplants.

The best-known immunodeficiency disorder is acquired immunodeficiency syndrome (AIDS), which is caused by the human immunodeficiency virus (HIV). AIDS often leads to various otherwise rare diseases, such as *Pneumo-*

cystis carinii pneumonia and Kaposi's sarcoma (a form of cancer). These diseases are called opportunistic diseases because they rarely occur in people with healthy immune systems, but occur more in people with weakened immune systems, in whom conditions for development are favorable. HIV infection also damages the central nervous system (the brain and the spinal cord), which leads to dementia (progressive deterioration of mental functioning).

HIV infection may cause no symptoms in the early stages or can produce flu-like symptoms, including fever, chills, fatigue, sweating at night, and a dry cough. Other symptoms include sudden unexplained weight loss and chronic diarrhea. Although some infected people may have no symptoms, they still can transmit the virus to others.

HIV is transmitted by sexual contact or by direct contact with infected blood or body fluids. HIV can be transmitted from an infected woman to a fetus during pregnancy or to an infant during childbirth or through breast milk. HIV also can be transmitted by sharing needles during intravenous drug use. In the past, some people were infected with HIV through blood transfusions or contaminated blood products. Today, however, all donated blood is routinely screened for HIV, and the blood supply in the United States is safe.

At present there is no cure for AIDS. Early diagnosis and treatment are vital. Certain medications that are currently available, when used in combination, seem to slow development of the disease. These medications include nucleoside analog reverse transcriptase inhibitors (such as zidovudine, also called AZT), which interrupt an early stage of virus replication, and protease inhibitors (such as indinavir, ritonavir, and saquinavir), which interrupt the same process at a later stage. Although these "cocktail" drug regimens typically cause unpleasant side effects such as nausea and diarrhea, when started early, they are enabling many people infected with HIV to live longer, more productive lives. Other drugs designed to combat the virus, bolster the immune system, and prevent or treat opportunistic infections that result from HIV infection are now being tested. Research on an AIDS vaccine is also under way. For more information on HIV and AIDS, see page 186.

Immunodeficiency can be an unwanted side effect of certain medications, such as those used to treat cancer. Anticancer drugs used during chemotherapy affect cells that divide rapidly, including the white blood cells (lymphocytes) that fight infection. Because of this, people undergoing chemotherapy may become more susceptible to opportunistic infections.

Airborne Allergies

An allergy is an exaggerated or inappropriate response of the immune system to a substance that is harmless to most people. Substances that can cause such reactions are called allergens. Common allergens include pollen, dust particles, certain foods, insect venom, mold, and medications. Doctors think that the reason some people are allergic to a particular substance is because they have inherited a tendency to be allergic (although not necessarily to that particular substance). Being exposed to a potential allergen when the body's defenses are lowered or weakened—such as during a viral infection—seems to contribute to the development of an allergy. People with allergies are often sensitive to more than one allergen.

During an allergic reaction, the immune system is responding to a false alarm. When a person comes into contact with an allergen, the immune system launches an inappropriate immune response by releasing large amounts of an antibody (a disease-fighting protein) called immunoglobulin E. Each time the person encounters an allergen, these antibodies signal the body to produce powerful chemicals, such as histamine, that travel to where the allergen is located (such as the airways, the skin, or the surface of the eye) and cause inflammation. Symptoms of inflammation include redness, swelling, pain, and warmth. When pollen, dust, or other airborne allergens cause inflammation of the mucous membrane that lines the nose, the condition is known as allergic rhinitis. Common symptoms include runny nose, coughing, nasal congestion, and sneezing.

One of the most common allergies is pollen allergy. Each spring, summer, and fall, trees, weeds, and grasses release tiny particles called pollen, which ride on currents of air. The pollen enters the nose and throat, triggering allergic reactions in susceptible people. Among North American plants, weeds, especially ragweed, are the most prolific producers of pollen. In fact, the popular term "hay fever" typically refers to allergy to ragweed pollen. Other important pollen-producing weeds include sagebrush, redroot pigweed, tumbleweed, and English plantain. Trees that produce allergic pollen are oak, ash, elm, hickory, pecan, box elder, and mountain cedar. Although a wide variety of grasses grow in North America, only about seven types produce pollen that causes allergic responses.

Each plant has a pollinating period that is the same from year to year. The relative lengths of night and day seem to be the trigger for pollination, so the farther north you live, the later (and shorter) the pollinating period and the later (and shorter) the allergy season. A pollen count measures how much pollen is in the air at a given time. Pollen counts tend to be highest early in the morning on warm, dry, breezy days and lowest on chilly, wet days. If you have allergic rhinitis, try to stay indoors as much as possible on high-pollen-count days, especially in the morning. If you work outdoors, wear a face mask that filters out pollen. If possible, take your vacation at the height of pollen season and go to a location, such as the beach, where pollen counts are minimal.

House dust probably is the most common cause of airborne allergies, producing symptoms of allergic rhinitis. House dust is a mixture of potential allergens. It often contains fabric fibers, cotton lint, feathers and other stuffing materials, bacteria, mold, food particles, bits of plants and insects, and dust mites (microscopic insects). Dust mites live in bedding, upholstered furniture, and carpets. They thrive in summer, and they can live all year in warm, humid houses. The mites produce waste-containing proteins, which are the actual causes of the allergic reaction. Waste products of cockroaches also are are an important cause of allergy symptoms in infested households, especially in urban areas.

If you have a dust allergy, take the time to dustproof your home, especially your bedroom. Eliminate as many dust-gathering and dust-producing items—such as wall-to-wall carpeting, blinds, down-filled blankets, feather pillows, forced-air heating vents, pets, and closets full of clothing—as you can. Encase your mattress in a zippered, plastic, dustproof cover. Wash all of your bedding once a week in water hotter than 130 degrees Fahrenheit. Frequently wipe with a damp cloth all surfaces where dust accumulates.

Many people are allergic to animals, particularly household pets. Pet allergy is not triggered by the dander or hair of dogs or cats but rather by proteins in their saliva, which they transmit to their hair through licking. An animal allergy can take 2 or more years to develop and may not subside until 6 or more months after contact with the animal has ended. The best way to avoid an allergic reaction is to stay away from animals—even if it means finding a new home for a beloved pet. To decrease the level of cat allergens, try bathing the cat weekly, which neutralizes the protein on the fur. And keep the animal out of the bedroom.

Mold is a type of fungus that grows seasonally and causes allergic reactions in some people. Mold levels peak in late summer but, in warmer climates, molds thrive all year and can cause allergic symptoms year-round. Molds can be found wherever there is moisture. Outside, they grow on rotting logs and decomposing leaves. In the house, molds thrive in basements, bathrooms, damp closets, refrigerator drip trays, houseplants, air conditioners and humidifiers, garbage cans, mattresses, and old foam rubber pillows. When inhaled, tiny mold spores often evade the protective mechanisms of the nose and upper airways and reach the lungs. There they can cause bronchospasm (temporary narrowing of the airways in the lungs) or trigger an asthma attack (see page 245) in a person who has asthma.

To minimize your contact with allergy-triggering molds, have someone else mow your lawn and rake leaves, or wear a tight-fitting mask when you do these chores. Clean and disinfect your bathroom fixtures regularly, and be sure to air out closets, mattresses, pillows, and garbage cans. Regularly clean your air-conditioner filter and your humidifier filter and water reservoir according to the manufacturer's instructions. A dehumidifier can help dry out your basement, but you must clean the machine frequently to prevent mold buildup.

In addition to sneezing, coughing, runny nose, and nasal congestion, people with allergic rhinitis also may have itchy, watery eyes and conjunctivitis (an inflammation of the lining of the eyelids). Dark circles typically appear under the eyes, caused by increased blood flow near the sinuses. Some people with allergies may develop asthma, a serious and potentially life-threatening respiratory disorder that causes tightness in the chest, wheezing, and sometimes severe shortness of breath.

Your health history (see page 82) is an important tool that can help your doctor diagnose a potential allergy. While taking your medical history, he or she can determine whether your symptoms recur at the same time each year, which suggests a seasonal allergen such as pollen. The doctor also will ask questions to determine what substances seem to trigger your allergies. To confirm this information, the doctor may perform skin testing, in which tiny amounts of suspected allergens are applied to, injected under, or scratched onto the skin. A small, reddened area will appear in the area where any substance to which you are allergic was applied. Blood tests also may be performed to detect blood levels of antibodies to a specific allergen.

Doctors generally recommend three approaches to the treatment of allergies: avoidance, medication, and allergy injections. For some people, complete avoidance of an allergen such as pollen or mold may require moving to a location where the allergen does not grow. Others may need to give up a favorite pet. If you have allergies, you may not be able to completely avoid the substances that provoke an allergic reaction. That is why doctors try to control allergic symptoms with medications, sometimes in combination. The most common medications prescribed for this purpose include antihistamines, which counter the effects of histamine, the inflammation-inducing chemical released by the body during an allergic reaction. Nasal corticosteroids, which are sprayed into the nose, combat inflammation, swelling, and mucous secretion. Another nasal spray, called cromolyn sodium, prevents allergic reactions from starting. Effective antihistamines and decongestants also are available over the counter. Ask your doctor for recommendations.

Taking a series of allergy injections (immunotherapy) is the only method of reducing your allergy symptoms over the long term. This treatment usually is given over the course of 2 or 3 years. The doctor injects you with gradually increasing doses of the allergen. In response, your body decreases production of antibodies to that substance and begins producing protective antibodies instead. About 85 percent of people with allergic rhinitis experience a substantial reduction in their symptoms within 2 years of beginning their allergy injections.

Allergies to Medications

Drug allergies arise from a complicated response by the immune system to a specific medication. A person usually goes through three stages when developing an allergy to a medication. First, he or she must be exposed to the drug by taking one or more doses. Next, the person's immune system identifies the drug as harmful and begins producing antibodies to fight it. Finally, the person takes another dose of the drug, and the allergy symptoms appear. The symptoms may appear immediately, within 1 to 2 hours, or within a few days to a week after taking the drug. Common symptoms of drug allergy include skin rash or hives, difficulty breathing, and itching. Severe drug allergies may cause seizures, loss of consciousness, or shock (see box below). If you have had a previous severe allergic reaction, you will need to carry an injecting device that contains epinephrine with you at all times, so you can inject yourself immediately if you have another allergic reaction. An injection of epinephrine can save your life.

Anaphylactic Shock

Anaphylactic shock is a severe, life-threatening allergic reaction. The reaction usually occurs after an insect sting or bite or after injection of a specific drug such as penicillin. Occasionally the reaction occurs after eating a particular food or taking a specific medication. Anaphylactic shock is a medical emergency that requires immediate medical treatment.

During an anaphylactic reaction, the body releases massive amounts of histamine and other powerful chemicals in response to the presence of the allergen. The blood vessels widen, causing a sudden, severe decrease in blood pressure. Other symptoms can include hives (itchy, raised, red patches on the skin); swelling of the lips, tongue, and throat; abdominal pain; diarrhea; and difficulty breathing due to bronchospasm (narrowing of the airways in the lungs).

If you or someone you know has an anaphylactic reaction, call 911 or your local emergency number. While waiting for emergency help to arrive, have the person lie down, with face up, head low, and legs raised about a foot high to improve blood flow to the upper body. An injection of epinephrine is needed as soon as possible to counteract the allergic reaction. If you or the person has had a severe allergic reaction before and carries an injecting device that contains epinephrine, use it as soon as symptoms appear.

Medications that typically produce an allergic reaction include antibiotics (such as penicillin), sulfa drugs, insulin that contains pig or ox protein, vaccines, and aspirin. If you are allergic to any medications, be sure to tell your doctor and other healthcare providers who are treating you, such as a nurse or a dentist. Also, in case of emergency, you should always wear a medical identification bracelet or necklace and carry a wallet card that informs people of your allergy. This will help ensure appropriate medical treatment.

Warning Signs of Allergy to Medication

Always report any unpleasant or unexpected side effects of medication to your doctor.

The following symptoms may indicate an allergy to medication:

• rash
• hives (itchy, raised, red patches on the skin)
• itching
• swollen lips

If you experience any of these symptoms after taking medication, contact your doctor. If you experience more serious symptoms—such as nausea and vomiting, difficulty breathing, confusion, loss of consciousness, swollen tongue or throat, or slurred speech—seek emergency medical help immediately. A severe allergic reaction is a medical emergency that can lead to respiratory failure and shock (see "Anaphylactic Shock," previous page).

Allergies to Food

A food allergy is a reaction of the immune system to a food or food ingredient that most people find harmless. If you eat a food that produces an allergic reaction, your immune system responds by releasing numerous chemicals that cause allergic symptoms. A food allergy is different from a food intolerance, which does not trigger an immune response. A food intolerance (such as lactose intolerance, see page 266) usually arises from an enzyme deficiency and produces symptoms such as stomach cramps, gas, or diarrhea. Food intolerances are relatively common, but a true food allergy is rare, affecting only about 1 percent of the population.

The most common foods that cause allergies in adults are fish and shellfish, eggs, and nuts—such as peanuts, walnuts, and pecans. Symptoms of food allergy can include skin reactions such as hives or rashes, nasal congestion, asthma attacks (see page 245) in people who have asthma, and gastrointestinal problems such as nausea, gas, or diarrhea. Because both food allergies and food intolerances can cause intestinal symptoms, the two disorders are easily confused and must be diagnosed by a doctor.

Food allergy symptoms can appear immediately after eating or may develop over time—within hours or even days. In severe cases the food can provoke a serious reaction known as anaphylaxis (see "Anaphylactic Shock," previous page), which can be life-threatening. Signs and symptoms of anaphylaxis include hives, difficulty breathing, a drop in blood pressure, and loss of consciousness.

To determine whether you have a true food allergy, your doctor probably will perform one of two tests: a skin prick test or a blood test called the radio-allergosorbent test (RAST). During the skin prick test, the doctor deposits a small amount of the suspected food allergen onto your forearm and then pricks the skin beneath it with a needle. A small red bump will appear at the site if you are allergic to that particular food. For the RAST, a sample of your blood is taken and sent to a laboratory for analysis to determine whether your body has formed antibodies to the food in question. Your doctor also may ask you to record everything you eat in a food diary for a couple of weeks to help in the diagnosis.

Many people will outgrow food allergies, except allergies to nuts, fish, and shellfish. The best treatment for a food allergy is to avoid eating the food that causes the allergic reaction. You will need to read food labels carefully and ask questions when dining out to make sure that the foods you eat do not contain the allergen. Severe allergic reactions are life-threatening. If you have had a previous severe allergic reaction, you will need to carry an injecting device that contains epinephrine with you at all times, so you can inject yourself immediately if you have another allergic reaction.

Warning Signs of Food Allergy

If you have a food allergy, your immune system mistakenly regards a particular food as harmful and begins producing antibodies to that food. Each time you eat that food, your immune system releases various chemicals to protect your body. These chemicals produce symptoms that can affect your airways, skin, or intestinal tract. Symptoms of food allergy can include:

- skin reactions such as hives or rashes
- nasal congestion
- nausea, diarrhea, or gas
- shortness of breath, or asthma attacks in people who have asthma

If the reaction is severe, you may experience life-threatening symptoms within minutes of eating. A severe allergic reaction can rapidly cause difficulty breathing, lowered blood pressure, and loss of consciousness (see "Anaphylactic Shock," page 383). If you or a person you are with has these symptoms, seek emergency medical help immediately.

The Common Cold and the Flu

The common cold and the flu (influenza) are both caused by viruses. The viruses that cause colds and the flu are transmitted when an infected person coughs or sneezes into the air and another person inhales the infected droplets. You can also catch a cold or the flu by kissing an infected person or by touching your mouth after touching the other person's hands or an object he or she has touched. Each cold is caused by a different virus, and there are nearly 200 different cold viruses. Adults average about two to four colds per year. The virus that causes the flu changes from year to year; that is why a flu immunization is good for only a year. When these viruses enter your body, they multiply rapidly. Your immune system tries to fight them, producing symptoms that include coughing, sneezing, and a runny nose.

The flu is a viral infection of the nose, throat, and lungs. It is usually mild in young and middle-aged adults but can be life-threatening in older people and people who have a chronic illness such as heart disease, emphysema, asthma, bronchitis, kidney disease, or diabetes. The flu also can lead to more serious, potentially life-threatening infections such as pneumonia (see page 250). Because pneumonia is one of the five leading causes of death among older people, it is important for older people to take steps to prevent the flu. The best preventive measure is a flu shot (see page 93), given each fall at the beginning of the flu season. A pneumonia shot (see page 252) is another preventive measure available for older people and people who have a chronic illness; the pneumonia shot is given only once.

Many people confuse the common cold with the flu, but there is one easy way to tell the difference: the flu usually causes a fever, while a cold does not. Also, a cold causes nasal congestion more often than the flu. In general, cold symptoms are milder than flu symptoms and do not last as long.

The flu is very contagious. Symptoms differ from person to person, but common symptoms include weakness, body ache, headache, and sudden fever. The fever can last from 1 to 6 days. People with the flu also have a cough, chills, and reddened, watery eyes. If the flu progresses to pneumonia, symptoms become more severe, and chest pain may occur as the lungs become inflamed. If the pneumonia was caused by a bacterial infection, it can be treated with antibiotics. Antibiotics are not effective for treating viral infections, including the common cold.

There is no cure for the common cold, and many of the over-the-counter remedies available at your local pharmacy (such as pain relievers and decongestants) treat only the symptoms of a cold. Most colds will clear up within a week or so. The usual treatment for the flu is to take aspirin, acetaminophen, or ibuprofen to reduce the fever and body aches, drink plenty of liquids, and rest in bed until after the fever has been gone for 1 to 2 days. Antiviral medications such as amantadine, rimantadine, zanamivir, and oseltamivir are available by prescription to prevent and treat many types of influenza.

CHAPTER 20
Eyes

The eye is the organ of sight. Light rays enter the eye through the pupil (the circular opening in the center of the iris). The cornea (the tough, transparent, dome-shaped covering of the front of the eyeball) and the lens (the transparent, internal optical component of the eye) focus the light rays on the retina (the light-sensitive membrane that lines the back of the eye) to form an image. The image is converted to electrical impulses that move along the optic nerves to the visual cortex (the area of the brain that is concerned with vision), where the image is perceived.

Although many vision problems are minor and may be easy to treat, others may cause serious complications that, if left untreated, can lead to vision loss or even blindness. Most vision problems are detected during a routine eye examination. That is why it is important for you to have regular eye examinations, especially as you get older.

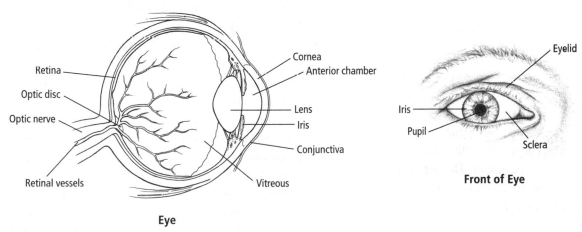

Eye

Front of Eye

Glaucoma

There are two major types of glaucoma—chronic open-angle glaucoma and acute closed-angle glaucoma. Chronic open-angle glaucoma is the most common. It usually develops gradually over a number of years. In chronic open-angle glaucoma, the normal pressure of the fluid in the eyes slowly rises. At the front of your eyes lies a small space known as the anterior chamber. A clear fluid called the aqueous humor flows in and out of the chamber to deliver nutrients to nearby tissues and remove wastes. In people with chronic open-angle glaucoma, the drainage angle (the channel through which fluid leaves the eyeball) does not function normally and the fluid does not drain properly. As the fluid builds up, the pressure inside the eyes increases, potentially causing irreversible damage to the optic nerve. Because it transmits visual images to the brain, damage to the optic nerve produces vision loss that can result in blindness.

In acute closed-angle glaucoma, the drainage angle becomes completely blocked and there is a sudden, very high increase in pressure inside the eyes that can quickly lead to blindness. In a less common type of glaucoma, called normal tension glaucoma, the optic nerve is damaged, even though pressure inside the eyes is within the normal range. This type of glaucoma is poorly understood.

About 3 million people in the United States have glaucoma; it is the third most common cause of blindness in Americans. Anyone can develop the disorder, but some people are at higher risk than others, including people with a family history of glaucoma; people who are nearsighted, have diabetes, or are over age 60; and African Americans over age 40. In fact, glaucoma is five times more likely to occur in African Americans than in whites, and the disease causes blindness more often in African Americans.

Chronic open-angle glaucoma usually produces no symptoms until the optic nerve has been damaged. Blind spots may gradually develop, especially in the peripheral (side) vision. Objects in the front of the field of vision still may be seen clearly, but those at the side may be missed. As the disease progresses, the person's field of vision becomes increasingly narrow until total blindness occurs. Acute closed-angle glaucoma comes on suddenly and usually without warning (see box). Symptoms may include blurred vision, severe eye pain, headache, halos around lights, nausea, and

Warning Signs of Acute Glaucoma

Chronic open-angle glaucoma, the most common type of glaucoma, develops gradually and usually produces no symptoms until blind spots begin to appear in peripheral (side) vision. Acute closed-angle glaucoma occurs suddenly and causes the following symptoms:

- blurred vision
- severe eye pain
- headaches
- halos or rainbows around lights
- nausea and vomiting

Acute closed-angle glaucoma is a medical emergency that requires immediate medical treatment. If you suddenly experience any of these symptoms, call your doctor immediately or go directly to the nearest hospital emergency department. Do not delay. If not treated promptly, acute closed-angle glaucoma can cause blindness.

vomiting. This type of glaucoma is a medical emergency that requires immediate medical treatment.

Because chronic open-angle glaucoma causes no symptoms, it is usually detected during a routine eye examination performed by an ophthalmologist, a physician who specializes in treating disorders of the eyes. The doctor will examine your eyes to determine if the disease has affected them. He or she also will test your peripheral vision to determine the extent and the stability or progression of any damage caused by glaucoma. This is done by performing a visual field test, in which you cover one eye and look straight ahead while an object is shown in different areas of your field of vision. You will be instructed to give a response when you see the object. Your responses will be recorded and used to evaluate your field of vision.

In a computerized visual field test, you sit facing a screen, place your chin on a chin rest, and press a button each time you see a tiny flashing light. A computer printout of your responses allows your doctor to evaluate your field of vision. A similar test that does not use a computer can also be performed.

To measure the pressure inside your eyes, the doctor will perform a test called applanation tonometry. After he or she puts a drop of a local anesthetic on each cornea, the doctor puts a drop of an orange fluid called fluorescein in each eye. Then the doctor gently places an instrument called a tonometer against the cornea to measure pressure in each eyeball. The test is safe and painless. You will not feel the tonometer against your eyeball, but you will see a bright blue circle of light moving toward your eye. The test takes only a few seconds. (In a similar, though less accurate, procedure called air tonometry, a gentle puff of air is directed onto the cornea to measure the pressure inside your eyes. Anesthetic is not needed because the tonometer does not touch the cornea.) The doctor then places eyedrops in your eyes to dilate (widen) the pupils. Once the pupils are dilated, the doctor can examine the insides of your eyes with an ophthalmoscope (a handheld viewing instrument that projects a very bright light onto the back of the eye) to assess the condition of the optic nerves. After the examination your eyes will be sensitive to light for a while, so try to arrange in advance for someone to drive you home.

Additional tests may include gonioscopy, in which the ophthalmologist anesthetizes the eyes with eyedrops and places a special contact lens called a gonioscope on the cornea to examine the drainage angle of each eye for any changes or signs of blockage. The doctor also may take special photographs (called disc photos) of the optic nerves at various intervals so that he or she can monitor any changes or damage due to progression of the disease.

Glaucoma usually cannot be cured because damage to the optic nerve is irreversible. However, the disease can be controlled with medication and surgery. Medication prescribed to treat glaucoma is usually given as eyedrops. Some glaucoma medications reduce the pressure in the eyes by slowing the flow of fluid into the eyes. Other medications help to improve fluid drainage. Although regular use of these medications will control the fluid pressure inside your eyes, the drugs may lose their effectiveness over time. Also, some medications may cause unwanted side effects. In such cases, the ophthalmologist may alter the dosage, change medication, or suggest other ways to solve the problem. You will need to take the medication for the rest of your life.

The goal of eye surgery in treating glaucoma is usually to make it easier for fluid to drain from the eye. For acute closed-angle glaucoma, the doctor performs a surgical procedure called an iridotomy. In this procedure, a laser (a highly concentrated, powerful beam of light) is used to make a small hole in the iris to relieve pressure inside the eyeball. The procedure is brief and is usually performed in the doctor's office or in an outpatient facility. For chronic open-angle glaucoma that cannot be controlled with medication, the doctor performs laser surgery to change the structure of the drainage angle to allow for better fluid drainage. This type of surgery is also performed in the doctor's office or in an outpatient facility. Over time, the effects of this laser surgery may wear off, and additional treatment may be needed. Conventional eye surgery in an operating room may be performed for people whose glaucoma cannot be controlled with medication or laser surgery.

Early detection and treatment of glaucoma is the best way to control the disorder. If you are at high risk for developing glaucoma and are 40 or older, be sure to have your eyes thoroughly examined by an ophthalmologist at least every 2 years.

Cataracts

A cataract is a cloudy area in the normally clear lens inside the eye. The cloudy area worsens as protein fibers in the lens clump together, preventing light rays from passing through the lens and focusing on the retina, the light-sensitive membrane that lines the back of the eye. Cataracts usually develop very gradually, and early changes in the lens of the eye may go unnoticed. As the cataract continues to develop, symptoms begin to appear. The person may have blurred vision in one eye. Bothersome glare caused by bright sunlight or vehicle headlights is common. The person also may have poor night vision. Colors appear to be less bright. The person may experience increased nearsightedness that requires frequent changes in his or her eyeglass prescription. The person also may find it more difficult to see well enough to read and perform other daily tasks.

Cataracts in adults can be classified into three general types, depending on their location in the lens. The most common type is called a nuclear cataract or an age-related cataract and occurs in the center of the lens. The term "age-related" is somewhat misleading because people can have this type of cataract in their 40s and 50s. During middle age, most cataracts are mild and do not affect vision. After age 60, however, cataracts more commonly begin to interfere with vision. The second type of cataract is a cortical cataract, which starts as a wedge-shaped spoke at the outer layer of the lens. The spoke descends from the outer layer into the center, where it obstructs the transmission of light. This type of cataract can develop in people who have diabetes. The third type of cataract is called a subcapsular cataract. It starts as a small clouding at the back of the lens and develops slowly.

The exact cause of cataracts is unknown, although doctors have identified certain factors that may be involved in their development. Research has shown that people who live at high altitudes or who spend much time in the sun develop cataracts earlier than other people. Many ophthalmologists now advise people to wear sunglasses that protect against both ultraviolet A and B (UV-A and UV-B) rays and to wear a wide-brimmed hat to protect the eyes against sun exposure whenever they go outdoors. People who have diabetes also seem to have an increased risk of developing cataracts, as do those who take certain medications, such as corticosteroids. If you have any of these risk factors, talk to your doctor about your chances of developing cataracts.

To diagnose cataracts, an ophthalmologist will perform a thorough eye examination. He or she will dilate your pupils with eyedrops and will examine the inside of your eyes with a slit lamp microscope (a viewing instrument with a bright light and magnifying lenses) to detect any clouding of the lens. If a cataract is present, the doctor will determine the type, size, and location of the cataract.

At present there are no eyedrops or other medications that will eliminate cataracts. At first, your vision may be improved with prescription eyeglasses, bifocals, a magnifying glass for reading, or better lighting at home or at work. Once your vision becomes so poor that it affects your ability to function independently, you will probably need to undergo surgery to have the cataracts removed. However, you may not need surgery for many years; some people with cataracts never need surgery.

During cataract surgery the surgeon removes the clouded lens and usually replaces it with an artificial lens. Cataract surgery is one of the most common operations performed in the United States and also is one of the most successful. Good vision is restored in more than 90 percent of people who have cataract surgery. After surgery you will probably have to use eyedrops or wear protective eyeglasses for a time. Your vision may not become fully restored until a few weeks or months after surgery. Most people with a lens implant will need to wear bifocals.

In some cases the posterior capsule (the membrane at the back of the lens) may become cloudy months or even years after cataract surgery, causing blurred vision. This condition can be corrected with a surgical procedure that uses a laser (a highly concentrated, powerful beam of light). The procedure is brief and painless and can be performed in the doctor's office or in an outpatient facility.

If you are over age 60, the best way to protect your vision and to check for cataracts is to have your eyes examined by an ophthalmologist at least every 2 years. The examination should include dilation of the pupil so the doctor can see the lens and the back of the eyes. If a cataract is detected, your ophthalmologist will work with you to decide on the best course of treatment and will explain the risks and the benefits of cataract surgery.

Diabetic Retinopathy

Diabetic retinopathy is an eye disorder caused by diabetes (see page 365), a chronic disease that can damage blood vessels, including those in the eye. A leading cause of blindness in adults in the United States, diabetic retinopathy is caused by changes in the blood vessels of the retina, the light-sensitive membrane that lines the back of the eye. In some people, the blood vessels leak fluid. In others, abnormal new blood vessels grow on the surface of the retina. These abnormal blood vessels can bleed and leak into the vitreous humor (the jellylike substance that fills the center of the eye), preventing light from passing through to the retina. The abnormal blood vessels and bleeding also can produce scar tissue that pulls the retina away from the back of the eye, causing a detached retina. Anyone with diabetes can develop diabetic retinopathy, and the longer a person has diabetes, the more likely he or she is to develop this disorder. Nearly half of all people with diabetes will develop diabetic retinopathy.

There may be no obvious symptoms in the early stages of the disease, but some people with diabetic retinopathy experience blurred vision when the macula (the part of the retina that provides sharp central vision) swells because of the leaking fluid. Abnormal blood vessels that have grown on the surface of the retina can cause symptoms such as blurred vision, seeing spots, vision that alternates between being normal and diminished, pain in the eyes, and sudden loss of vision. If you experience any of these symptoms, contact your ophthalmologist immediately. In some cases, vision may not become impaired until the disease is severe. That is why regular (at least yearly, or more often if recommended by your physician) eye examinations performed by an ophthalmologist are so important for people with diabetes.

During the eye examination, the ophthalmologist will dilate your pupils with eyedrops and then examine your retina using an ophthalmoscope (a handheld viewing instrument that projects a very bright light onto the back of the eye). He or she will look for leaking fluid, abnormal bleeding, or new blood vessel growth on the retina. Early detection and treatment of diabetic retinopathy go a long way toward preventing vision loss and blindness and minimizing potential vision problems.

The best way to prevent diabetic retinopathy and to slow its progression is to consistently control the level of glucose in your blood (see page 368) through diet, exercise, medication, and insulin, if necessary. It also is important to keep your blood pressure within the normal range (see page 219). In some cases the ophthalmologist may recommend laser surgery in which a highly concentrated beam of light is directed onto the retina either to shrink abnormal blood vessels or to seal leaking blood vessels. This procedure can be performed in the doctor's office or in an outpatient facility. Laser surgery can reduce the risk of severe vision loss from diabetic retinopathy, but it may not restore vision that has already been lost.

A type of microsurgery (delicate surgery performed under a microscope) called vitrectomy may be used for advanced cases of diabetic retinopathy, in which the vitreous humor has become filled with blood. In this procedure the vitreous humor is removed and replaced with a clear solution. Vitrectomy may take several hours to complete and is performed in an operating room using either local or general anesthesia. The procedure can cause discomfort. Recovery time varies, depending on the extent of the problem.

Surgery to reattach the retina may be needed if scar tissue causes the retina to become detached from the back of the eye. The procedure is performed using either local or general anesthesia and may be combined with laser surgery or vitrectomy. Surgery may take several hours to complete and is performed in an operating room. The procedure can cause discomfort.

People who have diabetes are also at risk for other eye diseases. They are twice as likely to develop a cataract (see page 390) as people without diabetes, and the cataracts tend to develop at an earlier age. Glaucoma (see page 388) also occurs in people with diabetes twice as often as in other adults. The longer you have diabetes, the higher your risk of developing glaucoma.

Macular Degeneration

The part of the retina (the light-sensitive membrane that lines the back of the eye) that provides sharp sight in the center of the field of vision is called the macula. You need this sharp central vision to see fine details. It is essential for driving, reading, and recognizing faces. As you age, the tissue of the macula can become damaged, leading to a loss of central vision. Age-related macular degeneration is the leading cause of blindness in the United States.

There are two general types of macular degeneration: dry and wet. The dry form accounts for about 90 percent of all cases of the disorder. In this form, the macula slowly thins until vision becomes dimmed. Although only about 10 percent of all people with macular degeneration have the wet form, they are at much higher risk of losing their sharp central vision than are those with the dry form. New blood vessels grow under the retina in the wet form of the disease. These blood vessels bleed and leak fluid, creating a large blind spot in the center of the field of vision.

The greatest risk factor for macular degeneration is age. Although symptoms can appear when a person is in his or her 40s or 50s, they usually occur in people over age 60. Women tend to be at greater risk than men, and whites have a higher risk than people of other races. Smoking also appears to increase the likelihood of developing macular degeneration.

Neither form of macular degeneration causes pain. The most common early symptom is blurred vision. As fewer cells in the macula are able to function, affected people are less able to see details—for example, in faces or on printed pages. The blurred vision may lessen in more brightly lit areas, but once the light-sensing cells degenerate, a small but growing blind spot appears in the middle of the field of vision. Another symptom is that objects in straight lines, such as telephone poles or sentences on a page, appear crooked. This phenomenon can occur because fluid from the leaking blood vessels collects and lifts the macula, distorting vision.

To diagnose macular degeneration, an ophthalmologist will use eyedrops to dilate your pupils and an ophthalmoscope (a handheld viewing instrument that projects a very bright light onto the back of the eye) to view the retina. The doctor also may ask you to look at a pattern called an Amsler grid, which looks like a checkerboard. If your central vision is affected, the lines of the grid will appear wavy or distorted.

Currently there is no proven treatment for dry macular degeneration. Some doctors believe that taking antioxidant vitamins (see page 9), zinc supplements, or lutein (an antioxidant found in plants such as spinach, kale, and collard greens) may be helpful in slowing the progression of the disease. A number of low-vision aids, such as magnifying glasses or bright lights, can help affected people continue to participate in activities they enjoy and to lead independent lives.

Some cases of wet macular degeneration can be treated with laser surgery, in which a highly concentrated beam of light is used to destroy the new blood vessels under the retina. Laser surgery is less successful when the abnormal blood vessels have grown beneath the center of the macula. Laser surgery is usually performed in a doctor's office or in an outpatient facility, and the person is allowed to go home the same day.

Color Vision Deficiency

Color vision deficiency (color blindness) refers to abnormal color vision that causes a person to see colors differently than others see them or that causes problems distinguishing certain colors. The deficiency may range from difficulty telling the difference between shades of the same color to total inability to see any colors at all. Most people with this problem have a mild deficiency and have difficulty distinguishing shades of red and green.

Color vision deficiency is usually an inherited disorder. It is predominant in men, and about 8 percent of all males are affected, although women can carry the gene for defective color vision and pass it to their children. In people with color vision deficiency, receptor cells for color in the retina (the light-sensitive membrane that lines the back of the eye) malfunction, sending incorrect information about color to the brain. The severity of the disorder varies from person to person. Color vision deficiency is diagnosed according to the person's symptoms and the results of color vision testing.

Some people have defective color vision that is not inherited. Aging can cause the lens of the eye to darken, affecting a person's ability to differentiate colors. Certain drugs and eye diseases also can disturb normal color vision.

There is no cure for inherited color vision deficiency, but affected people can take steps to counteract the problem. Some people learn to compensate by developing their own methods of distinguishing different colors—for example, by brightness or location. Tinted prescription eyeglasses may help some people who have red-green color vision deficiency.

If you have a family history of color vision deficiency and work in an occupation that requires distinguishing colors, or if you are having trouble identifying colors, see an ophthalmologist to be tested for color vision deficiency. He or she can recommend steps you can take to compensate for the problem.

CHAPTER 21
Ears

The ear is the organ of hearing and balance. It has three main parts: the outer ear, the middle ear, and the inner ear. Sound waves enter the outer ear and proceed to the middle ear, where they cause the eardrum to vibrate. The vibrations move through three tiny bones—the malleus (hammer), incus (anvil), and stapes (stirrup)—in the middle ear and proceed into the inner ear, where they are changed into nerve impulses. These nerve impulses are transmitted by way of the vestibulocochlear nerve to the brain, where they are perceived as sound.

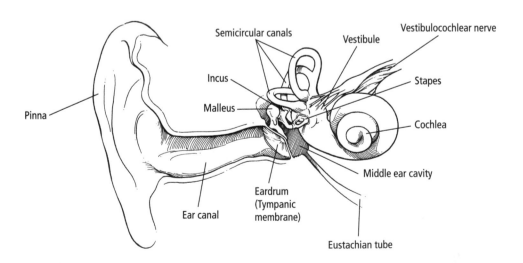

Ear

Hearing loss can interfere with your ability to communicate and can compromise your safety. Other ear disorders can cause unpleasant symptoms such as ringing in the ears (tinnitus), dizziness, and loss of balance. Tiny, fluid-filled structures in the inner ear help you keep your balance.

Hearing Loss

Aging and excessive exposure to loud noise are the most common causes of hearing loss. Other factors—such as viral or bacterial infections, an inherited disorder, or a benign tumor in the ear—also can produce hearing loss. One in 10 people in the United States has a hearing loss severe enough to affect his or her ability to hear normal speech. After age 50, most people have some degree of hearing loss. The changes occur very gradually and usually go unnoticed until a family member or friend mentions the person's hearing problems. Among older people, a third of those between ages 65 and 74 and half of those over age 85 have hearing loss.

There are two main types of hearing loss: conductive hearing loss and sensorineural hearing loss. Conductive hearing loss occurs when something, such as a buildup of earwax or an abnormality in the eardrum, prevents sound waves from being transmitted to the inner ear. This type of hearing loss can sometimes be corrected with medication or surgery. Sensorineural hearing loss refers to hearing problems that occur because of damage to the inner ear or the auditory nerve. Such damage can occur as a result of the aging process or because of exposure to loud noise. A hearing aid (see page 399) is most helpful for this type of hearing loss.

Exposure to loud noises—either a one-time exposure or repeated exposure over time—damages both the sensory hair cells of the inner ear and the auditory nerve. The longer you are exposed to loud noise and the closer you are to its source, the more damage it can cause.

The loudness of sound or noise is measured in units called decibels. A ticking watch is about 20 decibels, normal conversation is about 60 decibels, and city traffic noise is about 80 decibels. Sounds at 80 decibels or less are considered safe. Sounds between 90 and 100 decibels, such as a rock concert or a jet engine, may damage your hearing. Sounds that are between 120 and 140 decibels are usually painful and even a brief exposure can cause permanent hearing loss. Examples of things that can produce sounds over 120 decibels include motorcycles, snowmobiles, jackhammers, firecrackers, woodworking tools, and firearms.

Exposure to loud noise can occur in the workplace, in recreational settings, and at home. Some people are more sensitive to noise than others. In general, however, noise is loud enough to affect your hearing if you have to shout over it to be heard or if the noise causes pain or ringing in your ears. Temporary hearing loss that lasts for a few hours after exposure to loud noise is a sign of damage to your hearing.

For some people with hearing loss, sounds may gradually become distorted or muffled. They may experience problems having a conversation, listening to music, or even hearing a ringing doorbell or telephone. Participating in daily activities may become more difficult and less enjoyable because the person cannot hear properly and feels left out. He or she also may hear a hissing or a ringing in the ears (tinnitus; see page 401). Hearing loss also may have psychological effects. The person may become a source of annoyance or frustration and be ridiculed or ignored by family and friends. He or she might become depressed or withdraw from others to avoid embarrassment.

Although noise damage to the inner ear is irreversible, there are steps you can take to prevent noise-induced hearing loss. The most important thing you can do to protect your hearing is to avoid loud noise whenever possible. It is a good idea, for example, to keep the volume low on your personal stereo. If other people can hear music coming from your headphones, the sound is probably loud enough to cause permanent damage to your hearing.

If you are exposed to loud noise in the workplace, be sure to wear appropriate ear protection. Using specially designed earmuffs is the most effective way to protect your hearing on the job. These earmuffs, which resemble stereo headphones, block out almost all sound. Usually they are worn by people who work around noisy equipment or under extremely noisy conditions, such as construction workers or airport baggage handlers.

Another effective form of ear protection (although less effective than earmuffs) is earplugs made of foam rubber, plastic, or wax. Earplugs are inserted into the outer ear canal and must fit snugly to provide optimal protection. They should be replaced promptly if they become soiled or worn, because they will quickly lose their effectiveness. Ordinary cotton balls cannot adequately protect your hearing. You can purchase earplugs in a variety of styles, shapes, and sizes at your local pharmacy.

If your workplace is very noisy, it is extremely important that you have your hearing checked regularly. If your employer does not have your hearing checked regularly, see your doctor, who will perform hearing tests (see "Diagnostic Procedures," page 404) to check for hearing loss. If hearing loss is detected early, you can take steps to prevent further damage to your ears. If noise levels at work seem too high, talk to your employer or your union representative. You may also contact your local health department or the local office of the Occupational Safety and Health Administration (OSHA) to report the problem.

If you think you may have hearing loss, see your doctor. He or she will perform audiometry (see page 404) using an instrument called a screening audiometer to test your hearing. This instrument produces a range of sound tones at various frequencies and volumes that are typically heard during speech. The doctor will ask you to raise your finger each time you hear a tone. The results of this test will determine whether your hearing loss is serious enough for your doctor to refer you to an audiologist, a health professional trained in evaluating hearing loss and fitting hearing aids (see below), or an otolaryngologist, a physician who specializes in treating disorders of the ear, nose, and throat.

Do You Have Hearing Loss?

Hearing loss is common, especially among older people. You may have some degree of hearing loss if any of the following apply to you:

- You have difficulty hearing over the telephone.
- You have difficulty following a conversation when two or more people are talking at the same time.
- Friends and family complain that you turn the TV up too loud.
- People often ask if you can hear them.
- You strain to understand conversations.
- You have difficulty hearing over background noise.
- You think that other people are mumbling when they speak.
- You have difficulty hearing someone who is whispering.
- You have difficulty hearing women or children talking.

If you have any of these problems, talk to your doctor. He or she can perform a simple hearing test to determine whether you have hearing loss and may refer you to an otolaryngologist or an audiologist for additional testing.

Hearing Aids

A hearing aid is a small, battery-powered device that fits in or over your ear and amplifies sounds. Although a hearing aid can be fitted to only one ear, hearing aids are usually placed in both ears to provide the best overall hearing. Amplification of sound in both ears allows the person to hear speech more clearly and helps him or her to distinguish where sounds are coming from, especially in noisy surroundings.

Although many models of hearing aids are available, most can be placed into one of the following categories. Behind-the-ear hearing aids fit over the ear and are connected to a custom-made earpiece. In-the-ear hearing aids sit inside the outer ear and the outer part of the ear canal. In-the-canal hearing aids are small, unobtrusive devices that fit inside the ear canal. The smallest and least visible devices are completely-in-the-canal hearing aids, which fit more deeply inside the ear canal. In-the-canal hearing aids and completely-in-the-canal hearing aids are the most cosmetically appealing because they provide powerful assistance to hearing without being visible. Many hearing aids also come with telephone pickup switches that provide special assistance while you are on the phone or listening to a public sound system. The type of hearing aid that is right for you depends on your degree of hearing loss, the size and shape of your ear and ear canal, your lifestyle, and your budget.

Custom-made hearing aids vary in price, depending on style and special features. Prices typically range from $500 for a standard hearing aid up to $2,500 for hearing aids that are fully computerized and programmable. However, price should not be your only consideration when choosing a hearing aid. You should also consider factors such as comfort, appearance, durability, reliability, and the service agreement.

Before choosing a hearing aid, you should have a thorough hearing evaluation (see "Diagnostic Procedures," page 404) performed by an otolaryngologist or an audiologist. You can purchase the hearing aid directly from the doctor or the audiologist or from an independent, licensed hearing aid distributor. A wax impression of your ear will be made so that the laboratory can create a hearing aid that fits your ear exactly. No matter where you purchase your hearing aid, however, it is essential to have it custom-fitted to your ear for best results. It is important to note that hearing aids purchased through mail order usually cannot be custom-fitted.

When you receive your hearing aid, you will be tested to determine how well you can hear and understand speech while wearing the device. You will also learn how to care for your hearing aid, how to insert and remove it, how to change the batteries, and how to use your hearing aid correctly. You will need to have your hearing aid tested and adjusted regularly to ensure that it is working properly. Once you begin wearing your hearing aid, give yourself time to adjust. You should begin by wearing the device first in quiet surroundings and gradually work up to noisier situations. Although a hearing aid cannot cure your hearing loss, it can allow you to hear sounds and voices more clearly so that you can communicate better and more easily participate in your usual activities.

Surgery to Correct Hearing Loss

Almost all people with hearing loss can benefit from using a hearing aid. Others, however, may need surgery to improve their hearing. Here are some surgical procedures that are performed to treat hearing loss:

- *Myringoplasty.* This procedure is used to repair a perforated eardrum (a hole in the eardrum) with a tissue graft (a transplantation of healthy tissue from one part of the body to another). The tissue is usually taken from another part of the ear, or from an area near the ear. The procedure is often performed using local anesthesia and causes a minimal amount of pain. The person may need to stay overnight in the hospital and will need to rest at home for about a week after surgery. In most cases, recovery is complete in about 6 weeks.

- *Tympanoplasty and stapedectomy.* These procedures are used to repair a perforated eardrum or to replace damaged bones in the middle ear. Damaged bones may be repaired, or they may be replaced with artificial implants, transplanted bones supplied by a donor, or bones constructed from cartilage. The procedure is performed using either local or general anesthesia and may cause mild pain for a few days. The person may not need to stay overnight in the hospital but will need to rest at home for about 7 to 10 days after surgery. In most cases, recovery is complete in about 2 months.

- *Cochlear implant.* This procedure involves implantation of an electronic device to treat severe sensorineural hearing loss (see page 397) that has caused total or near-total deafness. The implant changes sound waves into electronic impulses that are carried along the auditory nerve to the hearing center in the brain, enabling the person to distinguish different kinds of sounds and often to understand speech. The device has both internal and external components. The internal component (a special signal processor and electrodes) is surgically implanted into the ear while the person is under general anesthesia. The person usually needs to stay in the hospital for a couple of days. The ear will heal in about 4 to 6 weeks, after which the physician will fit the person with the external components (a microphone, a transmitting coil, a speech processor, and connecting wires). The person will then work with an audiologist to adjust the settings on the implant for the best hearing level and to learn how to use the device properly.

Tinnitus

Tinnitus is the medical term for ringing or other sounds in the ears that occur when there is no external source of these sounds. It is a very common condition, affecting an estimated 35 million people in the United States each year. It is estimated that 1 to 5 percent of these people have tinnitus so severe that it affects their ability to lead a normal life. Symptoms include ringing, hissing, buzzing, or whistling in one or both ears. The symptoms may be constant or come and go, the pitch can vary from high to low, and the sound can pulsate in time with the heartbeat. One type of tinnitus causes clicking or crackling sounds. These annoying sounds can be a major source of distraction and irritation, affecting performance at work and other daily activities. Tinnitus can make it difficult for the person to fall asleep.

Tinnitus is caused by hearing loss or by spasms (involuntary muscle contractions) in the muscles of the neck or jaw. The hearing loss, which may not be noticeable, may result from a variety of diseases and conditions, including stiffening of the bones in the middle ear, allergies, high blood pressure, diabetes, a tumor, a thyroid condition, or head or neck injury. Certain medications—such as anti-inflammatory drugs, antidepressants, aspirin, or antibiotics—can trigger tinnitus. However, most cases of tinnitus result from damage to the sensory hair cells and the microscopic endings of the auditory nerve, which are in the inner ear. This damage is common in older people. In younger people the damage usually results from continual exposure to loud noise. Hearing loss typically accompanies tinnitus, but one often becomes apparent before the other.

If you hear ringing in your ears or other unusual or unwanted sounds, see your doctor. He or she will probably refer you to an otolaryngologist, who will first administer a hearing test. Additional tests, such as a computed tomography (CT) scanning or magnetic resonance imaging (MRI), a test for balance, and blood tests, may be performed to determine the cause of your tinnitus. Possible causes may include infection, obstruction, or Ménière's disease (see below). If the tinnitus is caused by an infection, your doctor will probably prescribe antibiotics. If there is an obstruction, such as a buildup of earwax or dirt, your doctor will remove it. In many cases, however, a cause cannot be identified.

There are a number of steps you can take to reduce the severity of your tinnitus, depending on its cause. The most important thing you can do is to avoid loud noises. Some people also find that relaxation exercises (see page 119) help to relax their muscles, improve circulation, and reduce the ringing in their ears. If your tinnitus is caused by high blood pressure or poor circulation, you should have your blood pressure checked regularly and work with your doctor to control it. Reduce your intake of stimulants such as coffee, tea, colas, and tobacco products. Exercise regularly to promote good circulation.

Some doctors recommend using a technique called masking to relieve the effects of tinnitus. Because the condition is more noticeable in quiet surroundings, you can try to mask the unwanted sounds in your ears by listening to a competing sound, such as a radio or television, an air conditioner, a ticking clock, or radio static. Tapes that play "white noise" can also distract you from the annoying sounds of tinnitus. Your doctor may recommend a tinnitus masker, which is worn like a hearing aid and gives off a more pleasant sound that masks the tinnitus. A hearing aid sometimes helps mask tinnitus, even if your hearing seems adequate. Before trying any of these techniques, however, talk to your doctor about which methods are best for you. Most people will learn to tolerate their tinnitus. Some people benefit by joining a support group where they can share experiences and information with other people who have tinnitus. Others may find that counseling helps them to cope with the condition. Ask your doctor for a referral.

Ménière's Disease

Ménière's disease is an abnormality in the inner ear that causes a number of symptoms—dizziness, tinnitus (see page 401), hearing loss that comes and goes, and pressure in the affected ear. The symptoms of Ménière's disease appear suddenly and can occur daily or as seldom as once a year. The dizziness can lead to nausea, vomiting, and sweating and can become so severe that the person has to lie down. Ménière's disease usually affects only one ear and is a somewhat common cause of hearing loss. At first the person's hearing returns to normal between episodes, but over time the hearing worsens. Ménière's disease affects about 3 million to 5 million people in the United States, with about 100,000 new cases diagnosed each year. The cause of the disease is unknown.

A part of the inner ear known as the labyrinth is necessary for hearing and balance. The labyrinth contains a fluid called endolymph. When you move your head, the fluid moves within the labyrinth, causing nerves in the labyrinth to send signals to the brain about the movement of your body. Symptoms of Ménière's disease occur when excess fluid builds up in the labyrinth.

To diagnose Ménière's disease, a doctor first takes a medical history and performs a thorough physical examination. The doctor is usually able to diagnose the condition on the basis of the person's symptoms. Hearing tests (see "Diagnostic Procedures," next page) and balance tests help to confirm the diagnosis and rule out other possible causes of the symptoms. The most common hearing test used to diagnose Ménière's disease is audiometry, in which a person's ability to hear sounds of varying frequencies and volumes is evaluated.

To assess the person's balance, the doctor may perform a test that includes flooding the person's ears with water. This produces rapid eye movements that help the doctor evaluate balance. Because a brain tumor can produce symptoms similar to those of Ménière's disease, the person may need to have a scan of the brain to rule out a possible tumor.

There is no cure for Ménière's disease, but certain treatments can help manage the symptoms. Some doctors recommend dietary changes. Eliminating salt (sodium), caffeine, and alcohol relieves the frequency and intensity of episodes in some people. Stopping the use of tobacco (see page 107) and reducing stress (see page 118) also may lessen the severity of symptoms. Your doctor may prescribe diuretics to help your body eliminate excess fluid, thereby decreasing the severity and frequency of episodes. Medications that control allergies also can be helpful. The dizziness typically stops after 10 to 20 years, but the hearing loss will persist.

Three types of surgery have been developed to correct the disorder, but their effectiveness has been difficult to establish. Another important factor to consider is that all surgery on the ear carries a risk of hearing loss. The most commonly performed surgical treatment for Ménière's disease is insertion of a shunt (a tiny tube) into the inner ear to drain excess fluid. In another type of surgery, called vestibular neurectomy, the nerve responsible for balance is cut so it can no longer send distorted messages to the brain. Because this nerve lies close to the nerves that are responsible for hearing and facial muscle control, this type of surgery carries a risk of loss of hearing or facial movement. Older people often have difficulty recovering from this type of surgery. During a third type of surgery called a labyrinthectomy, the surgeon removes the membrane inside the labyrinth to eliminate the dizziness caused by Ménière's disease. This procedure is irreversible and produces a total loss of hearing in the affected ear. People considering this type of surgery need to know that their other ear may someday also be affected by Ménière's disease, which means that total deafness is a possibility in the future. In rare cases, labyrinthectomy and vestibular neurectomy may cause permanent balance problems, especially in older people.

Diagnostic Procedures

The following procedures are used to test for hearing loss and to diagnose or rule out certain possible underlying causes of hearing loss:

- *Audiometry*. This is the most commonly used hearing test. The first part measures how well you can hear sounds conducted through the air and indicates the condition of your overall hearing. The test is usually administered in a soundproof room using a machine called an audiometer. Through headphones, you listen to a series of sound tones that range from high to low, one tone at a time. Each tone begins at an easily audible sound level. You indicate with a prearranged signal when you hear the tone. The sound level decreases gradually until you are no longer able to hear the tone; this point is your hearing threshold for that frequency. The second part of the test measures how well you can hear sounds conducted through your head and indicates whether your hearing loss is conductive or sensorineural (see page 397). The procedure is the same as for the first part of the test, but this time you wear special vibrating headphones. Next you are tested for words to establish the lowest threshold at which you can hear two-syllable words (called your speech-reception threshold) and to determine the percentage of one-syllable words you can repeat back correctly (called speech discrimination). Your hearing thresholds for all parts of the test are recorded on a graph called an audiogram.
- *Impedance audiometry*. This hearing test measures how well your eardrums reflect sound waves. During the test, a probe that is covered with soundproof material is placed into your outer ear canal, sealing off the entrance to both sound and outside air pressure. The probe then transmits a continuous sound as air is pumped into the ear canal through the probe at various pressure levels (from low to high), and a microphone in the probe measures reflected sound waves. These reflections are recorded on a graph called a tympanogram. This test is used to detect fluid in the middle ear, a perforated eardrum, and disorders of the three tiny sound-conducting bones (the malleus or hammer, the incus or anvil, and the stapes or stirrup) of the middle ear.
- *Auditory evoked response testing* (also called auditory brain stem response testing). This computerized hearing test is used to measure the electrical activity of the vestibulocochlear nerve by determining how long it takes nerve impulses traveling along the nerve to reach the brain stem. During the test, electrodes are placed on your scalp to analyze your brain's response to sound

stimulation produced by an audiometer. This test is sometimes used to rule out an acoustic neuroma (a noncancerous tumor in the ear canal).

- *Electrocochleography.* This hearing test measures the electrical activity of the sensory hair cells in the inner ear in response to sound waves. During the test, the eardrum is anesthetized and a very fine needle is passed through the eardrum until it is very near the sensory hair cells. Sound tones of varying frequency (low to high) and loudness are then transmitted into the ear through headphones, while the needle detects the electrical activity of the sensory hair cells. The electrical activity is recorded on a graph called an electro-cochleogram. This test is sometimes used to diagnose Ménière's disease (see page 402).

CHAPTER 22

Teeth and Gums

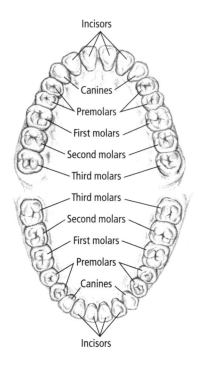

Incisors

Canines

Premolars

First molars

Second molars

Third molars

Third molars

Second molars

First molars

Premolars

Canines

Incisors

Your Teeth

Most of us have 32 permanent teeth. Teeth start the digestive process when we eat food. Incisors have a sharp edge for cutting food, the canines tear food, and the premolars and molars grind food.

You can keep your teeth and gums healthy by brushing and flossing every day. And be sure to visit your dentist regularly for examinations and cleanings. Good oral healthcare will help ensure strong teeth and good overall health for years to come.

Keeping Your Teeth and Gums Healthy

Having a clean mouth is good for you in many ways. Not only does it give you fresh breath and a nice smile, but it also gives your self-esteem a lift. Thorough daily cleaning of your teeth and gums helps prevent tooth decay and periodontal disease (gum disease). Keeping your teeth and gums healthy also can improve your overall health. Periodontal disease may be a factor in the development of chronic conditions such as heart disease.

The best way to ensure oral health is to brush your teeth at least twice a day and to floss them daily. Brushing and flossing remove the thin sticky layer of bacteria that grows daily on your teeth. This layer of bacteria is called plaque, and it is responsible for both tooth decay and periodontal disease. When you eat, the bacteria in plaque produce acids that attack the teeth and irritate the gums, making them inflamed. Over time, the gums may bleed and pull away from the teeth. Bacteria and pus accumulate in the pockets that form in the

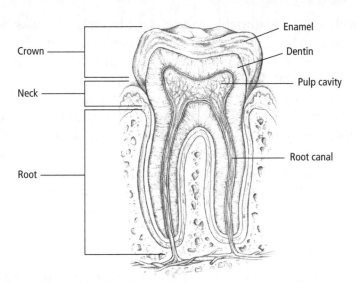

Crown

Neck

Root

Enamel

Dentin

Pulp cavity

Root canal

Structure of a Tooth

A tooth is living tissue. The crown is the part of the tooth that shows above the gums. Dentin, a tissue that is harder than bone but sensitive if its enamel covering is broken, makes up most of the tooth. Teeth contain one to three roots, which are embedded in bone. The pulp cavity at the core of a tooth contains nerves, connective tissue, and blood vessels and lymphatic vessels (which provide nourishment and disease protection).

spaces between the gums and the teeth. Eventually the bone around the teeth deteriorates, and the teeth loosen and fall out.

Flossing your teeth every day helps to remove the plaque that accumulates between your teeth, where your toothbrush cannot reach. It is also important to see your dentist for a thorough teeth cleaning twice a year, assuming that your gums are healthy. A professional cleaning helps to remove calculus (commonly known as tartar), a hard mineral deposit that forms on the teeth, providing an additional surface to which plaque can adhere. If you have periodontal disease or tend to accumulate calculus faster than normal, your dentist may recommend more frequent cleaning.

When you brush your teeth, be sure to use a soft-bristled brush. Brushes with medium or hard bristles are too abrasive and can make your gums recede from your teeth. Your teeth can then become sensitive to cold liquids because the roots of the teeth, which are normally covered by the gums, have been partially exposed. Place the toothbrush against your teeth at an angle and brush back and forth gently in short strokes. Brush the outer and inner tooth surfaces and the chewing areas of the teeth. Be sure to brush your tongue to remove bacteria and to freshen your breath.

To floss your teeth properly, use about 18 inches of floss and wind some of it around one of the middle fingers on each hand. Hold the floss between the thumb of one hand and the index finger of the other hand, or use both index fingers, or whatever feels most comfortable to you. Gently slide the floss between your teeth, up to the gum line. Do not snap the floss into your gums. Move the floss up and down between your teeth, and repeat this procedure on the rest of your teeth. If you find dental floss to be too unwieldy, try using another kind of dental cleaner, such as a pick, to clean between your teeth. Ask your dentist to show you how to use the device properly so you do not injure your teeth or gums.

Sugary and starchy foods—such as sweets, bread, crackers, and cereal—are more likely to cause plaque buildup than other foods. Try to limit your intake of these foods between meals, or brush your teeth soon after eating them. Better yet, snack on fresh fruit, raw vegetables, or plain yogurt. It will be better for your overall health as well.

Corrective Dentistry

To treat damage caused by tooth decay and gum disease, your dentist has a wide array of techniques available. He or she also can replace or repair teeth lost or damaged because of an injury to the mouth or the jaw. Extraction (pulling) of a tooth is now a last resort. Sometimes the line between corrective and cosmetic dentistry blurs when cosmetic techniques are used to repair or replace lost or damaged teeth. Remember to see your dentist twice a year for a thorough cleaning and checkup so that he or she can detect and treat any tooth or gum problems early. Common corrective dental techniques include:

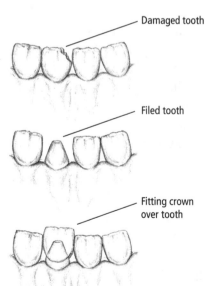

Damaged tooth

Filed tooth

Fitting crown over tooth

Fitting a Crown

For a crown, your dentist first makes an impression of the natural shape of your damaged tooth. He or she then files the tooth down to a stub in preparation for fitting the crown. The crown has a hollow core that fits precisely over the filed-down tooth. The crown is cemented in place over the tooth.

- *Silver amalgam fillings.* Silver fillings consist of an alloy of several metals—such as silver, zinc, or tin—and mercury. Dentists use silver fillings to fill a tooth after all of the decayed material has been removed. Although it is a matter of some controversy, no proof exists that dental amalgam containing mercury poses any threat to your health.
- *Crowns.* Sometimes called caps, crowns are placed over a tooth that does not have enough tooth structure left for more conservative treatment, such as a veneer.
- *Bridges.* Dentists use replacement teeth called bridges to fill in the spaces left by one or more missing teeth to prevent the teeth adjacent to the space from shifting out of their normal position. The bridge is cemented to the adjacent teeth, which are fitted with crowns or caps.
- *Implants.* Implants are also used to replace missing teeth by placing a "substitute" root form into the jawbone. Crowns, caps, or bridges can then be attached to the implants without involving adjacent teeth.

- *Root canal therapy*. During root canal treatment, the dentist or oral surgeon first administers a local anesthetic and removes the infected nerve tissue from the tooth. Then he or she prepares the root canal to accept the filling material. At the next visit, the dentist will fill and seal the root canal with a plastic material that prevents future infection. The tooth may then require a crown or a cap.

Cosmetic Dentistry

Today there are a number of techniques that can improve the appearance of your teeth and brighten your smile. These cosmetic dental techniques vary in price. Some are simple and others are complex. Your dentist can advise you about the best cosmetic dental procedures for your situation. The most common cosmetic dental procedures are:

- *Tooth whitening or bleaching*. Bleaching is simple and effective and has few side effects. The dentist makes a mold of your teeth, from which rubber mouth guards are made. At home, you place the tooth-whitening solution into the mouth guards and wear the guards for an hour each day, for 2 to 4 weeks.
- *Cosmetic contouring*. In this process, the dentist reshapes the front teeth, using a hand-held instrument, to create a more pleasing appearance.
- *Veneers*. A veneer is a porcelain laminate shell used to make a new front surface for a tooth that is misshapen, darkened, or spaced too far from a neighboring tooth.
- *White fillings*. These white plastic fillings, called inlays or onlays, are used instead of silver fillings to treat dental cavities in a more aesthetically pleasing way.
- *Crowns*. Sometimes called caps, crowns are placed over a tooth that does not have enough tooth structure left for more conservative treatment, such as a veneer.
- *Braces*. Orthodontic appliances, commonly called braces, straighten teeth that are crowded or crooked. Braces can be made with metal or plastic brackets and wires.
- *Aligners*. Aligners are clear, removable pieces of plastic molded to fit over the teeth to straighten them without wires and brackets. An aligner is worn day and night for about 2 weeks and is then replaced with the next one in the series. Unlike braces, aligners can be removed for eating, brushing, and flossing.

Periodontal Disease

Periodontal disease, also known as gum disease, is inflammation of the gums and other tissues surrounding the teeth that is caused by a bacterial infection. The disorder affects as many as 75 percent of adults over age 35. It is the main cause of tooth loss in adults.

The earliest stage of periodontal disease is called gingivitis. The main symptom of gingivitis is gums that bleed when you brush or floss your teeth. At this stage, gum disease is both preventable and reversible because the plaque buildup has not yet extended below the gum line to the roots. Brushing your teeth daily is not enough to prevent gingivitis. The only way to stop gingivitis and to prevent further inflammation is to brush your teeth consistently twice a day, floss your teeth daily, and have a professional tooth cleaning at least twice a year. You should also maintain a balanced diet and avoid smoking or chewing tobacco.

Left untreated, the gums begin to pull away from the teeth, and pockets form between the teeth and the gums. The pockets may become filled with pus, and the gums may recede farther. Plaque spreads to the roots of the teeth, and the infection begins to damage the bone and other supporting tissue. The teeth begin to shift and loosen and either fall out or have to be extracted (pulled) by the dentist.

Warning Signs of Periodontal Disease

Periodontal disease, also known as gum disease, is the number one cause of tooth loss in American adults. It may also be a risk factor for heart disease or other medical conditions. An estimated 75 percent of adults over age 35 in the United States have some form of periodontal disease, but the disorder is easily reversed in its early stages by consistent, daily toothbrushing and flossing. Because periodontal disease is painless, you may not know that you have it. If you notice any of the following signs of periodontal disease, see your dentist right away:

- gums that bleed when you brush or floss your teeth
- red, swollen, or tender gums
- gums that have pulled away from your teeth
- bad breath or a bad taste in your mouth that does not go away
- pockets of pus around your teeth and gums
- loose teeth
- pain when chewing

Not only is periodontal disease damaging to your teeth and gums, it also may adversely affect your overall health. Periodontal disease may contribute to the development of heart disease, the number one cause of death in the United States. Doctors are still not sure why there appears to be a connection between periodontal disease and heart disease, but research has shown that the bacteria responsible for periodontal disease can enter the bloodstream and cause plaque buildup in the arteries leading to the heart. Periodontal disease also has been implicated in the development of stroke, pneumonia, and peptic ulcers.

It is important to have regular dental checkups to prevent and detect periodontal disease. If you think you have the condition, see your dentist right away. He or she will perform a thorough examination of your mouth, teeth, and gums. If the condition is present, the dentist will probably assess the severity of the disorder by checking for bleeding with a probe, measuring the depth of any pockets, assessing how well each affected tooth is still attached, and evaluating bone loss through dental X rays. He or she will develop a treatment plan that is tailored to your needs, depending on the extent of the periodontal disease.

Dentists use a variety of therapies to treat periodontal disease, but all focus on the removal and control of the infectious bacterial plaque. In a process known as scaling, the dentist uses handheld instruments to remove the hardened plaque and calculus from above and below the gum line. During root planing, the dentist smoothes out the surface of the root by removing the bacteria and toxins that lead to periodontal disease. Ultrasonic scaling involves use of an instrument that converts a high-frequency electrical current into mechanical vibrations, which remove plaque and calculus. The dentist may also use a technique called subgingival debridement to remove tooth surface irritants from below the gums so that infection will not occur at the treated site.

If periodontal disease has progressed to an advanced stage, the dentist may have to treat it with one of two surgical techniques. Both procedures attempt to remove diseased tissue so that new replacement tissue can grow. The first technique is called resective surgery, in which the dentist lifts the gum away from the tooth and bone to remove diseased tissue and reshape infected bone. The dentist then repositions the gum and stitches it back into place. Another type of surgery, known as regenerative surgery, attempts to actually regrow the jawbone and supporting tissue by using special inserts that help new tissue grow.

Dentists are beginning to use some new therapies to fight periodontal disease. Inserts containing antibiotics or anti-inflammatory drugs are available that can be placed directly into infected pockets to destroy bacteria. Mouth rinses or toothpastes containing drugs or antimicrobial agents that can destroy the microorganisms responsible for periodontal disease also have been developed. Ask your dentist to recommend one.

Temporomandibular Disorder

Temporomandibular disorder (TMD) is a phrase that refers to a group of painful disorders affecting the jaw and the muscles that control chewing. The temporomandibular joint connects the lower jaw, called the mandible, to the temporal bone at the side of your head. The discomfort may be occasional and temporary, often occurring in cycles, and may eventually stop with no treatment. Some people will develop long-term symptoms. The disorder affects men only half as often as it does women.

There are three main forms of TMD. The most common form is called myofascial pain, in which the muscles that control jaw function and the neck and shoulder muscles become painful. Another form is called internal derangement of the joint, which includes dislocation of the jaw and displacement of the soft, shock-absorbing disk in the jaw. TMD can also be caused by degenerative joint disease, such as arthritis in the jaw joint. A person may have more than one form of TMD at the same time.

TMD can produce a range of symptoms, most commonly pain in or around the jaw joint. Other symptoms include limited movement or locking of the jaw; pain that radiates to the face, neck, or shoulders; a painful clicking, popping, or grating sound in the jaw joint when the mouth is opened; and a sudden change in the way the upper and lower teeth fit together. Headaches, earaches, hearing problems, and dizziness also may sometimes be linked to TMD.

Severe injury to the jaw or temporomandibular joint is a leading cause of TMD. A heavy blow to the jaw can fracture the bones of the joint or damage the disk of the jaw, interfering with the normal movement of the jaw and causing the jaw to lock or be painful. An injury also can lead to arthritis in the jaw joint. Some doctors think that stress can cause or aggravate TMD, especially when the affected person clenches or grinds his or her teeth at night. No evidence exists that gum chewing, an overbite or underbite of the teeth, or orthodontics such as braces directly cause TMD. Many people experience clicking of the jaw, but if no pain or locking is present, they probably do not need treatment.

There is currently no widely accepted test that correctly diagnoses TMD. Most doctors arrive at a diagnosis based on the person's description of his or her symptoms and a physical examination of the face and jaw. During the physical examination, the doctor will feel the joints to detect any pain or tenderness, listen for any popping or clicking of the joint, and check for limited motion or locking of the jaw joint. The doctor will review the person's medical and dental history to pinpoint any past conditions that could have produced the current symptoms. If the doctor thinks that arthritis may be causing TMD, he or she may order X rays.

For some affected people, the discomfort of TMD will eventually go away on its own. Because many cases of TMD are temporary and do not get worse, doctors usually prescribe simple and conservative treatments for the disorder. Eating soft foods, applying heat or ice packs, and avoiding extreme jaw movements such as wide-mouthed yawning often produce favorable results. Stress-reducing relaxation techniques (see page 119) also can improve symptoms. Doctors sometimes enlist the help of a physical therapist, who can provide gentle muscle-stretching exercises. The doctor may recommend using nonsteroidal anti-inflammatory drugs such as aspirin or ibuprofen for a short period. He or she may prescribe muscle relaxants. A dentist may recommend that you wear a plastic appliance called a splint or bite guard, which fits over your upper or lower teeth. This device can help prevent you from grinding your teeth at night.

Dental procedures used to adjust and balance the bite (how the upper and lower teeth come together when the jaw is shut)—such as braces, crowns, and bridges, and grinding down portions of the teeth—may help relieve symptoms of

TMD. Surgery to replace the jaw joints with artificial implants is necessary in only a small percentage of affected people.

Oral Cancer

Oral cancer is one of the most debilitating and disfiguring types of cancer. Tumors affecting the lip, mouth, tongue, and soft palate (the part of the throat at the back of the mouth) can interfere with swallowing and speech. If the cancer spreads to other parts of the body, it can cause disability and even death. But if oral cancer is detected and treated early, it has a very high cure rate. More important is the fact that oral cancer is highly preventable.

Tobacco use is the number one cause of oral cancer. A smoker's risk of oral cancer is two to four times higher than that of nonsmokers. In fact, people who are most at risk of developing oral cancer are men over age 40 who smoke cigarettes, cigars, or a pipe, or who use smokeless tobacco (chewing tobacco or snuff). Smokeless tobacco is particularly dangerous because it contains 100 times the amount of cancer-causing compounds found in other forms of tobacco. This fact is especially disturbing because the use of smokeless tobacco continues to rise, primarily among adolescent boys.

Heavy alcohol consumption increases the risk of developing oral cancer for smokers and nonsmokers alike, but heavy drinking increases the risk by 15 times for heavy smokers. This suggests that smoking and alcohol consumption somehow work together to produce oral cancer by increasing each other's harmful effects. Even high alcohol-content mouthwashes have been implicated in the development of oral cancer.

A type of cancer known as Kaposi's sarcoma develops in about 30 percent of people who have acquired immunodeficiency syndrome (AIDS). The disease produces red or purple patches (lesions) on the skin or the mucous membranes that line the mouth, nose, and anus. This type of cancer can be the first sign of AIDS and is often first detected during a dental examination. Lip cancer has been linked to long-term sun exposure and pipe smoking.

Most oral cancers develop on the surface layer of tissue and are called squamous cell carcinoma. Symptoms that can indicate the presence of oral cancer include:

- a sore on the lip or in the mouth that does not heal
- a lump on the lip or in the mouth or throat
- a white or red patch on the gums, tongue, or lining of the mouth (which may be painless in the early stages)
- unusual bleeding, pain, or numbness in the mouth
- a feeling that something is caught in the throat
- difficult or painful chewing or swallowing
- swelling of the jaw that causes dentures to fit poorly

- a change in the voice
- pain in the ear

These symptoms may be caused by other, less serious problems, but they should always be brought to the attention of a physician or a dentist, who can make a firm diagnosis and provide appropriate treatment.

If an abnormality is found in the mouth, the doctor will perform a biopsy, in which a sample of the abnormal tissue is removed and examined under a microscope. Once cancer is diagnosed, the doctor will attempt to stage the cancer. This means that he or she will try to find out the extent to which the cancer has developed and possibly spread. Cancer can travel through the lymph system and spread to other parts of the body. Oral cancer usually spreads first to the neck. Staging tests may include dental X rays and X rays of the head and chest, a computed tomography (CT) scan (a series of X rays transmitted to a computer that forms detailed pictures of the body), and magnetic resonance imaging (MRI; which links a powerful magnet with a computer to make cross-sectional images of the body). The doctor also will examine the lymph nodes in the neck to check for swelling.

After diagnosing and staging the cancer, the doctor will develop an individualized treatment plan. Treatment for oral cancer depends on a number of factors, including the location, size, type, and extent of the tumor. The doctor also will consider the person's age and general health when developing a treatment plan. Oral cancer treatment generally consists of surgery to remove the abnormal tissue, and radiation therapy to stop the cancerous cells from growing. These treatments may be used alone or in combination. Chemotherapy (treatment with powerful anticancer drugs) also may be used in conjunction with surgery and radiation therapy to relieve pain in advanced stages of the disease.

The doctor will try to plan therapy to minimize side effects, but most oral cancer treatment produces side effects, some temporary and some permanent. Surgery to remove cancerous tissue may require removal of part of the soft palate, tongue, or jaw. Such surgery is likely to affect the person's ability to chew, swallow, or talk. He or she may also look different, prompting depression (see page 345) or lowered feelings of self-worth. Weight loss may become a problem because eating may be difficult. Radiation therapy can cause fatigue, along with red, dry, tender skin that "weeps" fluid. The person's skin also can become darker and more sensitive to the sun.

The most important steps you can take to reduce your risk of developing oral cancer are to stop using tobacco (see page 107) in any form and to drink alcohol only in moderation. To lessen the risk of developing lip cancer, use a lotion or lip balm that contains a sunscreen and wear a hat with a brim outdoors to block the sun's harmful rays.

CHAPTER 23

Skin and Hair

Your skin is your largest organ. It covers your body tissues and internal organs and protects them from injury and infection. Skin is made up of two layers: a thin outer layer called the epidermis and a thicker inner layer called the dermis. Under the dermis is a layer of fat called subcutaneous tissue. The outer part of the epidermis is made up of dead cells and keratin (a tough, fibrous type of protein), which form a protective covering. These dead cells are constantly shed and then replaced by new cells. The inner part of the epidermis is made up of living cells that divide rapidly to produce those new cells. Certain cells in the epidermis produce the pigment known as melanin, which protects your skin and determines your skin color.

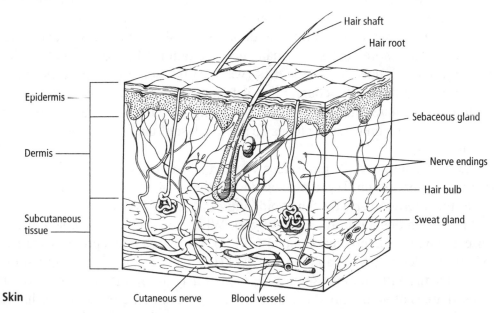

Skin

The dermis is made up of connective tissue and contains structures such as hair follicles, sweat glands, sebaceous glands (which produce an oily substance called sebum), blood vessels, lymph vessels (which carry lymph into and out of the lymph glands), and nerves. Your skin also has some other important roles, including sensation—such as touch, temperature, and pain—and regulation of body temperature through perspiration and dilation (widening) and constriction (narrowing) of blood vessels.

Your hair is an extension of your skin. Hair is made up of dead cells and keratin. Each hair shaft has a spongy core (medulla), a surrounding layer of thin fibers (cortex), and a thin covering of overlapping cells (cuticle). Each hair is rooted in a hair follicle (a tiny pit in the surface of the skin), from which it grows. While a hair is growing, the hair root is surrounded by live tissue called a bulb, which supplies keratin to the hair. Certain cells at the base of the hair follicle produce melanin, which determines your hair color. The main function of hair is protection.

Sunburn and Protecting Your Skin from the Sun

Too much exposure to ultraviolet rays from the sun, sunlamps, or tanning beds produces sunburn. The most common symptom of sunburn is red, swollen, and painful skin that can blister. If the sunburn is severe and covers a large portion of your body, you may also experience chills, fever, nausea, and vomiting. Repeated sun exposure also can produce harmful long-term effects, including wrinkling, premature aging of the skin, and skin cancer (see page 428). The most serious type of skin cancer, malignant melanoma (see page 428), is often fatal.

People who are most likely to be sunburned and who are most at risk for sun-induced skin cancer are those with fair skin, blue eyes, and red or blond hair, although anyone who spends time outdoors is at risk. The more sun exposure you receive, the more your skin is damaged. Certain medications—such as the antibiotic tetracycline, some diuretics (water pills), some tranquilizers, birth control pills, and over-the-counter antihistamines—make the skin more sensitive to the sun, increasing the likelihood of being sunburned. You are at risk for sunburn even on cloudy days; clouds do not block sunlight—they merely scatter the sun's rays.

There are a number of simple steps you can take to protect yourself from the harmful rays of the sun. Try to plan outdoor activities for early in the morning or late in the afternoon so you can avoid being in the sun between 10:00 AM and 3:00 PM, when the sun's rays are strongest. When you are out in the sun, use a sunscreen with a sun protection factor (SPF) of 15 or higher that protects against both ultraviolet A (UV-A) and ultraviolet B (UV-B) rays. The lighter your skin, the higher the SPF number should be. Generously apply the sunscreen to all exposed areas of your skin at least 30 minutes before going outdoors so that it has time to be fully absorbed. Always reapply sunscreen immediately after swimming or every few hours if you are perspiring. Remember to put sunscreen on your ears, the back of your neck, and any bald spots on your head. Use a lip balm that contains sunscreen. Wear a wide-brimmed hat, and always wear sunglasses that filter at least 90 percent of both UV-A and UV-B rays. Check labels for this information when you are shopping for sunglasses.

If you get a sunburn, cover the burned area with cool, clean, wet cloths or gauze, or take a cool bath or shower. Take an over-the-counter anti-inflammatory drug such as aspirin or ibuprofen to relieve pain, fever, and inflammation. Do not use a spray that numbs the burned area because it may cause an allergic or irritant reaction. Drink plenty of liquids and rest in a cool room for several hours. Before you expose your skin again, make sure that the inflammation is gone, and put extra sunscreen on the previously burned areas so you do not get burned again.

Atopic Eczema

Atopic eczema is a recurrent inflammatory skin condition that produces redness, itching, and scaly patches. People who have atopic eczema also often have other allergic conditions, such as allergic rhinitis (see page 379) or asthma (see page 245), or are allergic to penicillin or sulfa. Atopic eczema is a very common condition that affects about 3 percent of Americans. The disorder can occur at any age but typically appears between infancy and young adulthood. The condition often improves on its own before puberty but also can persist throughout life.

Most people have dry skin at some point, but people with atopic eczema have periodic eruptions of red, scaly patches of skin. In adolescents and young adults the patches usually appear inside the elbows and behind the knees and at the ankles and wrists; in children they appear on the face and neck. But the eruptions can occur anywhere on the body and may not follow a pattern. The itching produced by the eruptions can be severe and prolonged.

People who have atopic eczema seem to have easily irritated skin, so anything that dries or irritates the skin may trigger a flare-up. They are often sensitive to low levels of humidity, and their skin condition may worsen in the winter. If this is true for you, try to bathe no more than once a day, avoid using very hot water, and use the mildest soap you can find. After bathing, pat your skin dry; do not rub it. Immediately apply a moisturizing lotion or oil to your skin, before it has completely dried. Avoid dressing in clothes made of rough or scratchy fabrics, which can aggravate the condition. Sweating also can make the condition worse.

Depending on the severity of the condition, your doctor may refer you to a dermatologist (a doctor who specializes in treating disorders of the skin). To distinguish atopic eczema from other types of skin conditions, the dermatologist will examine the skin eruptions, noting where on your body they appear and how often they occur. To control atopic eczema, the dermatologist probably will prescribe a cream or ointment containing a corticosteroid, a drug that relieves inflammation. If any of the inflamed patches have become infected because of overly aggressive scratching, the doctor also may prescribe an antibiotic. Severe cases of atopic eczema may require treatment with ultraviolet light or oral corticosteroid medication.

Allergic Contact Dermatitis

Allergic contact dermatitis is a skin condition that occurs when your skin comes into contact with allergens, substances to which you are allergic but that are harmless to most people. This condition is not triggered by harsh soaps or acids, for example, because these substances are irritants that will produce a rash on anyone's skin, given enough exposure.

Upon contact with an allergen, the skin reddens and swells and may blister. The blisters may burst, leaving scaly patches. The condition is sometimes difficult to distinguish from other skin conditions, such as atopic eczema (see previous page).

Substances that can trigger allergic contact dermatitis include nickel or nickel-plated items, rubber, hair dyes, and cosmetics such as perfumes and lotions. (Some people are allergic to the chemicals used to preserve cosmetics, while others are allergic to the fragrances used in these products.) Rubber can cause a more serious allergic reaction that goes beyond a simple rash. Some people who are allergic to rubber (including the latex rubber used in rubber gloves) experience itchy, watery eyes and, in some cases, shortness of breath that could lead to anaphylactic shock (see page 383), a potentially fatal allergic reaction. Chromium contained in cement, leather, paints, and antirust products also can produce allergic contact dermatitis. Rashes produced by plants such as poison ivy, poison oak, and poison sumac also are considered allergic contact dermatitis. People who are sensitive to poison ivy, oak, and sumac also may be allergic to the oils contained in mango skins and cashew nut shells.

To diagnose allergic contact dermatitis and to determine its cause, your doctor will examine your rash and ask questions about the materials you use at home and at work. He or she may perform a patch test, in which small amounts of suspected allergens are applied to your skin for a couple of days. If an area of skin becomes inflamed, that substance may be an allergen for you.

The rash produced by allergic contact dermatitis will usually clear up on its own once the allergen has been removed. The only way to prevent the condition from recurring is to avoid all contact with the allergen. A dermatologist can help you identify your allergens.

Seborrheic Dermatitis

Seborrheic dermatitis is a common skin disorder in which red, scaly, itchy patches of skin appear where the sebaceous (oil) glands are located in the skin—

on the scalp, eyebrows, sides of the nose, behind the ears, and in the middle of the chest. The patches also can occur in the navel, under the arms, in the groin area, and on the buttocks. Extensive scratching of the itchy patches can damage the skin, producing an infection that causes the skin to become crusty and drain pus.

The disorder most commonly occurs during three stages of life: infancy (when it is known as cradle cap), middle age, and old age. People with oily skin or oily hair are susceptible to seborrheic dermatitis, and infrequent shampooing can increase the likelihood of developing the disorder. People who have acne (see below) also may develop seborrheic dermatitis. The condition seems to occur in people who have other illnesses, such as Parkinson's disease or immune system problems. Some researchers think that a yeastlike organism may cause seborrheic dermatitis.

If you have seborrheic dermatitis, a dermatologist will identify the condition based on its appearance. There is no cure for seborrheic dermatitis, but it usually improves with treatment. Your doctor may recommend nonprescription medicated shampoos that contain tar, zinc pyrithione, selenium sulfide, sulfur, or salicylic acid. A corticosteroid cream or lotion applied directly to the affected areas may also be helpful. Be sure to keep the affected areas clean and dry. Seborrheic dermatitis can recur, even with appropriate treatment.

Acne

Acne is a chronic skin disorder caused by inflammation of the hair follicles and the sebaceous (oil) glands in the skin. The disorder produces skin blemishes commonly called pimples. The blemishes usually appear on the face, neck, back, chest, and shoulders. Although it is not a serious condition, acne can cause scarring that can affect your appearance.

Acne occurs when hair follicles become blocked by plugs of sebum, the oily secretion produced by the sebaceous glands that lubricates the skin and hair. Bacteria then grow in the blocked follicles, causing inflammation. People with acne usually have a number of different types of blemishes, including whiteheads, which appear on the skin as small, white bumps, and blackheads, which look like black spots. Other blemishes include papules, which are inflamed pink bumps that are tender to the touch, and pustules or pimples, which are inflamed, pus-filled bumps that are red at the base. Painful, inflamed, pus-filled bumps that are lodged deep in the skin are known as cysts; they can produce scarring.

People of any age can develop acne, but it most commonly occurs in adolescents. Almost 85 percent of all teenagers and young adults between ages 12 and 24 have some acne. Acne usually clears up by the time a person reaches his or her 30s, but some people in their 40s and 50s still have the condition. Acne is more common among whites.

A number of factors can contribute to the development of acne. Rising levels of male sex hormones called androgens during puberty cause the oil-producing sebaceous glands to make more sebum. Another factor appears to be heredity. The tendency to develop acne seems to run in families. Stress can aggravate the condition, as can perspiration and high levels of humidity. Friction from tight collars, backpacks, or bike helmets also can make acne worse. Picking at the blemishes can produce scarring. Certain drugs, including lithium and barbiturates, may cause outbreaks of acne. Contrary to popular belief, chocolate and greasy foods seem to have little effect on the development of acne in most people.

There is a wide range of nonprescription acne-treatment products available. Most limit the formation of new blackheads and whiteheads and reduce inflammation. The most common over-the-counter drugs used to treat acne are benzoyl peroxide, resorcinol, salicylic acid, and sulfur. These medications can produce side effects, including skin irritation, burning, or redness, but the side effects disappear when the person stops using the product.

By the time a person decides to see a doctor, he or she has probably tried several over-the-counter medications and seen little improvement. Acne may be treated by a dermatologist, but family physicians and internists also treat people who have acne. The main goal of treatment is to prevent scarring, but doctors also seek to reduce the number of blemishes and minimize the embarrassment felt by people affected with a skin disease. Drugs prescribed to treat acne address several causes: clumping of cells in the hair follicles, increased oil production, bacterial infection, and inflammation. Your doctor may recommend a combination of medications to reach these goals.

Topical (applied to the skin) prescription drugs used to treat acne include benzoyl peroxide, clindamycin phosphate, erythromycin, adapalene, azelaic acid, and tretinoin. Tretinoin is a vitamin A derivative and is very effective for treating whiteheads and blackheads. Side effects from these drugs can include stinging, burning, redness, peeling, scaling, and discoloration of the skin. If you experience side effects, tell your doctor as soon as possible.

For people with moderate or severe acne, doctors may prescribe oral antibiotics in addition to a cream, lotion, or gel. Antibiotics help control acne by checking the growth of bacteria and reducing inflammation. They must be taken for at least 4 to 6 weeks to be effective. Some of these antibiotics may make the skin more sensitive to the sun, so you will need to take extra precautions (see page 416) when in sunlight. They also can cause upset stomach, dizziness, and skin discoloration. A doctor may prescribe a powerful medication called isotretinoin for people who have severe acne that has not responded to treatment with other acne medications. Isotretinoin can produce a number of unwanted side effects, some of which—such as increased blood cholesterol, abnormal liver enzyme levels, and birth defects—can be serious. While you are taking the drug, your doctor will monitor the levels of glucose, cholesterol, triglycerides (fats), and liver enzymes in your blood. Discuss the risks and the benefits of taking isotretinoin with your dermatologist, who can help you decide whether use of this drug is the best treatment for you.

Other treatments for acne include removal of individual blemishes, injection of a corticosteroid drug into a cyst, or a chemical peel. Cosmetic surgery (see page 439) is sometimes used to treat scarring caused by acne.

If you have acne, do not attempt to stop an outbreak or reduce oil production by aggressively scrubbing your skin or using strong soaps. This will only make the problem worse. Instead, gently wash your skin with a mild soap whenever it feels oily or greasy. And always wash your face after exercising. Your doctor can recommend the best soap or cleanser to use. Avoid squeezing, picking, or pinching your skin because doing so could cause even more inflammation and eventual scarring. Soften your beard with soap and water before shaving, and shave lightly to avoid nicking the blemishes. Do not try to dry out your skin or hide the blemishes by getting a suntan, because the benefits are temporary at best. Exposure to the sun can seriously damage your skin, can promote premature aging of your skin, and can cause skin cancer. Also, many drugs used to treat acne make your skin more sensitive to the sun.

Shaving Bumps

Shaving bumps or razor bumps (known medically as pseudofolliculitis barbae) is a common skin condition in the beard area of black men and others who have curly hair. The condition occurs when the sharp ends of shaved hairs grow back into the skin, causing inflammation. Eventually these ingrown hairs can cause scars, which resemble hard bumps, to form on the face and neck.

The only sure way to avoid developing shaving bumps is to grow a beard. If this is not practical, follow these shaving tips:

- Shave every day with a safety razor.
- Be sure to use sharp blades; replace the blades after every two shaves.
- Before shaving, gently wash your face with mild soap and a warm, soft washcloth; rinse your face thoroughly; and leave your face wet.
- Apply a nonirritating shaving cream or gel. Ask your doctor to recommend one.
- Always shave in the direction of hair growth.
- Do not pull or stretch your skin.
- Do not shave too closely. Press lightly with the razor. It is better for your skin if you press less firmly and shave more often.
- Do not keep going over the same spot. This can irritate your skin.
- Do not attempt to remove ingrown hairs with a tweezers. This can irritate your skin and may lead to infection.
- After shaving, rinse your face thoroughly and pat it dry.

If the condition does not clear up after trying these at-home tips, see your doctor. He or she may prescribe a cream or gel that includes a vitamin A–containing drug called tretinoin or an oral antibiotic to treat the condition.

Warning: Do not share razors. Doing so places you at risk of contracting a bloodborne infection such as hepatitis B or HIV (human immunodeficiency virus).

Psoriasis

Psoriasis is a persistent skin disorder that produces red, itchy, dry patches of skin with silvery scales. The disorder often begins in childhood and comes and goes throughout a person's life. The areas most commonly affected are the scalp, elbows, arms and legs, knees, groin and genitals, fingernails and toenails, and lower back. There are several different types of psoriasis, distinguished by the shape and pattern of the scales. The most common type begins as small, red patches that grow larger and form scales.

The cause of psoriasis is unknown, but it may be linked to an abnormality in the function of white blood cells that somehow triggers inflammation in the skin and causes it to shed too quickly. The condition seems to run in families. Four million to 5 million people in the United States have psoriasis. Factors that can trigger the condition include bacterial or viral infections, certain drugs, dry and cold weather, sunburn, skin injury, drinking alcohol, and stress.

Doctors can diagnose psoriasis by examining the skin or by taking a sample of the skin and examining it under a microscope. The goals of treatment are to lessen inflammation and slow skin cell growth. A variety of different treatments—topical (applied to the skin) creams or lotions, light therapy, and oral medication—have been developed to reach these goals. If you have psoriasis, the treatment your doctor recommends will depend on your age, your overall health, and the severity of your condition. No treatment can cure psoriasis, but symptoms can be improved or controlled.

A common type of cream or ointment prescribed for the treatment of psoriasis is a corticosteroid preparation (such as hydrocortisone), which is used in a weak formula for sensitive areas such as the face or the groin and in a stronger formula for other areas. Side effects of these preparations include thinning of the skin, dilation (widening) of the blood vessels, bruising, and skin-color changes. The doctor may inject a corticosteroid drug into areas that are difficult to treat. Topical retinoids (such as tazarotene) are vitamin A–like medications that may be prescribed to treat mild to moderate psoriasis. Other topical psoriasis preparations include those that contain a drug called anthralin, synthetic vitamin D, or coal tar. Many nonprescription shampoos, oils, and sprays are available to treat psoriasis on the scalp.

Both natural sunlight and artificial ultraviolet light from light boxes alter the growth of skin cells, so doctors can use light therapy to treat psoriasis. Light therapy must be used under the supervision of a doctor because excessive exposure to sunlight or artificial ultraviolet light can cause skin wrinkling, skin cancer, damage to the eyes, or a flare-up of psoriasis. A treatment that combines light therapy with coal tar dressings is helpful for treating severe cases of psoriasis. Another effective treatment, called PUVA (psoralens and ultraviolet A), combines ultraviolet light therapy with the oral medication psoralen.

Other medications that may be prescribed to treat psoriasis include methotrexate and oral retinoids. Methotrexate is a powerful but effective anticancer drug that can cause serious side effects, such as liver disease. Before a doctor prescribes methotrexate, he or she will have the person undergo a liver biopsy (a small sample of liver tissue is obtained and examined under a microscope) to make sure that the person's liver is healthy. After the person begins taking methotrexate, the doctor carefully monitors blood levels of the drug to prevent potential problems. Retinoids (such as acitretin) may be taken alone or in combination with light therapy. Possible side effects include dryness of the skin, lips, and eyes; increased cholesterol levels; and formation of bone spurs.

Jock Itch

Jock itch (known medically as tinea cruris) is a fungal infection of the groin. The fungus also can infect other areas of the body, such as the feet and the area between the toes, where it causes athlete's foot (see next page). The infection begins as small, red spots that enlarge to form rings. At the edge of the ring the skin is raised, red, and scaly.

Jock itch is common in men who perspire heavily, who exercise vigorously in hot weather, or who are overweight. The infection can be transmitted to your groin from your feet if you have athlete's foot and you scratch both areas. Like all tinea infections, jock itch is somewhat contagious. You can get a tinea infection from wet surfaces (such as a shower stall), from another person, or even from an animal. Men who wear athletic protectors or equipment can develop a case of jock itch, especially in hot, humid weather.

If you think that you may have jock itch, see your doctor. The condition may be hard to distinguish from other skin problems that have different causes and treatments. The doctor may scrape off a small sample of affected skin and examine it under a microscope to confirm the diagnosis. Jock itch is treated by applying an antifungal cream to the groin area daily for at least a month. Other tinea infections may be more difficult to clear up and may require treatment with an oral antifungal medication. You will need to use all of the antifungal medication prescribed—even if your skin looks and feels better—to be sure the infection has been completely eliminated.

Athlete's Foot

Athlete's foot (known medically as tinea pedis) is a common fungal infection of the foot. It affects mainly adolescent and adult males. The tinea fungus readily grows in moist, damp areas such as shower stalls and floors. Sweating and inadequate ventilation of the feet provide ideal conditions for growth of the fungus.

The fungus can affect the skin between the toes or on the soles or sides of the feet. The affected skin itches, peels, cracks, and forms scales or blisters. Athlete's foot also can affect the toenails, making them thicken, scale, and crumble. Fungal infections of the toenail can be very difficult to treat. Untreated athlete's foot can cause breaks in the skin, leading to a bacterial infection.

To diagnose athlete's foot, your doctor will examine the affected areas of your skin and may remove a small sample of skin to examine under a microscope. The doctor will prescribe an antifungal cream to be applied to your skin. If the athlete's foot is severe, he or she may prescribe oral antifungal medication. You will need to use all of the antifungal medication prescribed—even if your skin looks and feels better—to be sure that the infection has been completely eliminated.

To prevent athlete's foot, keep your feet as clean and as dry as possible. Follow these useful tips to help prevent athlete's foot:

- Dry your feet thoroughly, especially between your toes.
- Take your shoes off at home to expose your feet to the air.
- Wear sandals during the summer.
- Wear absorbent cotton socks and change them every day.
- Do not walk barefoot in locker rooms or at poolside. Wear thongs or reef shoes.
- Never share shoes.
- Shake an antifungal powder into your shoes in hot weather.

Boils and Carbuncles

A boil is a collection of pus beneath the top layer of skin. It is caused by bacterial infection of a hair follicle, the tiny pit in the surface of the skin in which a hair grows. Boils can cluster under the skin; such a cluster is known as a carbuncle. Boils may result from infection of a cut or scrape in the skin, poor hygiene, cosmetics that clog the pores, exposure to chemicals, and friction from tight clothing or shoes. Perspiration contributes to the development of boils and carbuncles and can make them worse. Boils and carbuncles usually appear on the scalp, beard area of the face, arms, legs, underarms, and buttocks.

Boils begin as tender, inflamed, solid, sometimes painful bumps under the skin that enlarge as they fill with pus. Sometimes the nearby lymph nodes also become enlarged. Boils grow larger for a few days until they rupture, draining pus onto the surface of the skin. Carbuncles discharge their contents through a number of openings in the surface of the skin. Once they have ruptured, boils and carbuncles are less painful, but inflammation may persist for a few days or weeks. Scarring occurs in most cases.

You may be able to detect a boil on your own. Avoid squeezing or piercing a boil to open it up because the infection could spread. The best way to speed the opening of a boil is to apply warm, wet cloths to the area for 10 to 20 minutes several times a day. If you have a carbuncle or if the boil causes a fever or pain, see your doctor so he or she can prescribe oral antibiotics. In some cases, surgical drainage may be required.

To prevent the spread of boils and carbuncles, do not let others use your towels or washcloths, and be sure to change your clothes and bed linens every day. Launder these items in hot, soapy water before using them again. And always wash your hands after touching the affected area.

Common Noncancerous Skin Growths

A variety of spots or growths can appear on the surface of your skin—especially as you get older—but most are harmless and do not require treatment. The most common noncancerous skin growths are actinic (or solar) keratoses, cherry angiomas, skin tags, age spots (also called sun spots or liver spots), moles, seborrheic keratoses, and warts.

Actinic Keratoses

An actinic keratosis is a skin growth that has a rough surface and can be red, skin-colored, or white. It is also called a solar keratosis because it is caused by excessive exposure to the sun over time. Actinic keratoses usually develop on fair-skinned people during middle age or old age. They most commonly appear on the face, hands, forearms, and upper chest. In a small percentage of cases an actinic keratosis can develop into a form of skin cancer known as squamous cell carcinoma (see page 428), so even though it is a noncancerous skin growth, your doctor may remove it. Actinic keratoses can be permanently removed with surgery, including laser treatment.

Cherry Angiomas

A cherry angioma is a bright red spot that may be raised or flat and is composed of a collection of tiny, closely packed blood vessels near the surface of the skin. Cherry angiomas can develop on any part of the body but are most often found on the trunk. They increase in number after age 40. However, they do not become cancerous. Cherry angiomas that appear on the face can easily be removed for cosmetic reasons, but most are left untreated.

Skin Tags

Small flesh-colored or light brown flaps of skin that protrude from the surface of the skin are called skin tags. They most often occur on the neck, upper chest, and underarms and around the eyes. Skin tags are harmless but can be irritating if they are persistently rubbed. Doctors can easily remove skin tags that are irritating or unsightly by cauterizing (burning) them with heat, chemicals, or electric current, or by freezing them with liquid nitrogen.

Age Spots

Age spots (known medically as lentigines) are brown spots on the skin that resemble freckles and result from long-term exposure to sunlight. They are a sign that the skin is trying to protect itself from the sun by producing a pigment to help absorb the damaging sunlight. Age spots, also sometimes called sun spots or liver spots, appear in almost everyone as they get older, although they occur most frequently in fair-skinned people. Even people in their 20s or 30s can develop these spots—especially if they have fair complexions and have been exposed to excessive amounts of harmful sunlight. The spots most commonly occur on areas of the skin—such as the face, arms, hands, and tops of the shoulders—that are frequently exposed to the sun.

Treatment is usually not necessary unless you want to improve the appearance of your skin. You can purchase a nonprescription skin-bleaching cream at your local pharmacy to help fade the spots. There are a number of treatments available for age spots, including laser treatment to break up the pigment (color) in the spots, prescription skin creams, freezing with liquid nitrogen, or a chemical skin peel that uses a mild acid to remove the top layer of skin.

Moles

Moles are common skin growths that can appear on virtually any part of the body. Moles usually first appear as brown or black spots that enlarge slowly over time, becoming elevated and lighter in color. Moles can become flesh-colored, pink, tan, brown, or bluish black. Some eventually sprout hairs. Moles may darken with exposure to the sun.

Moles that are present from birth are known medically as congenital nevi. Moles that are larger than average or irregularly shaped or that have uneven color are called atypical or dysplastic moles. These types of moles have an increased likelihood of developing into the most serious form of skin cancer, malignant melanoma (see page 428). Any mole that changes, is asymmetrical, has an irregular border, displays an uneven color, or is larger than a pencil eraser should be examined by a dermatologist.

Most moles are harmless and require no treatment. However, some men may want to have a mole removed because of where it is located or because it is unsightly. A doctor can remove a mole by shaving or cutting it away and then stitching the nearby skin closed. Repeatedly shaving a mole will not cause it to become cancerous, but you may want to have a mole in the beard area removed because it is constantly irritated. Moles are usually removed in the doctor's office.

Seborrheic Keratoses

As they age, many people develop seborrheic keratoses, which are tan, brown, or black; raised; crusted; or waxy spots that have a "pasted-on" look. They most often appear on the chest, back, scalp, face, and neck and can occur alone or in clusters. Seborrheic keratoses are harmless and do not develop into skin cancer, although black seborrheic keratoses may be difficult to distinguish from skin cancer. A doctor can easily remove a seborrheic keratosis if it occurs in a location that affects your appearance. Doctors treat seborrheic keratoses by one of several methods: freezing them with liquid nitrogen, scraping them from the surface, burning them off using an electric current, or cutting them off with a scalpel or scissors.

Warts

Warts are skin growths caused by a viral infection. Warts usually are raised, rough, and flesh-colored but can also be dark, flat, and smooth. There are several different types of warts, including common warts, plantar (on the sole of the foot) warts, flat warts, and genital warts (see page 184). Common warts typically grow on the hands and fingers. They occur in areas where the skin has been broken, such as near bitten fingernails or picked hangnails. Plantar warts can be painful when walking. Flat warts are small and grow in clusters of 20 or more. They can appear anywhere, but in adult men they usually occur in the beard area and are thought to result from skin irritation from shaving. Genital warts are a sexually transmitted disease that occur on the genitals and anus or inside the rectum. They have been linked to the development of cervical cancer in women and other genital cancers.

Warts are contagious, which means that the virus that causes them can be passed from person to person. A doctor usually can diagnose warts based on their appearance. Warts should be treated promptly to prevent spreading them to another person. In some cases, common warts may clear up on their own or may be dissolved with an over-the-counter medication. The preferred method of removal for common warts is freezing with liquid nitrogen. Plantar warts may need treatment with acid plasters, liquid nitrogen, or medicated creams. Flat warts are removed by using a chemical skin peel or medicated creams. Genital warts can be treated with imiquimod cream or podofilox gel or may require freezing, acid treatments, or surgical removal.

Skin Cancer

Skin cancer is the most commonly occurring type of cancer in the United States. Experts estimate that 40 to 50 percent of Americans who live to age 65 will eventually develop some form of skin cancer. The risk is highest for people who have red or blond hair, light-colored eyes, and fair skin that freckles easily.

The two most common forms of skin cancer are basal cell carcinoma, which accounts for more than 90 percent of all skin cancers, and squamous cell carcinoma. Basal cell carcinoma is a slow-growing cancer, found in the base of the outer layer of skin, that rarely spreads to other parts of the body. Squamous cell carcinoma, which affects cells in the surface of the skin, also spreads infrequently, although it does so much more often than basal cell carcinoma.

A less common type of skin cancer, malignant melanoma, is the most serious form of skin cancer. It spreads quickly and can be fatal. The number of people with melanoma has more than doubled in the United States since about 1980, giving melanoma the fastest-growing incidence rate of all cancers. Melanoma begins in skin cells known as melanocytes, which produce melanin, the pigment

---

Warning Signs of Malignant Melanoma

Melanoma is the most serious and dangerous form of skin cancer. It quickly spreads to other parts of the body and can be fatal. The incidence of melanoma is increasing faster than any other type of cancer in the United States. The first sign of melanoma is often a change in the size, shape, color, or feel of an existing mole. Melanoma also can appear as a new black, blue-black, or red-bordered mole. Learn the warning signs of malignant melanoma so you can detect any changes in a mole early. Think of the letters "ABCD" to help you remember what to look for. (For pictures of suspicious moles, see page 92.)

- *A—Asymmetry.* Half of the mole does not match the other half.
- *B—Border.* The mole's edges are often ragged, notched, blurred, or irregular in outline. The pigment (color) may spread into the surrounding skin.
- *C—Color.* The color is typically uneven. Multiple colors—black, brown, tan, gray, red, pink, or blue—may be present.
- *D—Diameter.* The mole usually increases in size. Melanomas are typically larger than a pencil eraser (half an inch).

Melanomas vary greatly in appearance. Some have all of the above features; others may have only one or two. The most important thing to remember is to tell your doctor about any change you see in a mole as soon as possible so he or she can make a definite diagnosis. When detected and treated early, melanoma can be cured before it has a chance to grow and spread to other parts of the body.

that gives skin its color. When exposed to the sun, melanocytes produce more pigment, causing the skin to tan. Melanoma occurs when melanocytes become abnormal and begin to divide without control. The cancer cells then invade surrounding tissue and, in some cases, enter the bloodstream or lymph system to spread to other parts of the body. The first sign of melanoma is often a change in an existing mole (see box on previous page). In men, melanoma often appears on the trunk, head, or neck.

The leading cause of all types of skin cancer is excessive exposure to ultraviolet (UV) radiation from the sun, sunlamps, or tanning beds. The cumulative amount of exposure to UV radiation that you have had during your life determines your risk of developing skin cancer—the more exposure, the greater your risk. Most skin cancers appear after age 40, but the sun's damaging effects begin much earlier, in childhood. The most important thing you can do to reduce your risk of skin cancer is to limit the amount of time you spend in the midday sun.

The most common warning sign of skin cancer is a new growth or a sore that does not heal on your skin. The area may look like a small, pale lump or be firm and red. The lump may bleed or develop a crust. Skin cancer also can begin as a flat, red spot that is rough, dry, and scaly. Skin cancer typically appears on parts of the skin—such as the face, neck, hands, and arms—that have been repeatedly exposed to the sun, although it can appear on any part of the body.

Early detection and treatment increase the chances for a cure. That is why it is important to examine your skin regularly for any changes. The best time to perform a skin self-examination is after a shower or bath, using both a full-length mirror and a handheld mirror. Look for anything new—such as a change in a mole or a sore that will not heal. Check all areas of your body, including your face and neck, back, scalp, palms, forearms and upper arms, the backs and fronts of your legs, and your feet. Also check your genitals and the area between your buttocks. Use a comb to part your hair so you can examine your scalp. Examining your skin regularly will help you to become familiar with the normal moles, birthmarks, and blemishes that are present on your skin so you can tell if there is a change in them. Your doctor will check your skin for any "suspicious" growths during a routine physical examination.

Treatment for skin cancer usually involves some form of surgery and, in rare cases, may also require radiation therapy or chemotherapy (treatment with powerful anticancer drugs). Many skin cancers can be cut out of the skin easily in a doctor's office. After numbing the affected area with a local anesthetic, the doctor scoops out the cancer with a spoon-shaped instrument called a curette and then controls bleeding and kills any remaining cancer cells by using an electric current. Most people are left with a flat, white scar. Small skin cancers or precancerous conditions such as actinic keratoses (see page 425) can be treated using cryosurgery, in which the area is frozen with liquid nitrogen and then peeled away. Doctors can use laser treatment on cancer that has affected only the outer layer of skin. Laser treatment uses powerful, concentrated beams of light to destroy cancerous tissue.

When a large area of skin has been removed, the person who has been treated for skin cancer may need a skin graft to close the wound and fill in the area of missing tissue. To perform a skin graft, the doctor will take some skin and tissue from another part of the person's body and use it to replace the skin that was removed.

Doctors often use radiation therapy for cancers that appear in areas—such as the eyelid, ear, or tip of the nose—that are difficult to treat with surgery. Radiation therapy is very effective for treating skin cancer, especially in older people, who are less likely to experience any long-term effects. Doctors may treat cancers that are limited to the top layer of skin with creams that contain anticancer drugs such as fluorouracil. Intense inflammation can follow such treatment.

Follow-up care is extremely important because skin cancer can recur in the same general location. About 40 percent of people who have had skin cancer will develop a second skin cancer within 5 years. If you have had skin cancer, examine your skin regularly for any changes, see your doctor for regular checkups, and follow your doctor's instructions about preventing a recurrence. Also remember to stay out of the sun as much as possible.

Dandruff

Dandruff (known medically as seborrheic dermatitis), the scaling and sloughing of the skin on the scalp, usually occurs during adolescence and adult life, reaching its peak severity at about age 20. In a person with dandruff, small white or gray scales accumulate on the surface of the scalp. The scales detach from the scalp, falling among the hairs and on the shoulders. Doctors once suspected that a yeast infection may have been the cause of most cases of dandruff, but current evidence shows that no microorganisms have a role in its development.

The best method of treating dandruff is shampooing with an antidandruff shampoo that contains selenium sulfide, zinc, or tar. After removal with a shampoo, however, the scales often form again in 4 to 7 days. If your dandruff is severe, see your doctor, who may prescribe an antidandruff shampoo. Daily shampooing will help prevent dandruff. Ask your doctor to recommend an over-the-counter hydrocortisone cream or ointment to help relieve itching and redness.

Hair Loss

Our culture places great importance on hair and its appearance. Hair loss can cause embarrassment and loss of self-esteem. Your hair grows continually for 2 to 6 years, then rests for 2 or 3 months before falling out naturally. Shedding 50 to 100 hairs each day is a normal process, and each shed hair is replaced by a new hair that begins to grow out of the same follicle. Your hair grows about a half inch every month, but, as you age, your rate of hair growth slows.

There are many different types of hair loss, with a number of different causes. A high fever or severe infection can produce hair loss, as can an overactive or underactive thyroid gland. Other causes of hair loss include an inadequate amount of protein in your diet, iron deficiency, or cancer treatment. Certain prescription medications—such as those for gout, arthritis, depression, heart disease, or high blood pressure—can cause hair loss in some people. Large doses of vitamin A also can cause hair loss. If you notice that your hair is falling out in large amounts after you brush or comb your hair, see your doctor as soon as possible to determine the cause.

For men, the most common type of hair loss is male pattern baldness, in which hair sheds from the top of the scalp and the hairline at the same time. Most men will experience some degree of hair loss as they get older. Thinning hair and baldness in men are usually inherited. Hair loss can be treated and controlled. Some men compensate for their hair loss by styling their hair differently or by wearing hairpieces, but there are now a number of effective methods for treating male pattern baldness.

A nonprescription medication called minoxidil is somewhat effective for regrowing lost hair. The drug does not produce results right away, but after about 4 to 6 months you may be able to see soft, downy hair in the bald areas of your scalp. The new hair may become the same color and thickness as your existing hair. Minoxidil is not effective for treating hair loss caused by anything other than hereditary male pattern baldness. If you stop using the drug, the hair loss will begin again.

Another drug, called finasteride, has been shown to be effective against male pattern baldness. Available only in pill form, the drug was originally used as a treatment for an enlarged prostate gland (see page 170). During such treatment, doctors noticed that some men regrew hair in balding areas of the scalp. The drug appears to increase the number of hairs in thin or balding areas while also slowing hair loss. You will need to take finasteride every day for at least 6 months before seeing any results. The predominant, although rare (for fewer than 2 percent of men who use the drug), side effect is impaired sexual function. Neither finasteride nor minoxidil is effective for replacing lost hair in a receding hairline. As with minoxidil, if you stop using finasteride, you will continue to lose hair. (**Warning:** Women who could become pregnant must never use finasteride because the drug has been shown to cause birth defects.)

Hair replacement surgery (see page 442) can restore lost hair.

CHAPTER 24

Cosmetic Surgery

Men are changing the way they think about their appearance—some do not want to accept what nature has given them and are willing to use cosmetic surgery to look better. Men's attitudes about cosmetic surgery are changing, too. They no longer think of it as being for women only. Once thought of as a status symbol for the wealthy and famous, cosmetic surgery is now more accepted by the general public, including men. In fact, the number of cosmetic surgery procedures performed on men is increasing dramatically.

Liposuction, in which pockets of fat are suctioned from the body to improve the contour of the face, neck, trunk, or limbs, is the most common cosmetic surgery procedure performed on men. The second most common procedure among men is eyelid surgery, the third is nose reshaping, and the fourth is breast reduction surgery. Other types of cosmetic surgery performed on men include facelifts, facial resurfacing (skin-smoothing treatments for the face), facial implant surgery, abdominoplasty, chest implant surgery, calf implant surgery, and hair replacement surgery.

More and more men are having cosmetic surgery to look and feel younger and to give themselves a competitive edge in the workplace.

Choosing a Surgeon

If you are considering cosmetic surgery, it is important to find a well-trained and experienced plastic surgeon. The first step in this process is to assemble a list of qualified doctors; there are several sources from which you can develop such a list. For example, if a friend or family member has had cosmetic surgery and is pleased with the results, ask him or her for the surgeon's name. Your doctor also may be able to recommend some plastic surgeons in your area. Local hospitals can provide the names of plastic surgeons on staff. However, the best way to locate a qualified plastic surgeon in your area is to contact a local or national professional association of plastic surgeons or your state medical society. These organizations also can tell you whether the doctors on your list are board-certified (see page 94).

Once you have narrowed your choices to two or three doctors, schedule an interview with each one so you can discuss his or her approach to the procedure and ask about fees. Because health insurance plans do not usually cover the cost of cosmetic surgery, you will need to determine whether the surgeon offers payment plans or whether he or she accepts credit cards. When you call for an appointment, ask for brochures about the surgery in question and read through them before your visit so you can ask informed questions about the procedure and its risks and possible outcomes. Write down your questions in advance. Make sure that the surgeon provides you with realistic expectations about the potential results of the surgery. Ask to see photographs of other patients who have had the procedure you are considering. Ask the surgeon to explain any terms you do not understand. After the interviews, you will be in a good position to make an informed decision.

Preparing for Surgery

Once you have decided on a cosmetic procedure and have selected a qualified surgeon, you are ready to begin preparing for surgery. During your first meeting with the surgeon you have selected, he or she probably will ask you to explain your reasons for wanting to have the procedure and how you expect to look and feel after surgery. Open communication between you and the surgeon is crucial when planning your surgery, so be candid about what you hope to achieve through surgery. The surgeon will explain whether you will have surgery in the doctor's office, at an outpatient surgery center, or at a hospital. He or she also will discuss the type of anesthesia that will be used. Any type of surgery carries risks, so make sure that you ask questions to help you fully understand the risks of the surgery you are considering. Although complications do not occur very often and usually are minor, the outcome of surgery is never fully predictable. The risks of cosmetic surgery include injury to the skin or a nerve, infection, or an adverse reaction to anesthesia or medication. Serious complications also can include formation of fat or blood clots that could travel to the lungs and cause injury or even death. There also is the possibility that you will be disappointed with the cosmetic results of the surgery. You can lower your risk of complications by following your surgeon's instructions carefully.

The surgeon will take photographs of you before and after surgery so the two of you can evaluate the results of the procedure. Before surgery the doctor will closely examine the part of your body to be altered and will discuss a number of issues related to the specific type of surgery you wish to have. For example, if you are planning to have a facelift, the doctor will closely evaluate your head and neck, checking to see if your hairline is receding, how far your beard grows up your cheeks and down your neck, and whether you have any facial scars or sun-damaged skin. He or she also will note whether your neck skin is loose or "jowly." The doctor will talk to you about the bruising and swelling that will occur after surgery. He or she also will discuss potential scarring.

The surgeon will ask whether you have any chronic diseases or conditions, such as high blood pressure or a blood clotting disorder, that could cause problems during surgery or affect the healing process. People with diabetes, chronic heart or lung disease, or poor circulation also have a higher risk of surgical complications. Tell the surgeon if you take any medication (prescription or nonprescription) or vitamins. Some drugs, such as aspirin, and some vitamins, such as vitamin E, can interfere with blood clotting. Also tell the doctor if you smoke. Smoking inhibits blood flow and can affect the way your skin heals after surgery.

There are no guarantees when it comes to the results of cosmetic surgery. Be sure that you have realistic expectations about how you hope to look and feel after the procedure. Discuss your expectations fully with your doctor and listen carefully to his or her description of the proposed outcome. Do not expect cosmetic surgery to stop or reverse the aging process. Although cosmetic surgery can enhance your appearance and increase your self-confidence, it will not necessarily match your ideal image or cause other people to treat you differently. The final result may differ from what you have in mind.

Recovery from cosmetic surgery takes time, and the signs of the surgery (such as swelling or bruising) may be visible for days or weeks after the procedure. Try to schedule your surgery during your vacation so the treated area will be fully healed by the time you return to work. Before surgery, be sure to closely follow your doctor's instructions about eating and drinking, smoking, and taking or avoiding certain drugs or vitamins. If you develop a cold or an infection before surgery, your procedure may need to be postponed.

You probably will be groggy from the anesthesia, so be sure to arrange in advance for someone to drive you home after surgery. Plan on taking it easy for the first few days after surgery. Depending on the type of procedure you have had, you may need to temporarily avoid strenuous activity. Follow your doctor's instructions about resuming your normal activities.

Liposuction and Abdominoplasty

Liposuction, the most common cosmetic surgery procedure performed on men, is a procedure that can improve the contour of your body by removing stubborn pockets of fat that you have not been able to remove through exercise or diet. During the procedure, the plastic surgeon uses a vacuum device to suction these unwanted fat deposits from specific areas of the body. For men, these areas are usually the abdomen, the flanks ("love handles"), or the chest. Other possible areas include the hips, buttocks, thighs, knees, upper arms, chin, cheeks, and neck. The best candidates for liposuction are men of normal weight with firm skin who have excess fat deposits in certain areas of the body. Liposuction is not a weight-loss method; you should be at or near your ideal weight before surgery.

Liposuction can be performed in a surgeon's office, in an outpatient surgery center, or in a hospital, depending on the amount of fat to be removed. If only a small amount of fat is to be removed, the procedure can be performed using a local anesthetic. Removing large amounts of fat from extensive areas of the body requires either regional anesthesia, which numbs a large area of the body, or general anesthesia. In some cases a surgeon may use general anesthesia if the person does not want to remain conscious during the procedure.

Before suctioning, the surgeon injects large volumes of saline solution that contains epinephrine. Epinephrine limits blood loss by constricting blood vessels and allows more fat to be removed. This technique, which also reduces post-operative bruising, is called tumescent liposuction. Some surgeons also may use high-frequency sound waves to help break up the fat before it is suctioned. This technique is called ultrasonic liposuction. It has not yet been shown that ultrasonic liposuction improves the results. During the procedure, the surgeon makes a small incision and inserts a narrow tube into the body. Attached to the other end of the tube is a vacuum pump or a large syringe used to suction out the fat. If the surgeon plans to suction fat from more than one area of the body, he or she will then repeat the procedure at the other targeted areas. To replace fluids lost along with the fat and to prevent shock, the surgeon or the anesthesiologist (a physician trained to administer anesthesia) gives fluids through a vein during and after surgery. When all targeted areas have been suctioned, the surgeon will close the incisions with sutures.

After surgery, fluid will drain from the incisions and, in rare cases, the doctor may insert a small drainage tube under the skin to prevent fluid from building up. You may have to wear a snugly fitting elastic garment over the treated area for a number of days to help control swelling. To prevent infection, the doctor may prescribe oral antibiotics. You will probably experience a modest amount of pain for the first week after surgery. The pain can be treated with pain relievers. You should be able to return to work within 3 days to a week, depending on the extent of the procedure and the type of work you do. Initially, the suctioned area will show significant bruising and swelling. The bruising usually clears up in about 2 to 3 weeks; the swelling generally clears up in about 3 months. Keep in mind that you will not be able to see the final results until the swelling has completely subsided. Final scarring is usually small and unobtrusive. A small percentage of people will experience minor irregularities and asymmetries in the suctioned area, which can be corrected with a second "touch-up" procedure.

Some men may request liposuction in the abdominal area and learn that abdominoplasty, commonly called a "tummy tuck," will more effectively help them reach their goal of a trimmer abdomen. Abdominoplasty is the operation of choice when the problem is excess abdominal skin, usually due to significant weight loss. Unlike liposuction, however, abdominoplasty leaves a permanent scar that stretches from one hip to the other. As with liposuction, for best results, candidates for abdominoplasty should be at or near their ideal weight.

During abdominoplasty, the surgeon removes excess skin and fat and repositions the navel before closing the incision. Abdominoplasty is major surgery, so you will need to stay home from work for 1 or 2 weeks, or possibly longer, to recover. Postoperative swelling will subside in several months; you will not be able to see the final results until then. It will take about a year to determine the final appearance of the scar. The good news is that the scar is low enough to be easily hidden beneath clothing, such as swimming trunks.

Facial Surgery

As they age, some men seek to improve the appearance of their face and neck through cosmetic surgery. Facial surgery covers a number of different procedures, including a facelift and forehead lift, eyelid surgery, nose surgery, facial implant surgery, and refinishing treatments for facial skin (such as chemical peels and dermabrasion). Sometimes two or more of these procedures are performed at the same time. Although facial surgery cannot reverse the aging process, it can give the face a younger, rejuvenated look that can increase your self-confidence and sense of well-being.

Facelift

With age, the muscles and skin of the face and neck begin to sag, and the skin begins to lose elasticity. A facelift can restore a more youthful appearance by removing excess fat, tightening underlying muscles, and repositioning the skin over the face and the neck. Most people who have a facelift are in their 40s, 50s, and 60s, but even older people can benefit from the procedure. Before deciding to have a facelift, discuss the procedure with a board-certified (see page 94) plastic surgeon to determine whether this type of surgery is right for you.

Before the procedure, your surgeon will evaluate your face and discuss your expectations about the surgery. He or she also will describe the risks and benefits of the surgery and discuss the costs involved. In addition, the surgeon will describe the procedure itself and the type of anesthesia to be used. You may want to grow your hair a bit longer before having surgery to help hide the scars afterward.

To perform a facelift, the surgeon makes an incision behind the hairline beginning at each temple, extending down in front of the ear, and continuing around behind the ear down to the lower scalp. He or she also may make a second incision, under the chin, if the neck is also being treated. Separating the skin from the fat and muscle below, the surgeon then trims or suctions fat from the areas around the neck and chin and tightens the underlying muscle. The skin is then pulled back over the face, and the excess skin is trimmed away. The surgeon closes the incisions with sutures. He or she may temporarily place a small tube under the skin behind the ear to drain any collected blood or fluid.

After surgery you probably will feel numbness and swelling in your face. These sensations are normal. Keeping your head elevated and still will minimize the swelling. Your face may look bruised and puffy, but it will look more normal after a few weeks. The surgeon will remove your stitches in about a week. Most people return to work in 1 or 2 weeks. The surgery causes mild pain that can be treated with pain relievers such as acetaminophen.

You may find that you have to begin shaving in new areas because beard-growing skin may have been repositioned to the back of your neck or behind your ears. Any scars from the facelift will most likely be hidden by your hair or by the natural creases in your face and neck. The scars will gradually fade. Your facelift will probably last about 10 years; to retain your youthful appearance, you may have to repeat the procedure.

Forehead Lift

A forehead lift, also called a brow lift, is designed to restore a more youthful appearance to the forehead and make the person look more rested and alert by smoothing out lines and raising the eyebrows. Although it can help people of any age with deep wrinkles in their foreheads, a forehead lift is most often performed on people between ages 40 and 70. It is often performed at the same time as a facelift.

Plastic surgeons can perform a forehead lift in either of two ways. In the traditional method, the surgeon makes an incision across the top of the forehead, under the hairline, from ear to ear. Next, the surgeon lifts away the skin of the forehead so he or she can remove or reposition the underlying muscle, which is the source of the wrinkles. He or she will then pull the forehead skin upward and trim away any excess skin and also may elevate the eyebrows before replacing the skin of the forehead and closing the incision with sutures or clips.

In an endoscopic forehead lift, the surgeon uses an endoscope (a flexible viewing instrument that transmits images to a video monitor). The surgeon inserts the endoscope under the skin of the forehead through four or five small incisions in the scalp. The endoscope allows the surgeon to see and work on the muscle and tissues beneath the skin. After completing the procedure, the surgeon will close the incisions with sutures or clips. This procedure is ideal for men with little hair because the scars are very small.

If you have undergone a traditional forehead lift, you probably will experience some pain, swelling, and numbness in the treated area. Keeping your head elevated and as still as possible will minimize swelling. The pain may be replaced by itching as the incision heals. The surgeon probably will remove the sutures or clips in 2 weeks. Recovery from an endoscopic forehead lift is quicker and less painful than recovery from a traditional forehead lift. Stitches or clips usually are removed within a week. You can return to work in about 10 days after either type of forehead lift.

Eyelid Surgery

The aging process causes the skin of the eyelids to droop, and fat often begins to accumulate above and below the eyes, producing "bags." Eyelid surgery (known medically as blepharoplasty) can be used to alleviate these age-related changes. Now the second most common type of plastic surgery performed on men, eyelid surgery can give you a younger appearance but will not remove crow's-feet or other wrinkles from around the eyes, eliminate dark circles, or raise sagging eyebrows. In some cases, eyelid surgery can actually improve vision if the eyelids droop and stretch so much that they cover part of the eyes. Most eyelid surgery is performed on people over age 35.

While planning your eyelid surgery, the surgeon will test your vision and check your ability to produce tears. Having dry eyes or not being able to produce enough tears can make the procedure more risky. Other disorders that increase the risks of eyelid surgery include a detached retina, glaucoma, thyroid problems, high blood pressure, heart disease, and diabetes. The surgeon will discuss the risks of the procedure and possible complications that can occur, such as temporary double or blurred vision, temporary swelling at the corners of the eyes, sensitivity to light, and the appearance of whiteheads near the surgical site. Some people may have difficulty closing their eyes while sleeping after eyelid surgery, but this complication is usually temporary.

Using local or general anesthesia, the surgeon will make incisions in the creases of your upper lids (and beneath the lashes of the lower lids if they are to be altered). The surgeon removes excess skin, trims excess fat, and closes the incisions with fine sutures. In some cases the incision is made inside the lower lid to avoid producing visible scars.

You will have to keep your head elevated for a few days after surgery. Cold compresses placed on your eyes will help to reduce swelling. The surgeon may prescribe eyedrops to keep your eyes moist. After 3 to 5 days, your sutures will be removed. Contact lens wearers can resume

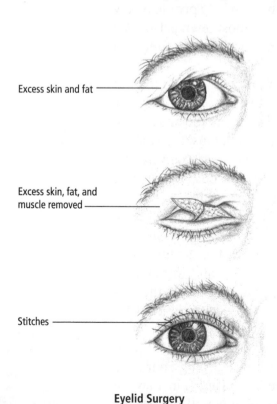

Excess skin and fat

Excess skin, fat, and muscle removed

Stitches

Eyelid Surgery

wearing their lenses in a week. Postoperative pain is minimal, and most people do not need pain relievers. Bruising is common and usually clears up in 1 or 2 weeks. Most people can return to work in a few days.

Nose Reshaping

Surgery to reshape the nose, known as rhinoplasty, can change the appearance of your nose in a number of ways. The surgeon can alter your nose's size, remove a hump, alter the tip, narrow the nostrils, or change its angle. Nasal surgery can even relieve some breathing problems, such as those caused by a deviated septum (crookedness of the thin wall of cartilage and bone that divides the nostrils).

When discussing nose-reshaping surgery, you and the surgeon will work together to develop a concept or goal for a new shape that will balance the rest of your face and enhance your appearance. How closely your final result resembles this goal is unpredictable. Your surgeon also will explain the risks and possible complications of nose reshaping, which, although rare, include infection, nose-bleed, and impaired breathing. In about one in 10 people, nasal surgery has to be repeated to correct a minor irregularity or problem with the cosmetic result.

During surgery, the surgeon separates the skin over the nose from the underlying supporting structures of bone and cartilage so he or she can reshape them. The skin is then replaced over the nose. After the procedure, the surgeon places a splint on the nose to help retain the new shape.

Following surgery, your face will be swollen and you may have slight pain in your nose along with a headache. Swelling and bruising also will appear around the eyes. You can reduce the swelling by applying cold, wet compresses over the areas. You will not be able to blow your nose for about a week to allow the area to fully heal. After 5 to 7 days the surgeon will remove the splint and any sutures or nasal packing; you can then return to work. Although you will be allowed to wear contact lenses, you will not be able to wear glasses for about 6 weeks, unless you tape them to your forehead to avoid direct pressure on the nose. In some cases it may take a year for the swelling to completely subside and reveal the final result.

Skin-Refinishing Techniques

Many people have skin-refinishing procedures to achieve smoother-looking skin. The most common types of procedures include chemical peeling, dermabrasion, and laser skin resurfacing. The main difference between a chemical peel and dermabrasion and laser skin resurfacing is that the two latter procedures use surgical instruments to remove the top layer of skin, while a chemical peel uses a chemical solution.

Chemical Peel   Doctors use chemical peels to enhance the texture of facial skin by creating a superficial, self-healing burn to remove damaged outer layers. A chemical peel may be recommended for men who have wrinkles or blemishes from sun exposure or who have uneven skin coloring. Sometimes doctors also use a chemical peel to remove precancerous skin growths, improve the appearance of acne scars, or control acne.

There are three main types of chemicals used in a chemical peel: alphahydroxy acids (AHAs), trichloroacetic acid (TCA), and phenol. Common AHAs include glycolic, lactic, and fruit acids. They are the mildest chemical peel formulas but usually have to be reapplied a number of times to achieve the best results. TCA is generally stronger than AHAs but still may require repeated treatments. Before the peel, the doctor may apply a vitamin A–containing cream (tretinoin) that enhances the results of the peel. AHA and TCA peels (light peels) require minimal recovery time. They refresh the skin by removing dead cells from the surface of the skin and stimulate formation of new collagen (a tough, fibrous, structural protein that is an important part of body tissues) to reduce future wrinkling. These peels do not remove existing wrinkles.

Phenol is the strongest chemical available for chemical peels and is used to minimize coarse wrinkles and scars from acne. Results are striking and longlasting, but healing can take up to several months. Phenol peels (deep peels) create a superficial burn that heals in about a week, revealing pinker skin. The pinker skin fades to a more normal tone in several months, but this tone may be lighter than the surrounding skin. Although the initial pinker skin is quite noticeable, it can easily be hidden with makeup. However, because most men are not willing to wear makeup, deep peeling is generally not a practical choice for men. Anesthesia is not required for a light peel, but it is required for the deeper, phenol peel. During a light peel you may feel some temporary stinging or burning as the doctor applies the solution to your face. After having the procedure you need to use a strong sunblock on your face to protect the sensitive skin from burning. Sunblock also helps to prevent the irregular skin coloring that can occur after a phenol peel.

Some states do not require that a chemical peel be done by a licensed physician, but it is important to find a doctor (or a registered nurse who works under a doctor's supervision) with experience in giving chemical peels because the procedure carries some risk of infection and scarring. After your treatment you will probably notice that the skin on your face is red and dry. It also may scale or flake somewhat. These conditions are only temporary. After a phenol peel your face may swell considerably—your eyes may even swell shut—and you may need someone to help out at home for a couple of days. The chemical peel will give your face a fresh, new look but will not prevent any future signs of aging or damage from sun exposure.

Dermabrasion   Dermabrasion helps to rejuvenate the skin by controlled surgical sanding of the face. Doctors use dermabrasion to treat skin that has been scarred by accidents or surgery or to smooth facial wrinkles. Neither procedure is recommended for people with dark skin because their complexions could become permanently blotchy or discolored. In fact, a change in skin color is the most common complication, even in light-skinned people.

It is best to seek dermabrasion from a qualified plastic surgeon or dermatologist; the technique is sometimes offered by inadequately trained nonphysicians. Dermabrasion requires local anesthesia, given along with a calming sedative. Serious cases of wrinkles or scarring may require general anesthesia. To perform dermabrasion, the doctor "sandpapers" away the top layer of skin, using a motorized wire brush device.

After surgery, your skin will be swollen and feel sore, as if you fell and scraped the side of your face. The skin on your face will scab over and, when the scab falls away, new, pinker skin will be revealed. You will not be able to shave for a while; follow your doctor's instructions about when to resume shaving. Your face will heal in about a week, but your skin will be pinker than usual for several months. You will need to use a strong sunblock to protect the sensitive skin from burning until the pink has faded to a more normal tone. This tone may be lighter than the surrounding skin; using sunblock also helps prevent this irregular skin coloring.

Laser Skin Resurfacing   Surgeons sometimes use lasers to treat fine lines, wrinkles, scars, and various skin lesions. Some surgeons believe that the precise nature of the laser makes it the treatment of choice. A laser is a device that focuses highly concentrated beams of light on the surface of the skin to create a controlled, superficial burn that heals on its own. Laser treatment requires either local or general anesthesia. Your face will heal in about a week, but your skin will be noticeably pinker for several months. You will need to use a strong sunblock to protect the sensitive skin from burning until the pink has faded to a more normal tone. This tone may be lighter than the surrounding skin; sunblock also helps prevent this irregular skin coloring. Resistance to wearing makeup to cover the pinker skin while it heals makes this procedure an impractical choice for most men.

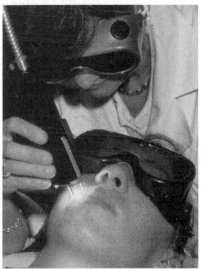

Laser Skin Resurfacing

Facial Implants

Facial implants can help make the contours of your face more pleasing by balancing your facial features. The most common types of facial implants are those of the cheeks, chin, and jaw. Facial implants are typically offered to men and women of any age who want to enhance the appearance of their face. Implants also can be used in other parts of the body—such as the chest or calves (see below)—to contour them and make them look more muscular.

Usually performed using local or general anesthesia, facial implant surgery can take 30 minutes to an hour. Most implants are made of solid silicone, which has not been shown to be harmful. Talk to your plastic surgeon if you have concerns about the safety of the implanted material. Various shapes and sizes of implants are available to simulate natural cheekbones and jawbones. During the procedure the surgeon will make an incision and insert the implant. The incision is often made inside the mouth, so the scar will not be visible. He or she will then close the incision with dissolving sutures.

Swelling can be significant after surgery, especially during the first 48 hours. The doctor probably will restrict your diet (to soft foods and liquids) and activities for a few days, depending on the type of surgery you have had. He or she also will give you instructions about cleaning your teeth. Complications are infrequent but can include infection. The implant also can shift out of place after surgery, requiring a second operation to correct its placement. Recovery time for a facial implant is usually minimal, but you should check with your surgeon before returning to work.

Chest Implants and Calf Implants

Implants can be used to augment the contours of the chest or calves. Surgery for either type of implant is performed under general anesthesia. For a chest implant the incision is made under the arm, and the implant is inserted over the pectoral muscles. For a calf implant the incisions are made behind the knees, and the implants are inserted over the calf muscles. Each operation lasts about 1 to 2 hours. Usually you can return to work about 1 week after surgery. You can begin exercising again about 1 month after surgery. Infection, although rare, is a possible complication of either surgery.

Hair Replacement Surgery

Hair replacement surgery for male pattern baldness is one of the most common cosmetic surgery procedures performed on men. Usually it involves grafting hair from the sides and back of the person's scalp (called the donor sites) to the bald area. Sometimes this technique is combined with another procedure called scalp reduction, in which the surgeon removes skin from bald areas of the scalp and uses elastic scalp extenders and expanders placed under the skin to stretch the remaining skin over the scalp. In another surgical procedure, called the flap technique, the surgeon moves areas of the scalp containing hair from the sides or back of the head to the top of the head. The flaps cover more area than the usual graft, and part of the flap remains attached to the original blood supply.

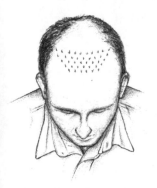
After the first grafting session

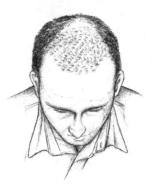
Grafted hair is growing

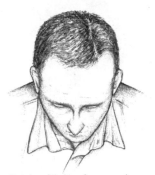
Hair has filled in after several grafting sessions

Hair Replacement

Hair replacement surgery is performed using local anesthesia. During the grafting procedure, long strips of scalp are harvested from the donor sites. The donor sites are then sutured. (Scars at the donor sites will be virtually invisible because they are hidden by surrounding hair.) The strips of scalp are then divided into hundreds of small grafts, each containing a few hairs. The grafts are then inserted into tiny openings that the doctor has made in the bald area. Although it will be several months before the grafts take hold and begin to grow hair, once hairs begin to grow, they are as permanent as the hairs at the donor sites.

After surgery you may experience aching, throbbing, and tightness in the scalp area. You will need to wear bandages over the grafted area overnight; the bandages will be removed the next day.

The doctor will tell you to avoid washing your hair for 2 days after surgery. When you wash your hair, wash it gently. Because strenuous activity increases blood flow to the scalp, you will need to avoid vigorous exercise and sexual activity until your doctor tells you otherwise. Avoid all contact sports and other activities that may cause damage to the treated area. Any sutures will be removed within 7 to 10 days. Several separate surgical procedures may be needed to complete the hair replacement, depending on the size of the bald area. A year may pass before the grafted hair is totally grown.

The type of hair replacement procedure you choose depends on the kind of hair loss you have. If you are considering hair replacement surgery, discuss your options with your plastic surgeon to determine the best choice to meet your needs.

GLOSSARY

This glossary defines terms that your doctor may have used or that you may have come across while reading this book. Italicized words within definitions refer you to other terms in the glossary for additional information.

abdominoplasty   Also known as a tummy tuck. A major surgical procedure, abdominoplasty is a type of *cosmetic surgery* in which excess fat and skin are removed from the abdominal area. Abdominoplasty usually is performed on people who have not been able to lose unwanted abdominal fat and skin through diet and exercise.

ACE inhibitor   See *angiotensin-converting enzyme inhibitor.*

acne   A common skin disorder caused by inflammation of the *hair follicles* and *sebaceous glands* and characterized by *pimples* that appear on the face, neck, back, chest, and shoulders.

acoustic nerve   See *auditory nerve.*

acquired immunodeficiency syndrome   A disorder of the *immune system* caused by infection with the *human immunodeficiency virus* (HIV).

actinic keratosis   Also known as solar keratosis (because it results from long-term exposure to excessive amounts of sunlight). A type of skin growth caused by overproduction of *keratin.* Actinic keratosis can develop into a form of skin cancer known as *squamous cell carcinoma.*

adenoma   A *benign* tumor that arises from glandular tissue.

adrenal gland   One of a pair of triangular glands located directly above each *kidney.* Adrenal glands produce a variety of *hormones* that affect nearly every system in the body.

adrenaline   See *epinephrine.*

advance directive   A legal document designed to help ensure that healthcare decisions made on a person's behalf are consistent with his or her preferences. See also *do-not-resuscitate order, durable power of attorney for healthcare,* and *living will.*

aerobic exercise   A physical exercise that requires your heart and lungs to work harder to meet your muscles' continuous demand for oxygen. Examples of aerobic exercise include brisk walking, dancing, step-aerobics, jogging, and biking.

age spots   Also known as liver spots, sun spots, or lentigines. Brown spots on the skin that resemble freckles and that are caused by long-term exposure to sunlight.

agnosia   The inability to recognize familiar faces, locations, or objects. Agnosia may result from brain damage due to head injury or *stroke*.

AIDS   See *acquired immunodeficiency syndrome*.

allergen   Any substance—such as pollen, animal dander, or a particular food—that produces an *allergic reaction* in some people.

allergic contact dermatitis   A skin condition that occurs when the skin comes into contact with an *allergen,* causing a *rash* that is characterized by redness, swelling, and blisters. Allergic contact dermatitis may be difficult to distinguish from other skin conditions (see *eczema, atopic*).

allergic reaction   An inappropriate *immune system* response that occurs when an *allergen* enters the body.

allergic rhinitis   Also known as hay fever. An inflammation of the *mucous membrane* lining the nose and caused by an *allergic reaction.* Symptoms include coughing, stuffy nose, and sneezing.

allergy   An abnormal sensitivity to an *allergen*.

alpha-blocker   A medication used to treat heart and circulation disorders such as *high blood pressure* and *peripheral vascular disease.*

ALS   See *amyotrophic lateral sclerosis.*

Alzheimer's disease   A progressive, incurable condition that destroys brain cells, gradually causing loss of intellectual abilities (such as memory) and extreme changes in personality and behavior.

amino acids   Chemical compounds that are the basic components of all *proteins.*

amnesia   Loss of the ability to store information in memory or to recall information already stored in memory. Amnesia can be caused by brain damage or disease and is a common symptom of various neurological disorders.

amyotrophic lateral sclerosis   Also known as Lou Gehrig's disease. This most common *motor neuron disease* is characterized by a progressive loss of muscle function, leading to paralysis.

anabolic steroids   Synthetic drugs that imitate the effects of *testosterone.*

anaphylactic shock   A severe, life-threatening *allergic reaction* that requires immediate medical treatment. Symptoms include a sudden, severe drop in *blood pressure* and difficulty breathing.

androgens   Male sex *hormones.*

anemia   A blood disorder caused by a deficiency of red blood cells or *hemoglobin;* anemia reduces the ability of the blood to supply oxygen to the tissues and to remove carbon dioxide from the body.

aneurysm   An abnormal ballooning of a weakened area in an *artery* wall. An aneurysm in the brain may rupture, causing a hemorrhagic *stroke.*

angina   A tight, heavy, squeezing pain sensation deep beneath the breastbone or in a band across the chest that results from a reduced supply of oxygen to the heart muscle, indicating *coronary artery disease.* The pain also may radiate to the left arm, shoulder, neck, jaw, or middle of the back and may be accompanied by nausea, sweating, or shortness of breath.

angiography   A diagnostic procedure for examining the inside of an *artery.* A *contrast medium* is injected through a *catheter* into the artery, and a rapid-sequence series of X rays is taken.

angioplasty   A surgical procedure used to clear a narrowed or blocked *artery.*

angiotensin-converting enzyme (ACE) inhibitor   An *antihypertensive* used to treat *high blood pressure* and *heart failure.*

ankylosing spondylitis   A form of *rheumatoid arthritis* that primarily affects the spine, shoulders, hips, and knees.

anorexia   A potentially life-threatening eating disorder (most frequently occurring in young women) that is characterized by an abnormal fear of being fat, prolonged avoidance of food, excessive weight loss, and obsession with exercise.

antibiotic   A medication used to treat bacterial infections.

antibodies   Also known as immunoglobulins. *Proteins* found in the blood and tissue fluids that protect the body from infectious organisms.

anticoagulant   A medication used to treat abnormal blood clotting.

antidepressant   A medication used to treat *depression.* Three commonly prescribed types of antidepressants are tricyclic antidepressants, monoamine oxidase inhibitors, and selective *serotonin* reuptake inhibitors.

antigens   *Proteins* such as microorganisms or toxins that trigger the *immune system* to produce *antibodies.*

antihistamine   A medication that blocks the effects of *histamine.*

antihypertensive   A medication used to treat *high blood pressure.* See also *alphablocker, angiotensin-converting enzyme (ACE) inhibitor, beta-blocker, calcium channel blocker,* and *diuretic.*

anti-inflammatory   A medication such as aspirin or ibuprofen that relieves the symptoms of inflammation.

antioxidant   A compound that protects against cell damage caused by *oxygen free radicals.*

anus   The opening at the *rectum* through which feces pass to the outside of the body.

aorta   The body's main *artery.*

aortic stenosis   The most common heart valve disorder. Aortic stenosis causes narrowing or stiffening of the *aortic valve* and can lead to *angina* and *heart failure.*

aortic valve   The valve between the *aorta* and the left *ventricle* of the heart.

aphasia   Loss of language skills (comprehension, expression, or both) due to a brain injury.

apraxia   The inability to perform tasks, such as dressing or tying one's shoes, because of loss of the ability to recall the sequence of necessary steps.

arrhythmia   An abnormally fast or slow *heartbeat* or an irregular heartbeat.

arteriole   A tiny branch of an *artery.*

arteriosclerosis   A term used to describe a group of disorders characterized by thickening and scarring of *artery* walls. See also *atherosclerosis.*

arteriovenous malformation   A *congenital* disorder in which there is a fragile, tangled web of *arteries* and *veins* in a particular part of the body, such as the brain, spinal cord, or *digestive tract.*

artery   A blood vessel that carries oxygen-filled blood away from the heart to the organs and tissues.

arthritis   A general term used to describe inflammation of a *joint* accompanied by swelling, stiffness, and pain. See also *osteoarthritis* and *rheumatoid arthritis.*

arthroplasty   A surgical procedure in which a damaged joint is replaced with an artificial joint made of metal and plastic. Arthroplasty is most often used on the knee and hip, but it is also performed on the ankles, hands, wrists, and toes.

arthroscopy   Examination of or surgery on a *joint* using a viewing tube called an arthroscope inserted through a small incision.

artificial crown   See *crown, artificial.*

asthma   A respiratory disorder characterized by reversible narrowing of the airways, causing wheezing, shortness of breath, chest tightness, and coughing.

asymptomatic   Without signs or symptoms of disease.

atheroma   Fatty deposits on the inner lining of an *artery* that can lead to *atherosclerosis.*

atherosclerosis   The buildup of fatty material called arterial *plaque* in the inner lining of an *artery;* atherosclerosis can narrow the blood vessels and reduce blood flow to the organs and tissues, increasing the risk of *myocardial infarction* (MI) or *stroke.*

athlete's foot   Also known as tinea pedis. A common contagious fungal infection of the foot that affects the skin between the toes or of the soles or sides of the feet. Athlete's foot causes the skin to itch, peel, crack, and, occasionally, form blisters.

atopic eczema   See *eczema, atopic.*

atria   See *atrium.*

atrial fibrillation   An abnormal *heartbeat* in which the *atria* beat rapidly and irregularly, and independently of the *ventricles.*

atrium   Singular of atria. One of the two small upper chambers of the heart.

audiogram   A graphic record of a person's hearing ability that is obtained during *audiometry.*

audiologist   A health professional trained to evaluate hearing loss and to fit *hearing aids.*

audiometry   Hearing tests performed to measure a person's hearing ability.

auditory nerve   Also known as the acoustic nerve. The part of the vestibulocochlear nerve (eighth cranial nerve) that carries sensory impulses from the *cochlea* in the inner ear to the hearing center in the brain, where the impulses are interpreted as sound.

autoimmune disease   A disease in which the *immune system* mistakenly attacks the body's own cells and tissues.

autologous blood donation   Donation of a person's own blood before scheduled elective surgery to make the blood available in case a transfusion is necessary during or after surgery.

"bad" cholesterol   See *low-density lipoprotein (LDL) cholesterol.*

B

balanitis   Inflammation of the head and *foreskin* of the *penis.*

basal cell carcinoma   A slow-growing form of skin cancer, found in the outer layer of skin, that rarely spreads to other parts of the body. Basal cell carcinoma accounts for about 90 percent of all skin cancers.

B cell   See *lymphocyte.*

Bell's palsy   A peripheral nerve disorder that causes one-sided weakness, twitching, or paralysis of the facial muscles.

benign Not cancerous.

benign prostatic hyperplasia Noncancerous enlargement of the *prostate gland* that obstructs the flow and passage of urine through the *urethra*.

beta-blocker An *antihypertensive* used to treat heart and circulation disorders such as *angina, high blood pressure,* and *arrhythmia*.

beta carotene An *antioxidant* found in orange and deep yellow fruits and vegetables that converts into *vitamin* A in the body.

bile A greenish yellow fluid secreted by the *liver* that removes waste products and helps break down fats during digestion.

biofeedback A relaxation technique in which a person learns to control involuntary body functions such as *heart rate*.

biopsy A diagnostic test in which a small sample of tissue is removed from the body and examined under a microscope.

bipolar disorder Also known as manic-depressive disorder. A mood disorder characterized by alternating episodes of deep *depression* and euphoria.

bite Also called occlusion. A term used to describe the contact between opposing upper and lower teeth.

bite guard Also called a splint. A plastic dental appliance that fits over the biting surface of the upper or lower teeth and helps prevent a person from grinding his or her teeth.

blackhead A dark-colored plug of *sebum* that blocks a *hair follicle.*

bladder A hollow, muscular organ in the *pelvis* that acts as a reservoir for urine.

blepharoplasty A *cosmetic surgery* procedure in which excess fat and skin are removed from the upper and lower eyelids.

blood clot A clump of coagulated blood.

blood pressure A measure of the force exerted against the walls of the *arteries* by the flow of blood as it is pumped throughout the body by the heart. See also *diastolic blood pressure* and *systolic blood pressure.*

B lymphocyte See *lymphocyte.*

BMI See *body mass index.*

body mass index A measurement used to determine whether your body weight falls in the healthful range.

boil A collection of *pus* beneath the top layer of skin caused by bacterial infection of a *hair follicle.*

bone density   A measure of the amount of *calcium* and other minerals in bone in relation to the width of the bone. A person's bone density is used to determine his or her risk of developing *osteoporosis.*

BPH   See *benign prostatic hyperplasia.*

bradycardia   A *heart rate* below 60 beats per minute.

bronchodilator   A medication that dilates (widens) constricted airways and is used to treat *asthma.*

bulimia   An eating disorder characterized by binge overeating followed by self-induced vomiting or laxative abuse.

bursa   A fluid-filled sac that acts as a cushion at a pressure point in the body, often near a *joint.*

bursitis   Inflammation of a *bursa,* attributable to *arthritis,* injury, or infection.

C

calcium   A mineral that is important for strong bones and teeth and also has an important role in muscle contraction, blood clotting, and nerve function.

calcium channel blocker   An *antihypertensive* used to treat heart and circulation disorders such as *angina* and *high blood pressure.*

calculus   A hard mineral deposit on teeth (also known as tartar), or a small, hard mass (such as a *gallstone* or a *kidney stone*) that forms in body tissues.

cap   See *crown, artificial.*

capillaries   Tiny blood vessels that carry blood between the *arterioles* and *venules.*

carbuncle   A cluster of *boils.*

carcinogen   Any substance, such as cigarette smoke, that can cause cancer.

cardiac catheterization   A diagnostic procedure in which a *catheter* is threaded through a blood vessel into the heart to monitor its function and to inject *contrast medium* for imaging.

cardiopulmonary resuscitation   A lifesaving procedure in which cardiac massage and artificial ventilation are performed on someone whose heart has stopped beating, in order to maintain the circulation of oxygenated blood to the brain.

cardiovascular system   Also known as the circulatory system. The network formed by your heart and blood vessels that pumps blood and carries it throughout your body.

carotid artery   One of the four major *arteries* that supply blood to the head and neck.

carotid endarterectomy   A surgical procedure to remove arterial *plaque* from the *carotid arteries*.

carpal tunnel syndrome   A common *repetitive stress injury* characterized by numbness, tingling, and pain in the wrist and hand. The injury results from compression of the *median nerve* where it enters the hand.

cartilage   A type of *connective tissue* that is an important structural component of certain parts of the skeletal system such as the *joints*.

cataract   A cloudy area in the normally clear *lens* of the eye that causes impaired vision.

catheter   A thin, flexible tube that is inserted into a vessel or body cavity to withdraw or instill fluids or to widen a passageway.

cecum   The large blind pouch that forms the beginning of the *large intestine*.

celiac disease   The inability to metabolize gluten, a *protein* found in most grains.

cerebrospinal fluid   The fluid that provides nutrition and support for the brain and the spinal cord.

cerebrovascular accident   See *stroke*.

chemical peel   A *cosmetic surgery* procedure that uses chemicals such as alpha-hydroxy acids, trichloroacetic acid, or phenol to remove damaged outer layers of skin, improving the skin's appearance and texture.

chemotherapy   Treatment of cancer using powerful drugs to destroy cancer cells throughout the body.

cherry angioma   A small, bright red, flat or raised spot made up of tiny, closely packed blood vessels near the surface of the skin. Cherry angiomas appear most often on the trunk but can appear anywhere on the body.

CHF   Congestive heart failure. See *heart failure*.

chickenpox   A common infectious disease caused by the *herpesvirus varicella-zoster virus* and characterized by a blistery *rash* and fever. Chickenpox is a mild disease in children but can lead to serious complications in adults.

chlamydia   A *sexually transmitted disease* (STD) caused by the microorganism *Chlamydia trachomatis*. Symptoms usually are mild, but some men with chlamydia may experience burning during urination and have a discharge from the *penis*.

Chlamydia trachomatis   A microorganism that causes *chlamydia, epididymitis,* and most cases of *nongonococcal urethritis (NGU)*.

cholesterol   A fatlike substance that is an important component of cells and is involved in the transport of fats in the blood. Types of cholesterol include *high-density lipoprotein (HDL) cholesterol* and *low-density lipoprotein (LDL) cholesterol*.

chordoma A type of slow-growing *malignant* tumor in the upper spinal cord.

chronic Describes a disorder or illness that persists for a long time.

circulatory system See *cardiovascular system.*

circumcision Removal of the *foreskin* of the *penis.* Although circumcision can be performed on adults, it is usually performed on newborns.

cluster headache See *headache, cluster.*

cochlea A coiled structure in the inner ear that changes sound waves into nerve impulses and transmits them to the brain through the *auditory nerve.*

cochlear implant An electronic device implanted in the *cochlea* in the inner ear that is used to treat *sensorineural hearing loss* that has resulted in deafness. A cochlear implant converts sound waves into electronic impulses that are transmitted to the hearing center in the brain via the *auditory nerve,* allowing the person to distinguish sounds and to understand speech.

cold, common A viral infection of the *mucous membrane* that lines the nose and throat. A cold causes a stuffy, runny nose, sneezing, and sometimes a cough and a sore throat.

colitis Inflammation of the *colon.*

colon The main section of the *large intestine,* extending from the *cecum* to the *rectum.*

colonoscopy An examination of the *colon* using a long, flexible, viewing instrument called a colonoscope.

color blindness See *color vision deficiency.*

color vision deficiency Also called color blindness. An eye disorder characterized by an inability to see colors as others see them or to distinguish colors.

colostomy A surgical procedure in which part of the *colon* is brought through an incision in the abdominal wall and an artificial opening is created through which feces can be discharged into a bag attached to the skin.

computed tomography A diagnostic technique that uses a computer and low-dose X rays to produce detailed cross-sectional images of body tissues that are displayed on a video monitor.

conductive hearing loss Impaired hearing caused by inadequate transmission of sound from the outer ear to the inner ear.

congenital Present from birth.

congestive heart failure See *heart failure.*

connective tissue A type of tissue, such as *cartilage* and *tendons,* that holds various body structures together.

contrast medium   A type of dye that is injected into an artery during diagnostic procedures such as *angiography* and *endoscopic retrograde cholangiopancreatography* (ERCP).

contusion   A bruise.

cornea   The tough, transparent, dome-shaped covering at the front of the eyeball that protects the eye and helps focus light onto the *retina*.

coronary artery bypass   A surgical procedure in which additional blood vessels are grafted onto obstructed coronary *arteries* so that blood can flow around (bypass) the obstructed areas and reach the heart.

coronary artery disease   Also known as heart disease or coronary heart disease. A condition in which one or more of the coronary *arteries* becomes narrowed or blocked, reducing or cutting off blood flow to the heart muscle. Coronary artery disease damages the heart, causing it to malfunction.

coronary heart disease   See *coronary artery disease*.

cosmetic surgery   *Plastic surgery* performed to improve a person's appearance.

CPR   See *cardiopulmonary resuscitation*.

crabs   See *pubic lice*.

Crohn's disease   A *chronic,* inflammatory, *digestive tract* disease of unknown cause.

crown, artificial   A substitute for the natural crown of a tooth (see next entry).

crown, natural   The uppermost, visible part of a tooth.

cryosurgery   See *cryotherapy*.

cryotherapy   Also known as cryosurgery. A procedure that uses low temperatures (such as those of liquid nitrogen) to destroy abnormal tissue by freezing.

CSF   See *cerebrospinal fluid*.

CT   See *computed tomography*.

cyanosis   Bluish coloring of the skin and *mucous membranes* caused by inadequate oxygen in the blood.

cyst   An abnormal lump or swelling that is filled with fluid.

cystitis   Inflammation of the inner lining of the *bladder,* usually caused by bacterial infection.

cystoscopy   Examination of the *bladder* and *ureters* using a viewing tube called a cystoscope.

cytomegalovirus   A *herpesvirus.* Infection with cytomegalovirus, in most cases, produces no symptoms. More serious infections can occur in those with an impaired *immune system,* such as people with *acquired immunodeficiency syndrome* (AIDS).

D

dandruff   Also known as seborrheic dermatitis. Scaling and sloughing of the skin on the scalp.

deep vein thrombosis   See *thrombosis, deep vein.*

defibrillator   A device that restores a normal *heartbeat* by delivering a brief electric shock to the heart muscle.

delirium   Sudden, temporary mental confusion.

delusional disorder   A mental disorder characterized by persistent belief in an irrational idea, such as persecution by others.

dementia   A progressive, permanent decline in mental abilities.

dentin   The hard tissue that surrounds the *pulp* of a tooth.

deoxyribonucleic acid   The structure inside every cell that carries genetic information.

depression   A mood disorder characterized by feelings of sadness, hopelessness, and helplessness, combined with apathy, poor self-esteem, and withdrawal from social situations.

dermabrasion   A *cosmetic surgery* procedure in which the outer layer of skin is sanded away to improve the appearance of scars or wrinkles or to remove tattoos.

dermatologist   A physician who specializes in treating disorders of the skin.

dermis   The thick inner layer of skin that is made up of *connective tissue* and contains structures such as *hair follicles,* sweat glands, *sebaceous glands,* lymph vessels, blood vessels, and nerves.

desensitization   A technique used to treat *phobias,* in which a person is gradually exposed to the object or the situation that he or she fears.

diabetes   The term commonly used to describe a disorder in which the body is unable to use *glucose* properly. Two forms of this disorder are type 1 diabetes and type 2 diabetes.

diabetic retinopathy   See *retinopathy, diabetic.*

dialysis   A technique used to filter waste products from the blood when *kidney* function is impaired.

diastolic blood pressure   The second, lower number in a *blood pressure* reading, indicating the pressure in the blood vessels when the heart rests between beats and fills with blood.

digestive tract   Also known as the gastrointestinal tract. The muscular tube through which food passes during digestion. The digestive tract consists of the mouth, throat, esophagus, stomach, and intestines.

digital rectal examination   An examination in which a doctor inserts a lubricated, gloved finger into the patient's *rectum* and feels the *prostate gland* for irregularities or for an increase in size. The examination is also performed to look for occult (hidden) blood and to evaluate the rectum.

diuretic   An *antihypertensive* that rids the body of excess water or salt by increasing the amount lost in urine. Diuretics are commonly used to treat *high blood pressure* and *heart failure.*

diverticula   See *diverticulum.*

diverticulitis   Inflammation or infection of *diverticula.*

diverticulosis   The presence of *diverticula* in the intestines.

diverticulum   Singular of diverticula. A small bulge or pouch protruding through the intestinal wall. Diverticula also can occur in the *urethra* and the esophagus.

DNA   See *deoxyribonucleic acid.*

do-not-resuscitate order   An *advance directive* that states that no one should perform heroic measures, including *cardiopulmonary resuscitation* (CPR) and the use of mechanical life support equipment, to restart a person's heart should it stop.

drainage angle   The tiny channel through which fluid leaves the eyeball.

DRE   See *digital rectal examination.*

duodenal ulcer   See *ulcer, duodenal.*

duodenum   The first section of the *small intestine,* beginning at the lower end of the stomach and extending to the *jejunum.*

durable power of attorney for healthcare   An *advance directive* in which a competent person gives another person the power to make healthcare decisions for him or her.

DVT   See *thrombosis, deep vein.*

dysthymia   A *chronic,* less intense form of *depression.*

E

ECG   See *electrocardiography.*

echocardiography   An *ultrasound* examination of the heart. The information recorded during the procedure is called an echocardiogram.

eczema, atopic   A recurrent, inflammatory skin condition that produces redness, itching, and scaly patches. Atopic eczema tends to run in families.

edema   Abnormal accumulation of fluid in the body tissues.

EEG   See *electroencephalography.*

ejaculation   Discharge of *semen* from the *penis* during *orgasm.*

electrocardiography   A procedure used to examine the electrical activity of the heart. The information recorded during the procedure is called an electrocardiogram.

electrocochleography   A hearing test that measures the sensitivity of the sensory hair cells in the inner ear in response to sound waves. The graphic record of the test is called an electrocochleogram.

electroencephalography   An examination of the electrical activity of the brain. The information recorded during the procedure is called an electroencephalogram.

electrolytes   *Sodium, potassium,* and other essential minerals that are involved in regulating various body processes.

embolism   Interruption of blood flow in a blood vessel by an *embolus.*

embolus   A plug of material (such as a *blood clot* or an air bubble) that can travel in the bloodstream and block a blood vessel.

enamel   The hard, thin covering of a tooth (see *crown, natural*).

encephalitis   Inflammation of the brain, often caused by a viral infection.

endocrine system   A network of glands, organs, and tissues that produce and secrete *hormones* directly into the bloodstream to regulate many essential body processes.

endocrine therapy   See *hormone therapy.*

endorphins   Chemicals in the brain that can improve mood and help control a person's response to pain and stress.

endoscopic retrograde cholangiopancreatography   An X-ray examination of the *gallbladder, bile* ducts, and *pancreas* using *endoscopy* and a *contrast medium.*

endoscopy   A procedure that uses a lighted viewing instrument called an endoscope to look inside a body cavity or organ to diagnose or treat disorders.

enzyme   A *protein* that controls chemical reactions in the body.

epicondylitis   Inflammation of the *tendons* that attach the forearm muscles to the elbow, usually caused by repetitive movement of the forearm. Golfer's elbow and tennis elbow are two types of epicondylitis.

epidermis   The thin outer layer of skin, made up of dead cells and *keratin,* which forms a protective covering. The epidermis also contains special cells that produce *melanin.*

epididymis   A long, coiled tube at the back of each *testicle* that collects *sperm* and stores them until they mature.

epididymitis   Inflammation of the *epididymis* caused by bacteria that are normally found in the intestine or by *Chlamydia trachomatis.*

epilepsy   A condition characterized by recurrent *seizures* caused by abnormal electrical activity in the brain.

epinephrine   Also known as adrenaline. A *hormone* produced by the *adrenal glands* that increases *heart rate* and blood flow and improves breathing.

Epstein-Barr virus   A *herpesvirus* that causes *mononucleosis.*

ERCP   See *endoscopic retrograde cholangiopancreatography.*

erectile dysfunction   Also known as impotence. The persistent inability to achieve and maintain an erection sufficient to complete sexual intercourse.

essential hypertension   See *primary hypertension.*

F

facelift   A *cosmetic surgery* procedure performed to tighten loose skin and muscles on the face, jaw, and neck.

fiber   The indigestible nutrient found in fruits and vegetables that passes through the *digestive tract* without being absorbed. Fiber provides bulk to help keep your digestive tract functioning properly and also helps protect against *colon* cancer.

finasteride   A medication for treating an enlarged *prostate gland* that is also used to treat *male pattern baldness.*

fistula   An abnormal channel between two internal organs or leading from an internal organ to the skin.

flu   See *influenza.*

folic acid   A B *vitamin* essential for cell growth and repair and for production of red blood cells.

follicle-stimulating hormone   A *hormone* produced in the *pituitary gland* that begins the production of *sperm* in the *testicles.*

foreskin   A loose fold of skin that covers the head of the penis. The foreskin is removed during *circumcision.*

fracture   A break in a bone.

free radicals   See *oxygen free radicals*.

FSH   See *follicle-stimulating hormone*.

G

gallbladder   A small, pear-shaped, muscular sac under the right lobe of the *liver*. The gallbladder stores *bile* secreted by the liver until the bile is needed for digestion.

gallstone   A small, hardened mass composed of *cholesterol, calcium* salts, and *bile* pigments. A gallstone can form in the *gallbladder* or in a bile duct.

gastric ulcer   See *ulcer, peptic*.

gastroesophageal reflux disease   A digestive disorder in which the valve connecting the esophagus and the stomach does not close properly, allowing stomach acids and other irritants to flow backward into the esophagus.

gastrointestinal (GI) series   Diagnostic procedures in which a series of X rays of the *digestive tract* are taken after a person swallows a barium mixture or receives a barium enema.

gastrointestinal tract   See *digestive tract*.

generalized anxiety disorder   A mental disorder characterized by persistent, unrealistic worry or fear about the common events of daily life such as work, health, and family relationships.

genital herpes   See *herpes, genital*.

genital warts   See *warts, genital*.

genitourinary tract   The organs concerned with sexual reproduction and with producing and excreting urine.

GERD   See *gastroesophageal reflux disease*.

gingivitis   Inflammation of the *gums,* usually caused by a bacterial infection that results from a buildup of dental *plaque*. An early stage of *periodontal disease*.

GI series   See *gastrointestinal (GI) series*.

glaucoma   Abnormally high pressure inside the eyeball that damages peripheral (side) vision, causing the visual field to become increasingly narrow until total blindness occurs.

glioma   A tumor that arises from the glial cells in the brain.

glomeruli   See *glomerulus*.

glomerulonephritis   Inflammation of the *glomeruli* in the *kidneys,* which can lead to impaired kidney function.

glomerulus   Singular of glomeruli. A tiny cluster of blood vessels inside the *nephrons* in the *kidneys.*

glucose   A simple sugar that is the body's main source of energy.

glucose meter   A device used by people with *diabetes* to measure blood *glucose* levels.

golfer's elbow   See *epicondylitis.*

gonioscopy   Examination of the *drainage angle* of the eyeball using a special contact lens called a gonioscope. Gonioscopy is used to diagnose *glaucoma.*

gonorrhea   A common *sexually transmitted disease* (STD) caused by the gonococcus bacteria and characterized by painful urination and discharge of *pus* from the *penis.*

"good" cholesterol   See *high-density lipoprotein (HDL) cholesterol.*

gout   A metabolic disorder characterized by high levels of uric acid in the blood, causing *joint* pain and inflammation, usually in a single joint.

granuloma   A tumorlike mass of cells.

gum   The soft tissue that surrounds the teeth.

gum disease   See *periodontal disease.*

H

hair follicle   A tiny pit in the surface of the skin from which a hair grows.

hay fever   See *allergic rhinitis.*

HDL cholesterol   See *high-density lipoprotein (HDL) cholesterol.*

headache, cluster   A series of recurring headaches that affects one side of the head and usually includes symptoms such as a runny nose and watery eyes.

headache, migraine   See *migraine.*

headache, muscle contraction   Also known as a tension headache. The most common type of headache, characterized by mild to moderate pain in the head or neck and muscle tenderness.

headache, tension   See *headache, muscle contraction.*

hearing aid   A small, battery-powered device that fits in or over the ear and amplifies sounds, improving hearing for people with certain types of hearing loss.

heart attack   See *myocardial infarction* (MI).

heartbeat   A contraction of the heart muscle that pumps blood into the *arteries* and throughout the body.

heart disease   See *coronary artery disease.*

heart failure   The inability of the heart to efficiently pump blood, leading to congestion of blood in *veins* and excessive accumulation of fluid in body tissues.

heart rate   The number of *heartbeats* per minute.

hematocele   A collection of blood in the *scrotum* that may result after injury or rupture of a *testicle.*

hematuria   The presence of red blood cells in the urine.

hemochromatosis   A hereditary metabolic disorder in which excessive amounts of iron accumulate in the body tissues.

hemodialysis   A form of *dialysis* in which blood circulates through a machine where it is filtered and purified before being returned to the body. Hemodialysis is used to treat *kidney* failure.

hemoglobin   The oxygen-carrying *protein* in red blood cells.

hemorrhoids   *Varicose veins* in the lining of the *anus* and *rectum,* often caused by straining during bowel movements.

hemospermia   Blood in the *semen.*

hemothorax   An accumulation of blood in the space between the chest wall and the lung, usually as a result of injury.

hepatitis   An inflammation of the *liver* that may be caused by infection, drugs, or toxins.

herniated disk   See *prolapsed disk.*

herpes, genital   A *sexually transmitted disease* (STD) caused by the *herpesvirus* herpes simplex virus 2 and characterized by recurrent outbreaks of small, red, painful blisters on the *penis, scrotum,* buttocks, *anus,* or thighs. There is no known cure. Herpes can be spread to another person between outbreaks, even if the infected person is symptom-free.

herpes simplex virus 1   A *herpesvirus* that usually affects areas of the body other than the genitals.

herpes simplex virus 2   A *herpesvirus* that causes genital herpes. See *herpes, genital.*

herpesvirus   Any of a group of viruses that includes *herpes simplex virus 1, herpes simplex virus 2, varicella-zoster virus, Epstein-Barr virus,* and *cytomegalovirus.*

high-altitude pulmonary edema   A life-threatening buildup of fluid in the lungs at high altitudes; can result from rapid ascent to high altitudes.

high blood pressure   Also known as hypertension. A condition in which *blood pressure* is persistently raised. See also *pulmonary hypertension, primary hypertension,* and *secondary hypertension.*

high-density lipoprotein (HDL) cholesterol   Also known as "good" *cholesterol.* HDL cholesterol is a type of fat carried in the bloodstream that protects against *coronary artery disease* by cleansing blood vessels of *low-density lipoprotein (LDL) cholesterol.*

hip replacement   See *arthroplasty.*

histamine   A chemical released by the body during an *allergic reaction* that produces symptoms of inflammation, including redness, swelling, heat, and pain.

HIV   See *human immunodeficiency virus.*

Holter monitor   A portable device worn around the neck or over the shoulder that records the electrical activity of the heart during a 24-hour period.

hormones   Chemicals, such as *testosterone,* that are produced by the body and released directly into the bloodstream to perform specific functions.

hormone therapy   Also known as endocrine therapy. Treatment of a disease, such as cancer, using *hormones* that affect the growth of cells in the body.

hospice   A philosophy of caring for people who are in the final phase of terminal illness that emphasizes comfort and quality of life and focuses on relieving pain and controlling other symptoms.

HPV   See *human papillomavirus.*

human immunodeficiency virus   A virus that infects the cells of the *immune system* and causes *acquired immunodeficiency syndrome* (AIDS).

human papillomavirus   Any of a number of strains of viruses that cause *warts.* HPV is also thought to be a cause of cancer of the *penis.*

hydrocele   A soft, painless swelling in the *scrotum* caused by accumulation of a watery fluid in the membrane covering the *testicles.*

hydrogenated fats   Vegetable oils that have been converted into a solid form, such as stick margarine or canned shortening. Hydrogenated fats can raise the level of harmful *low-density lipoprotein (LDL) cholesterol* in the blood.

hyperglycemia   An abnormally high level of *glucose* in the blood. Hyperglycemia usually occurs in people with untreated or improperly regulated *diabetes.*

hypertension   See *high blood pressure.*

hypoglycemia   An abnormally low level of *glucose* in the blood. Hypoglycemia usually occurs when a person with *diabetes* takes too much *insulin* or misses a meal. Hypoglycemia also can occur in people who do not have diabetes.

hypothalamus   A small structure at the base of the brain that regulates many body functions, including appetite and body temperature.

I

IBS   See *irritable bowel syndrome.*

IgA nephropathy   See *immunoglobulin A (IgA) nephropathy.*

ileostomy   A surgical procedure in which the *ileum* is brought through an incision in the abdominal wall and an artificial opening is created through which feces can be discharged into a bag attached to the skin.

ileum   The section of the *small intestine* that extends from the *jejunum* to the *cecum.*

immune deficiency   See *immunodeficiency.*

immune system   A network of specialized cells and organs that protects the body from infectious organisms and from cancer.

immunodeficiency   Also known as immune deficiency. Impaired effectiveness of the *immune system.*

immunoglobulin A (IgA) nephropathy   A *chronic* disorder of the *kidneys* caused by deposits of the *protein* IgA inside the *glomeruli* within the kidneys, which interferes with the blood-filtering process.

immunoglobulins   See *antibodies.*

immunotherapy   Treatment in which the body's *immune system* is stimulated to destroy cancer cells.

impotence   See *erectile dysfunction.*

incontinence, stress   See *stress incontinence.*

incontinence, urinary   See *urinary incontinence.*

inflammatory bowel disease   A term that refers to either of two *chronic* disorders of the intestine—*ulcerative colitis* or *Crohn's disease.*

influenza   Also known as the flu. A viral infection that causes a cough, fever, muscle aches, *joint* pain, headache, and fatigue.

insomnia   Difficulty falling asleep or staying asleep.

insulin   A *hormone* produced by the *pancreas* that is essential for the body's use of *glucose* as a source of energy.

interferon *Proteins* produced by the body that defend against viral infections and some types of cancer.

intracerebral hemorrhage Bleeding from a ruptured blood vessel into the tissues of the brain. See also *stroke*.

intravenous pyelogram (IVP) See *urography, intravenous*.

intravenous urography See *urography, intravenous*.

iris The colored part of the eye that lies behind the *cornea*.

irritable bowel syndrome An intestinal disorder characterized by recurrent abdominal pain and bouts of diarrhea and/or constipation. The condition occurs in otherwise healthy adults and usually is associated with stress.

ischemia A temporary decrease in the supply of oxygen to an organ or tissue.

IVP See *urography, intravenous*.

J

jaundice Yellowing of the skin and the whites of the eyes.

jejunum The section of the *small intestine* that extends from the *duodenum* to the *ileum*. Most digestion of nutrients occurs in the jejunum.

jock itch Also known as tinea cruris. A common, contagious, fungal infection that produces red, itchy, irritated skin in the groin area, inner thighs, or around the anus.

joint A point at which bone meets bone.

joint replacement See *arthroplasty*.

K

Kaposi's sarcoma A type of skin cancer characterized by small, reddish-purple tumors that first appear on the feet and ankles and later spread to other parts of the body. Kaposi's sarcoma affects many people who have *acquired immunodeficiency syndrome* (AIDS).

keratin A tough, fibrous *protein* that is present in skin, hair, and nails.

kidney One of a pair of abdominal organs that filter waste products and excess water from the blood. The kidneys have an essential role in maintaining *blood pressure*.

kidney stone A small, hard mass of mineral salts that can form in a *kidney*.

knee replacement See *arthroplasty*.

L

lactase An *enzyme* needed to break down *lactose* during digestion.

lactose One of the sugars found in milk.

lactose intolerance The inability to digest *lactose* due to a deficiency of *lactase*.

laparoscopy   Examination of or surgery in the abdomen using a viewing tube called a laparoscope and special instruments inserted through tiny incisions in the abdomen.

large intestine   The portion of the *digestive tract* that extends from the *small intestine* to the *anus.* The sections of the large intestine include the *cecum, colon,* and *rectum.*

laser skin resurfacing   A *cosmetic surgery* procedure in which a laser is used to treat wrinkles, scars, and various skin lesions.

LDL cholesterol   See *low-density lipoprotein (LDL) cholesterol.*

legionnaires' disease   A form of *pneumonia* caused by a bacterium that contaminates water and air-conditioning systems.

lens   The transparent, internal optical component of the eye.

lentigines   See *age spots.*

LH   See *luteinizing hormone.*

libido   Sexual desire.

ligament   Tough, fibrous tissue that connects bone to bone and provides stability in a *joint.*

light therapy   See *phototherapy.*

liposuction   A *cosmetic surgery* procedure in which unwanted pockets of fat are removed from the body using a special suction device. Liposuction is the most common type of cosmetic surgery performed on men.

lithotripsy   A procedure that uses ultrasonic shock waves to break up stones (such as *kidney stones)* that have formed in the urinary tract.

liver   An abdominal organ that produces chemicals needed by the body and controls the levels of many chemicals in the blood.

liver spots   See *age spots.*

living will   An *advance directive* prepared by a competent person that indicates his or her wishes regarding life-sustaining medical treatments. A living will goes into effect only after the person is unable to speak for himself or herself and can be revised or withdrawn by the person at any time.

Lou Gehrig's disease   See *amyotrophic lateral sclerosis.*

low-density lipoprotein (LDL) cholesterol   Also known as "bad" *cholesterol.* LDL cholesterol is a type of fat carried in the bloodstream that increases the risk of *atherosclerosis* and *coronary artery disease.*

lumbar puncture   A diagnostic procedure in which a hollow needle is used to remove *cerebrospinal fluid* from the lower part of the spinal canal for testing.

luteinizing hormone   A *hormone* produced in the *pituitary gland* that stimulates secretion of *testosterone* by the *testicles.*

Lyme disease   A bacterial infection transmitted by a tick bite that causes a *rash,* fever, and inflammation of the *joints* and the heart.

lymph nodes   Small glands clustered in the neck, armpits, abdomen, and groin that are part of the body's *immune system.* The lymph nodes supply infection-fighting cells to the bloodstream and filter out bacteria and other *antigens.*

lymphocyte   A specialized white blood cell that has an important role in the *immune system.* Lymphocytes protect the body from invading microorganisms and cancer cells. Two types of lymphocytes are B lymphocytes (B cells) and T lymphocytes (T cells).

M

macula   The part of the *retina* of the eye that provides sharp sight in the center of the field of vision. The macula is essential for seeing fine detail.

macular degeneration   Age-related damage to the *macula.* Macular degeneration leads to impaired vision.

magnetic resonance imaging   A diagnostic technique that uses a computer, a powerful magnetic field, and radio waves to produce detailed two- and three-dimensional images of body tissues that are displayed on a video monitor.

malabsorption disorders   Disorders characterized by impaired absorption of nutrients by the *small intestine.* Examples of malabsorption disorders include *celiac disease* and *lactose intolerance.*

male pattern baldness   A common inherited form of hair loss in which hair sheds from the top of the head and the temples at the same time. Male pattern baldness can be treated with drugs such as *finasteride* and *minoxidil.*

malignant   Describes an abnormal growth that is cancerous.

malignant melanoma   See *melanoma, malignant.*

manic-depressive disorder   See *bipolar disorder.*

median nerve   A nerve in the arm that controls movement of the forearm and hand and that transmits sensation from part of the hand to the brain.

melanin   The pigment that gives skin, hair, and eyes their color.

melanoma, malignant   The most serious form of skin cancer, the first sign of which is often a change in an existing *mole.* Malignant melanoma spreads quickly and can be fatal. The main cause of melanoma is overexposure to sunlight.

Ménière's disease   An inner-ear disorder characterized by dizziness, loss of balance, *tinnitus,* and hearing loss.

meninges   The membranes surrounding the brain and spinal cord.

meningioma   A rare, slow-growing, *benign* brain tumor that develops from the *meninges.*

meningitis   Inflammation of the *meninges,* usually as the result of an infection.

meniscus   A crescent-shaped disk of *cartilage* that reduces friction in *joints* such as the jaw, wrist, and knee.

metabolism   The chemical processes that take place in the body.

metastasis   The spread of cancer from its original location to another location in the body.

MI   See *myocardial infarction.*

microsurgery   Delicate surgery performed using a special binocular microscope.

migraine   A severe, persistent, sometimes disabling headache that occurs on one side of the head and may spread to the other side. A migraine is accompanied by symptoms such as nausea, vomiting, sensitivity to light and noise, fever, chills, aches, and sweating.

ministroke   See *transient ischemic attack* (TIA).

minoxidil   An *antihypertensive* that is also available in nonprescription lotion form to treat *male pattern baldness.*

mitral incompetence   See *mitral valve regurgitation.*

mitral insufficiency   See *mitral valve regurgitation.*

mitral valve   The valve in the heart that allows blood to flow from the left *atrium* to the left *ventricle.*

mitral valve prolapse   A common, usually minor defect of the *mitral valve* in which the valve does not close properly, allowing small amounts of blood to leak back into the left *atrium* from the left *ventricle.*

mitral valve regurgitation   Also known as mitral incompetence or mitral insufficiency. Leakage of blood back through the *mitral valve* into the left *atrium* each time the left *ventricle* contracts, leading to increased *blood pressure* in the blood vessels that carry blood from the lungs to the heart.

mitral valve stenosis   A narrowing of the *mitral valve* opening that increases resistance to blood flow from the left *atrium* to the left *ventricle.* Mitral valve stenosis can eventually lead to *heart failure.*

mole   A dark-colored growth on the skin that may be flat or raised and that may vary in size. Moles can appear anywhere on the body. In rare cases a mole may develop into a serious form of skin cancer known as malignant melanoma. See *melanoma, malignant.*

molluscum contagiosum   A common, *benign,* viral infection characterized by tiny lumps on the skin. Molluscum contagiosum is harmless and usually clears up without treatment in a few months. It is often a *sexually transmitted disease* (STD) in adults.

mononucleosis   An infectious disease caused by the *herpesvirus* Epstein-Barr virus and characterized by fever, sore throat, and swollen glands.

motor neuron disease   A group of rare disorders of unknown cause characterized by degeneration of nerves that control muscle activity in the brain and spinal cord, resulting in weakness and wasting of the muscles. See also *amyotrophic lateral sclerosis* and *Parkinson's disease.*

MRI   See *magnetic resonance imaging.*

MS   See *multiple sclerosis.*

mucous membrane   The thin, skinlike lining of the cavities and tubes in the body, such as the *digestive tract,* urinary tract, and respiratory tract.

mucus   A thick, slimy fluid secreted by a *mucous membrane* to lubricate and protect the part of the body it lines.

multiple sclerosis   A progressive, disabling disorder characterized by degeneration of the protective coverings of nerve cells, which interferes with normal functioning of the nervous system.

muscle contraction headache   See *headache, muscle contraction.*

myelography   A diagnostic examination of the spinal cord, nerves, and other tissues in and around the spinal canal, in which *contrast medium* is injected and X rays are taken. The information recorded during the procedure is called a myelogram.

myocardial infarction   Also known as a heart attack. Sudden death of a section of the heart muscle because of a loss of blood supply. The most common cause is blockage of blood flow in one of the coronary *arteries* by a *thrombus.* Symptoms include severe, constant chest pain; shortness of breath; nausea; vomiting; restlessness; cold, clammy skin; and loss of consciousness. Risk factors include high blood levels of *cholesterol, atherosclerosis, obesity, diabetes,* and *high blood pressure.*

myringoplasty   A surgical procedure used to repair a hole in the eardrum.

narcolepsy   A sleep disorder characterized by excessive daytime sleepiness, causing sudden, recurrent episodes of sleep throughout the day.

natural crown   See *crown, natural.*

nephron   The basic filtering unit of the *kidneys.*

nephrotic syndrome   A collection of symptoms and signs, including high levels of *protein* in the urine, high levels of *cholesterol* in the blood, low levels of protein in the blood, and swelling of body tissues, that together indicate *kidney* damage.

neuron   A nerve cell.

neurotransmitters   Chemical messengers in the brain.

nongonococcal urethritis   Inflammation of the *urethra* that is not caused by *gonorrhea* and is the most common type of *sexually transmitted disease* (STD). It can be caused by infection with *Chlamydia trachomatis* or a *herpesvirus.*

nonsteroidal anti-inflammatory drugs   Medications such as ibuprofen and naproxen that relieve pain and inflammation.

noradrenaline   See *norepinephrine.*

norepinephrine   Also known as noradrenaline. A *hormone* that helps regulate *heart rate* and *blood pressure* by narrowing blood vessels and increasing heart rate when blood pressure drops below the normal level.

NSAIDs   See *nonsteroidal anti-inflammatory drugs.*

oat cell cancer   See *small cell cancer.*

obesity   A condition in which a person weighs 20 percent or more over the maximum desirable weight for his or her build and height.

obsessive-compulsive disorder   A mental disorder characterized by persistent thoughts or impulses called obsessions that lead to repetitive, ritualized thoughts or behaviors (compulsions).

occlusion   See *bite.*

ophthalmologist   A physician who specializes in treating disorders of the eyes.

ophthalmoscopy   Examination of the inside of the eye with a handheld, lighted viewing instrument called an ophthalmoscope.

opportunistic infections   Infections that rarely occur in healthy people but frequently occur in people who have impaired *immune systems*—such as people with *acquired immunodeficiency syndrome* (AIDS).

optic nerve   One of a pair of nerves that transmit information about visual images received from the *retinas* of the eyes to the *visual cortex* of the brain.

orchiectomy   The surgical removal of one or both *testicles.*

orchitis   Inflammation of one or both *testicles*.

orgasm   Intensely pleasurable sensations caused by involuntary contractions of the genital muscles that occur at the peak of sexual excitement. In men, these muscle contractions lead to *ejaculation*.

osteoarthritis   Progressive, gradual thinning or destruction of *cartilage* in the *joints*, usually resulting from aging, injury, or overuse.

osteomalacia   Softening, weakening, and loss of minerals from the bones of an adult as a result of *vitamin* D deficiency.

osteoporosis   A disorder in which bones become thin, brittle, and more susceptible to *fracture*. Although osteoporosis is far more common in women, it also can occur in men.

otolaryngologist   A physician who specializes in treating disorders of the ear, nose, and throat.

oxidation   A damaging chemical reaction in the cells of the body caused by the actions of *oxygen free radicals*.

oxygen free radicals   Molecules produced in the body (by normal cell activity or by external agents such as radiation and cigarette smoke) that change, damage, or break down cells. Oxygen free radicals are a major cause of disease and aging.

P

pacemaker   An electronic device implanted in the chest to regulate the *heartbeat*.

Paget's disease   A *chronic* disorder of the bone formation process in which normal bone is replaced by weakened, thickened, deformed bone.

palpitations   An unusually strong, rapid *heartbeat*.

pancreas   A long, irregularly shaped gland located behind the stomach that secretes digestive *enzymes* and *hormones*, including *insulin*.

pancreatitis   Inflammation of the *pancreas*.

panic disorder   A mental disorder characterized by brief, intense episodes of high anxiety (called panic attacks) that occur without apparent cause.

paraphimosis   Constriction of the *penis* behind the head of the penis caused by an extremely tight, retracted (pulled back) *foreskin*. Paraphimosis causes swelling and pain. See also *phimosis*.

parathyroid glands   Two pairs of glands located near the *thyroid gland* in the neck. The parathyroid glands produce parathyroid *hormone*, which helps control the level of *calcium* in the blood.

Parkinson's disease   A *motor neuron disease* most common in people over age 60 that causes weakness, rigidity, and *tremors* in the muscles.

PCP   See *Pneumocystis carinii pneumonia.*

pelvis   The basin-shaped bony structure at the base of the spine, consisting of the ilium (part of the hipbone), the sacrum, and the coccyx (the tailbone). The pelvis protects organs such as the *bladder* and the *rectum.*

penis   The external male reproductive organ through which the *urethra* passes.

peptic ulcer   See *ulcer, peptic.*

pericarditis   Inflammation of the *pericardium* that often leads to chest pain and fever.

pericardium   The membrane that surrounds the heart.

periodontal disease   Also known as gum disease. Inflammation of the *gums* and other tissues surrounding the teeth, caused by a bacterial infection. See also *gingivitis.*

periodontitis   See *periodontal disease.*

peripheral vascular disease   Poor circulation in the legs (and sometimes in the arms) caused by narrowing of blood vessels in the affected area.

peritoneum   The membrane that lines the abdominal cavity and covers the abdominal organs.

peritonitis   Inflammation of the *peritoneum,* usually as a result of a bacterial infection of the abdominal cavity.

Peyronie's disease   A condition in which fibrous or scar tissue in the *penis* causes it to bend at an angle, especially during an erection.

phagocytes   Specialized white blood cells that have an important role in the *immune system.* Phagocytes surround and destroy invading microorganisms.

phimosis   Shrinking or tightening of the *foreskin* of the *penis* that prevents the foreskin from being drawn back over the head of the penis. Phimosis may interfere with urination or sexual activity. See also *paraphimosis.*

phlebitis   Also known as thrombophlebitis. Inflammation and *thrombus* formation in a *vein,* usually in the legs.

phobia   Persistent, irrational anxiety regarding a particular object, person, place, or situation.

phototherapy   Also called light therapy. Treatment using ultraviolet light. Phototherapy is often used to treat a form of *depression* called *seasonal affective disorder* (SAD) and skin disorders such as *acne* and *psoriasis.*

pimples   Acne skin blemishes such as *blackheads* and *whiteheads*.

pineal gland   A tiny area of the brain that may be involved in regulation of the 24-hour body cycles called biorhythms.

pituitary gland   A gland at the base of the brain that secretes *hormones* and regulates and controls other hormone-secreting glands and many body processes, including reproduction.

PKD   See *polycystic kidney disease.*

plaque, arterial   Fatty material that builds up inside *artery* walls. Arterial plaque can eventually lead to *atherosclerosis.*

plaque, dental   A sticky coating of saliva, bacteria, and food debris that forms on the teeth.

plastic surgeon   A physician who uses special surgical techniques to repair or reconstruct defects in or damage to the skin and underlying tissue.

plastic surgery   Surgery performed to repair or reconstruct skin and underlying tissue that is damaged or defective.

pleura   See *pleural membranes.*

pleural effusion   Accumulation of fluid between the *pleural membranes* that can cause difficulty breathing.

pleural membranes   The two membranes that line the chest cavity and cover the lungs.

pleurisy   Inflammation of the *pleural membranes* usually caused by a lung infection. Pleurisy causes chest pain that may travel to the tip of the shoulder on the affected side.

***Pneumocystis carinii* pneumonia (PCP)**   An *opportunistic infection* of the lungs caused by the microorganism *Pneumocystis carinii.* PCP affects many people who have *acquired immunodeficiency syndrome* (AIDS).

pneumonia   Inflammation of the lungs, usually caused by a viral or bacterial infection. Symptoms and signs include fever, chills, shortness of breath, and coughing up yellowish green sputum or sometimes blood.

pneumothorax   An accumulation of air in the space between the *pleural membranes* that causes the lung to collapse, leading to chest pain and shortness of breath.

polycystic kidney disease   A rare, inherited condition in which the *kidneys* are enlarged and contain multiple *cysts.*

polyp   A growth that projects, usually on a stalk, from a body membrane. Polyps sometimes can develop into cancer.

posttraumatic stress disorder   A persistent disturbance of emotions and behavior that develops after experiencing extreme trauma, such as witnessing a violent crime or participating in military combat.

potassium   An essential mineral that helps the body maintain water balance, conduct nerve signals, contract muscles, and maintain a normal *heartbeat.*

precancerous   Describes any condition that has the potential to become cancerous.

priapism   A persistent and painful erection that is not brought on by sexual arousal or stimulation. Priapism requires emergency medical treatment.

primary hypertension   Also known as essential hypertension. *High blood pressure* with no known cause.

primary sclerosing cholangitis   A rare condition in which the *bile* ducts become narrowed due to inflammation and scarring, causing bile to accumulate in the *liver* and damage liver cells.

proctitis   Inflammation of the *rectum,* causing soreness and bleeding and, in some cases, a discharge of *mucus* and *pus.*

proctoscopy   Examination of the *anus* and *rectum* with a viewing tube.

prolapsed disk   Also known as a herniated disk. A disorder in which one of the pads of *cartilage* between the vertebrae of the spine protrudes and presses on a *ligament* or nerve, causing back pain.

prostaglandins   Substances similar to *hormones.* Prostaglandins occur in many body tissues and produce a variety of effects throughout the body, such as pain and inflammation in damaged tissue.

prostatectomy   Surgical removal of all or part of the *prostate gland.*

prostate gland   The gland that produces *semen.*

prostate-specific antigen (PSA)   A *protein* produced only by the *prostate gland.* Because PSA is not normally found in the blood, high levels of the protein in the blood can indicate prostate cancer, but also can indicate less serious problems, such as an enlarged prostate gland.

prostate-specific antigen (PSA) test   A test to measure the levels of *prostate-specific antigen (PSA)* in the blood. The PSA test is used to detect possible cancer of the *prostate gland.*

prostatitis   Inflammation of the *prostate gland.* Prostatitis is usually caused by a bacterial infection.

prostatodynia   Pain in the *prostate gland.*

proteins   Complex substances composed of *amino acids.* Proteins are the basis of all living matter.

PSA   See *prostate-specific antigen (PSA).*

PSA test   See *prostate-specific antigen (PSA) test.*

pseudofolliculitis barbae   Also known as razor bumps and shaving bumps. A common skin condition in black men and other men with curly hair, in which ingrown hairs cause inflammation and scarring in the beard area.

psoriasis   A common, *chronic* skin disorder characterized by red, dry, itchy patches of skin with silvery scales. Psoriasis most often affects the scalp, nails, elbows, arms and legs, knees, groin area, and lower back.

psychiatrist   A physician who specializes in treating mental, emotional, and behavioral disorders.

psychologist   A nonmedical specialist who treats mental, emotional, and behavioral disorders. Psychologists cannot prescribe medication.

psychotherapy   Describes a variety of treatments for mental or emotional disorders. Psychotherapy is used to help people change their behavior through techniques such as talking, reinforcement, reassurance, and support.

pubic lice   Also known as crabs (because of their crablike appearance). Tiny insects that feed on blood and mainly live in pubic hair but that also can be found in hair on the legs and the trunk.

pulmonary embolism   A life-threatening condition that occurs when a *blood clot* forms in a *vein,* travels through the bloodstream, and blocks an *artery* in the lung.

pulmonary hypertension   *High blood pressure* in the *arteries* that supply blood to the lungs.

pulmonary rehabilitation   A comprehensive, multidisciplinary program of therapy to improve the comfort and functioning of a person who has *chronic* lung disease.

pulp   The soft tissue at the core of a tooth that contains nerves and blood vessels.

pulse   The rhythmic expansion and contraction of an *artery* as blood is pumped through it.

pupil   The circular opening in the center of the *iris* through which light rays enter the eye.

pus   A pale green or yellow creamy liquid composed of dead white blood cells, bacteria, and other substances and that forms at the site of an infection.

pyelogram, intravenous   See *urography, intravenous.*

pyelonephritis   Inflammation of the *kidney,* usually caused by a bacterial infection.

pylorus   A muscular valve at the lower end of the stomach that controls the passage of food into the *duodenum.*

radiation therapy   Also known as radiotherapy. Treatment using X rays or other forms of radiation to destroy or slow the spread of cancer cells.

radioallergosorbent test   A test that detects *antibodies* to specific *allergens.* RAST is used to diagnose *allergies.*

radionuclide scanning   A diagnostic imaging technique in which a radioactive substance is swallowed or injected into the bloodstream and collects in a target organ. A special camera is then used to produce images of the organ.

radiotherapy   See *radiation therapy.*

rash   An area of reddened, inflamed skin.

RAST   See *radioallergosorbent test.*

razor bumps   See *pseudofolliculitis barbae.*

rectal examination   See *digital rectal examination* (DRE).

rectum   The final section (about 9 inches long) of the *large intestine.*

remission   A partial or complete disappearance of the signs and symptoms of a disorder or disease.

repetitive strain injury   See *repetitive stress injury.*

repetitive stress injury   Also known as repetitive strain injury. An injury caused by persistent repetition of the same movement.

rest, ice, compression, and elevation (RICE)   Standard self-treatment routine for most *strains, sprains,* and muscle pulls.

restless legs syndrome   A sleep disorder characterized by unpleasant sensations in the legs.

retina   The light-sensitive membrane on which light rays focus. The retina lines the inside of the back of the eye.

retinoids   *Vitamin* A–like medications that are used to treat skin conditions such as *acne* and *psoriasis.*

retinopathy, diabetic   Damage to the blood vessels of the *retina.* Diabetic retinopathy is the most common eye disease caused by *diabetes.*

rheumatoid arthritis   A *chronic, autoimmune disease* that causes pain, swelling, and stiffness in the affected *joints*. In severe cases the joints are completely destroyed. Rheumatoid arthritis also can affect the heart, lungs, and eyes.

rhinoplasty   A type of *cosmetic surgery* performed to reshape a person's nose.

RICE   See *rest, ice, compression, and elevation (RICE)*.

root canal therapy   A dental procedure in which infected or dead nerve tissue is removed from a tooth and replaced with a special filling material. The tooth is sealed to prevent infection and may then be covered with an artificial crown. See *crown, artificial*.

rotator cuff   The arrangement of muscles and *tendons* surrounding the shoulder *joint* that provides movement and stability.

S

SAD   See *seasonal affective disorder (SAD)*.

salt-sensitive   A term used to describe a person whose *blood pressure* goes up or down in relation to the amount of *sodium* in his or her diet.

saturated fat   A type of fat in the diet, found in meat and dairy products, that can raise the level of *cholesterol* in the blood and increase the risk of *coronary artery disease* and some forms of cancer. See also *unsaturated fat*.

schizophrenia   A serious, disabling mental disorder characterized by distorted thoughts, emotions, and behavior.

schwannoma   A *benign* tumor of the central nervous system that develops from the Schwann cells, the cells that form a protective sheath around *neurons*.

sclerotherapy   A procedure for treating *varicose veins* in which an irritant solution is injected into an affected vein, causing its walls to stick together and block the flow of blood through the vein. Nearby veins then take over the work of the treated vein.

scrotum   The external pouch of skin and muscular tissue that contains the *testicles*.

seasonal affective disorder (SAD)   A form of *depression* that tends to occur during the fall and the winter, when there are fewer hours of sunlight.

sebaceous glands   Tiny glands in the skin that produce *sebum*.

seborrheic dermatitis   See *dandruff*.

seborrheic keratosis   Harmless common skin growths caused by overproduction of *keratin*. Seborrheic keratoses may be covered by a waxy crust and may be tan, brown, or black; flat or raised; and smooth or rough.

sebum   An oily substance secreted by the *sebaceous glands* that lubricates the skin and hair.

secondary hypertension   *High blood pressure* that can be cured by successfully treating its underlying cause.

seizure   Excessive electrical activity in the brain that causes temporary loss of consciousness, memory, or movement. See also *epilepsy.*

semen   Also known as seminal fluid. A fluid produced by the male reproductive organs that contains *sperm* and that is discharged from the *penis* during *ejaculation.*

seminal fluid   See *semen.*

seminal vesicle   One of a pair of glands at the top of each *vas deferens.* The seminal vesicles produce most of the fluid in *semen.*

sensorineural hearing loss   Deafness caused by damage to the inner ear or the *auditory nerve.* The damage may be caused by a congenital defect, disease, or trauma.

serotonin   A substance present in the brain and other body tissues that acts as a *neurotransmitter.* Serotonin is involved in regulating mood.

sexually transmitted disease   An infection transmitted primarily through sexual contact with an infected person.

shaving bumps   See *pseudofolliculitis barbae.*

shin splints   Pain in the front and sides of the lower part of the leg. Shin splints are caused by *strain* or damage to underlying structures and worsen during exercise.

sickle-cell disease   An inherited blood disorder characterized by deformed, sickle-shaped red blood cells that contain an abnormal form of *hemoglobin.* These fragile blood cells break up easily, blocking and damaging blood vessels and reducing the supply of vital oxygen to organs and tissues.

sigmoid colon   The section of the *colon* that connects with the *rectum.*

sigmoidoscopy   Examination of the *rectum* and *sigmoid colon* using a viewing instrument called a sigmoidoscope that is passed into the body through the *anus.*

sinoatrial node   The heart's internal pacemaker, which sends out electrical impulses that tell the heart when to contract.

skin patch test   A test in which a doctor attaches patches of material containing possible *allergens* to a person's skin and observes the skin's reactions.

skin prick test   A test in which a doctor scratches a person's skin with needles that have been dipped into possible *allergens* and observes the skin's reactions.

skin tag   A small, harmless, flesh-colored or light brown flap of skin that sticks out from the surface of the skin. Skin tags usually appear on the neck, chest, and underarms and around the eyes.

sleep apnea   A potentially life-threatening sleep disorder characterized by brief, involuntary interruptions of breathing during sleep.

sleep disorders   See *insomnia, narcolepsy, restless legs syndrome,* and *sleep apnea.*

small cell cancer   Also known as oat cell cancer. A fast-growing, highly *malignant* cancer that affects the lungs but that spreads to other parts of the body.

small intestine   The longest portion of the *digestive tract,* extending from the stomach to the *large intestine.* It has three sections—the *duodenum,* the *jejunum,* and the *ileum.*

snap gauge   A device used to diagnose *erectile dysfunction* by measuring erections that occur during sleep.

sodium   An essential mineral (salt) that helps the body maintain water balance and *blood pressure.*

solar keratosis   See *actinic keratosis.*

sperm   The male sex cell that fertilizes the female cell of reproduction called the egg or ovum.

spermatic cord   A structure from which each *testicle* is suspended. The spermatic cord is made up of blood vessels, nerves, and the *vas deferens.*

spermatocele   A painless cyst on the *epididymis* that is filled with fluid and *sperm.* Spermatoceles usually require no treatment.

SPF   See *sun protection factor.*

sphygmomanometer   An instrument—made up of an inflatable cuff, a rubber bulb, and a gauge, glass column, or digital readout display—used to measure *blood pressure.*

spirometry   A test that measures the volume of air entering and leaving the lungs. Spirometry is performed to diagnose or monitor lung disorders. The instrument used to perform the test is called a spirometer.

spleen   An organ in the upper abdomen that is part of the body's *immune system* and that controls the quality of circulating red blood cells. The spleen also produces *antibodies, lymphocytes,* and *phagocytes.*

splint, dental   See *bite guard.*

sprain   Stretching or tearing of *ligaments* in a *joint.*

squamous cell carcinoma   A common type of skin cancer that develops in cells on the surface of the skin. Squamous cell carcinoma is usually caused by long-term overexposure to sunlight and is most common in light-skinned, fair-haired people more than 60 years old.

stapedectomy   A surgical procedure used to repair or replace the innermost bone of the middle ear.

STD   See *sexually transmitted disease.*

stenosis   Narrowing of a duct, canal, body passage, or tubular organ. See also *aortic stenosis* and *mitral valve stenosis.*

stent   A tiny device made of metallic or plastic wire mesh that is used to keep an *artery* open after *angioplasty.*

stoma   A surgically constructed opening, especially in the abdominal wall.

stomach ulcer   See *ulcer, peptic.*

stones, gallbladder   See *gallstones.*

stones, kidney   See *kidney stones.*

strain   Stretching or tearing of *tendons* and their attached muscles.

strain gauge   A device used to diagnose *erectile dysfunction* by measuring erections that occur during sleep.

stress fracture   A *fracture* caused by repeated trauma or overuse of a bone.

stress incontinence   The involuntary leaking of urine during activities (such as coughing, sneezing, or jogging) that increase pressure inside the abdomen.

stroke   Also known as a cerebrovascular accident. Sudden damage to part of the brain caused by an interruption in blood flow to the area. Ischemic stroke, the most common type of stroke, results from blockage of a blood vessel in the brain. Hemorrhagic stroke results from a ruptured blood vessel in the brain (see also *intracerebral hemorrhage).*

sunburn   Inflammation of the skin caused by overexposure to sunlight. Overexposure to sunlight increases the risk of malignant melanoma. See *melanoma, malignant.*

sun protection factor (SPF)   A number assigned to a *sunscreen* that indicates the level of protection it provides from the sun's damaging ultraviolet rays. The higher the number, the greater the level of protection. Doctors recommend that people use a sunscreen with an SPF of 15 or greater.

sunscreens   Preparations applied to the skin that help protect it from the damaging ultraviolet rays in sunlight. Sunscreens are added to many suntan lotions to help prevent *sunburn.* Doctors recommend that people use a sunscreen with a *sun protection factor (SPF)* of 15 or greater.

sun spots   See *age spots.*

syphilis   A *sexually transmitted disease* (STD) caused by infection with a bacterium that enters the body through broken skin or through the *mucous membranes* in the genitals, *rectum,* or mouth. If untreated, the disease can cause serious damage to tissues and organs throughout the body.

systolic blood pressure   The first, higher number in a *blood pressure* reading, indicating the pressure in the blood vessels when the heart beats and pumps blood through the *arteries.*

T

tachycardia   An unusually rapid *heart rate* of more than 100 beats per minute.

tartar   See *calculus.*

T cell   See *lymphocyte.*

temporomandibular disorder   A term used to describe a painful group of disorders that affect the jaw *joints* and their supporting muscles and *ligaments.*

tendinitis   Inflammation of a *tendon,* usually caused by excess friction between a tendon and a bone.

tendon   Strong, fibrous tissue that connects muscle to bone.

tennis elbow   See *epicondylitis.*

tension headache   See *headache, muscle contraction.*

testes   See *testicles.*

testicles   Also known as the testes. The pair of male sex organs that produce *sperm* and *testosterone.*

testosterone   The key male sex *hormone,* which stimulates muscle growth and the development of male sex characteristics.

thrombi   Plural of *thrombus.*

thrombolytics   Medications used to dissolve *blood clots* in cases of *embolism, thrombosis,* and *myocardial infarction* (MI).

thrombophlebitis   See *phlebitis.*

thrombosis   Formation of a *blood clot* inside an intact blood vessel.

thrombosis, deep vein   Formation of *blood clots* in veins deep inside the legs, usually resulting from sluggish blood flow caused by lack of activity.

thrombus   A *blood clot* that forms inside a blood vessel. A blood clot that breaks off and travels through the bloodstream is called an *embolus.*

thymus gland   A gland in the upper chest that has an important role in the *immune system.*

thyroid gland   A gland in the neck that secretes *hormones* essential to the regulation of various processes that occur in the body, including *heart rate* and *blood pressure.*

TIA   See *transient ischemic attack.*

tic   Involuntary, repetitive muscle movements.

tinea cruris   See *jock itch.*

tinea pedis   See *athlete's foot.*

tinnitus   A very common ear disorder characterized by persistent ringing, hissing, or other sounds in the ear when there is no external source of these sounds.

tissue plasminogen activator   A *thrombolytic* medication used in the treatment of ischemic *stroke.*

T lymphocyte   See *lymphocyte.*

TMD   See *temporomandibular disorder.*

tonometry   A procedure for measuring fluid pressure in the eye using a device called a tonometer. Tonometry is used to detect and monitor *glaucoma.*

torsion of the testicle   A condition in which a *testicle* turns on its *spermatic cord,* sometimes cutting off the testicle's blood supply.

Tourette's syndrome   An inherited disorder characterized by involuntary movements and uncontrollable vocal sounds.

tPA   See *tissue plasminogen activator.*

trans fatty acids   Synthetic fats produced during food processing.

transient ischemic attack (TIA)   Also known as a ministroke. A brief interruption in blood flow to the brain, causing temporary symptoms such as impaired vision, sensation, movement, or speech. See also *stroke.*

transurethral incision of the prostate   A surgical procedure to treat *benign prostatic hyperplasia* (BPH) in which tiny cuts are made in the *prostate gland* to relieve pressure on the *urethra* and allow urine to flow more easily.

transurethral resection of the prostate   A surgical procedure to treat *benign prostatic hyperplasia* (BPH) in which excess tissue is removed from the *prostate gland* to allow urine to flow more easily through the *urethra.*

tremor   Involuntary, rhythmic muscle movement, most commonly in the hands, feet, jaw, tongue, or head, caused by alternating contraction and relaxation of the muscles.

trichomoniasis   A *sexually transmitted disease* (STD) that usually occurs in both men and women but usually does not cause symptoms in men. If symptoms occur, they may include a discharge from the *penis* and painful or frequent urination, especially in the morning.

triglycerides   The major fats in the blood. A high level of triglycerides indicates an increased risk of *coronary artery disease, high blood pressure,* and *diabetes.*

trigger finger   A *repetitive stress injury* characterized by inflammation of the *tendons* and surrounding tendon sheaths in a finger and that prevents the finger *joint* from moving smoothly.

tuberculosis   An infectious disease caused by a bacterium that is transmitted from person to person through inhalation of infected airborne droplets. Tuberculosis primarily affects the lungs.

TUIP   See *transurethral incision of the prostate.*

tummy tuck   See *abdominoplasty.*

TURP   See *transurethral resection of the prostate.*

tympanoplasty   A surgical procedure used to repair a hole in the eardrum.

U

ulcer   An open sore on the skin or on a *mucous membrane.*

ulcer, duodenal   A peptic ulcer in the *duodenum.* See *ulcer, peptic.*

ulcer, gastric   Also known as a stomach ulcer. A peptic ulcer in the stomach. See *ulcer, peptic.*

ulcer, peptic   A hole or a break in the *mucous membrane* lining the *digestive tract* that occurs in the presence of stomach acid.

ulcer, stomach   See *ulcer, peptic.*

ulcerative colitis   *Chronic* ulceration and inflammation of the lining of the *mucous membrane* of the *colon* and *rectum.*

ultrasound   A diagnostic imaging procedure that uses high-frequency sound waves to create a picture of internal body structures on a video screen.

ultraviolet light therapy   See *phototherapy.*

unsaturated fat   A type of fat found in most vegetable oils that does not raise *cholesterol* levels in the blood. See also *saturated fat.*

urea   A waste product of the breakdown of *protein* in the body.

uremia   A toxic condition in which excess *urea* and other waste products are in the blood. Uremia is caused by *kidney* failure.

ureters   The two long, narrow tubes that carry urine from the *kidneys* to the *bladder.*

urethra   The narrow channel through which urine passes from the *bladder* to outside the body.

urethral stricture   Narrowing or blockage of part of the male *urethra* by scar tissue from an injury or infection. A urethral stricture causes difficult, sometimes painful urination.

urethritis   Inflammation of the *urethra.*

urinalysis   Testing of a sample of urine for diagnostic purposes.

urinary incontinence   The inability to control the passage of urine.

urography, intravenous   Also known as intravenous pyelogram (IVP). A diagnostic examination of the urinary tract in which *contrast medium* is injected into the bloodstream and X rays are taken.

urology   The branch of medicine concerned with the study, diagnosis, and treatment of diseases of the *genitourinary tract* in men (and the urinary tract in women).

varicella-zoster virus   A *herpesvirus* that causes *chickenpox* and shingles.

varicocele   A mass of *veins* like *varicose veins* in the *scrotum* caused by a malfunction of the valves within the veins of the *spermatic cord.*

varicose veins   Enlarged, twisted *veins* just beneath the skin that result from weakening of the valves in the veins. Varicose veins most commonly occur in the legs.

vas deferens   One of a pair of tubes that store *sperm* and carry it from the *testicles* and *epididymis* to the *urethra* during *ejaculation.*

vasectomy   A male sterilization procedure in which each of the *vas deferens* is cut and tied to prevent *sperm* from reaching the *urethra.*

vasodilators   Medications that widen blood vessels. Vasodilators are used to treat such conditions as *angina* and *heart failure.*

vein   A blood vessel that carries blood from the organs and tissues to the heart.

vena cava   One of a pair of major *veins* that carry deoxygenated blood to the right side of the heart.

veneer   A porcelain laminate shell that is used to make an artificial front surface for a tooth.

ventricle   One of the two large lower chambers of the heart. The left ventricle is the main pumping chamber of the heart.

venules   Small *veins.*

villi   Tiny fingerlike projections lining the *mucous membrane* of the *small intestine.* Villi absorb nutrients into the bloodstream.

visual cortex   The area of the brain that is concerned with vision.

vitamin   A chemical essential for normal functioning of the body.

vitrectomy   A type of *microsurgery* used in advanced cases of diabetic retinopathy. See *retinopathy, diabetic*. During vitrectomy, the *vitreous humor* is replaced with a clear solution.

vitreous humor   The jellylike substance that fills the center of the eye.

warts   Harmless, contagious growths on the skin or *mucous membrane* caused by a viral infection. See also *warts, genital*.

warts, genital   A common *sexually transmitted disease* (STD) caused by the *human papillomavirus* (HPV). Genital warts grow in and around the *anus* or on the *penis*.

weight-bearing exercise   Any exercise, such as jogging, brisk walking, or stair climbing, that works the large muscles of the lower body, stimulating bone growth and building *bone density*.

whitehead   An *acne* skin blemish that looks like a small white bump. Whiteheads usually occur in clusters on the cheeks and nose and around the eyes.

INDEX

replacement surgery, 431, 432, 442–43
shaving bumps, 421–22
hair dyes, 418
hallucinations, 357, 359, 360
hallucinogens, 23, 24, 100, 110–11
hamstring pulls, 64
hands, 308, 311–13
hangovers, 26
hay fever, 380
HDL. *See* high-density lipoprotein (HDL) cholesterol
headaches, 339–41, 412
brain tumors, 328–29
caffeine withdrawal, 11
food sensitivities, 53
hangovers, 26
migraines, 53, 330, 339–40
stress, 119
Health and Human Services Department, U.S., 6
healthcare proxies, 134
hearing aids, 90, 397, 399–400, 402
hearing loss, 397–405
brain tumor, 328, 329
heart, 203–35
alcohol consumption, 22, 101
cardiac catheterization, 228, 229
cardiopulmonary resuscitation, 210
echocardiography, 210, 213, 226–29, 234
electrocardiography, 227–29, 231, 249–50
enlarged, 218, 229
exercise, benefits of, 55, 56
Holter monitor, 212, 231, 233
medical checkup, 87
transplants, 235
valve disorders, 226–29, 230
See also coronary artery disease; high blood pressure
heart attack, 29, 89, 204, 207–12, 214
atherosclerosis, 218
blood clots, 206, 207, 222
diabetes, 369
mitral valve regurgitation, 227
warning signs, 66, 206, 208–9, 264
heartbeat
arrhythmia, 208, 212–14, 230–33, 235
atrial fibrillation, 227, 228
defibrillators, 233
pacemakers, 90, 231–33, 343
palpitations, 11, 226, 227, 231
heartburn, 262, 263, 265

heart disease. *See* coronary artery disease
heart failure, 212, 218
alcohol consumption, 3, 23
congestive, 225, 227–30, 233–35, 292, 354
emphysema, 247
insomnia, 355
mitral valve regurgitation, 227
sleep apnea, 71
heart murmurs, 226, 227, 228
heart rate, 87, 117, 211, 214, 230
exercise and, 12–13, 57
hyperthyroidism, 374
heat injuries, 65–66
heat stroke, 66
heat treatment, 64, 307, 308, 315, 319
microwave thermotherapy, 173
pacemakers and, 233
Helicobacter pylori, 261, 265
hematocele, 164
hematuria, 290, 291, 296
hemochromatosis, 279, 282
hemodialysis, 191, 293
hemoglobin, 49, 88, 238–41, 368
hemophilia, 187
hemorrhagic stroke, 323, 325
hemorrhoids, 237, 239, 271–72
hemothorax, 254
heparin, 211, 250, 301
hepatitis, 23, 191–92, 279–82, 422
immunization against, 93–94, 142
substance abuse risks, 14, 24, 100, 109, 110, 191, 281
hepatoma, 280
hermaphroditism, 165
herniated disks, 307
heroin, 23, 24, 99, 110, 147
herpes, genital, 112, 183–84, 186, 192
herpes simplex virus, 183
herpesvirus, 188
heterosexuality, 141
hiatal hernias, 262–63
high-altitude pulmonary edema, 256
high blood pressure, 217–25, 354, 401, 431
congestive heart failure, 235
diabetes, 221, 225, 369, 371, 393
diet and nutrition, 43, 220–23
exercise and, 13, 55, 220–21
eyelid surgery risks, 438
gout, 311
as heart disease factor, 204, 217
kidney disease, 217–19, 288, 292, 293, 296

medications, 149, 224–25
meditation's effect, 117–18, 224
portal hypertension, 279, 280
prevention of, 219–24
pulmonary hypertension, 225, 234, 249
risk factors, 219
sleep apnea, 356
smoking, 27, 219, 222
stress, 119, 223–24
stroke, 217, 219, 323, 324
tinnitus, 402
weight and, 17, 18, 52, 67, 69–70, 219–21
high-density lipoprotein (HDL) cholesterol, 28, 43, 89, 101, 215, 222
hips, 301, 305, 308, 310, 316
Hispanic Americans, 367
histamines, 380, 382, 383
HIV. *See* AIDS/HIV
hives, 383, 384, 385
HMG CoA reductase inhibitors, 215
Holter monitor, 212, 231, 233
home nursing care, 133
home safety, 33–34
homicide, 25, 39, 98, 116, 127
homosexuality, 72, 141–43
hormone implants, 196
hormones, 219
adrenal gland, 117, 144, 175, 365
aging and, 144
bipolar disorder, 348
digestive system, 259, 260, 263
endocrine system, 364–65
erectile dysfunction, 147, 151, 152
heart rate, 230
stress, 118–19
thyroid gland, 151, 374–75
See also specific hormones
hormone therapy, 175, 294
estrogen replacement, 143–44
hospice, 133
hot flashes, 176
human immunodeficiency virus. *See* AIDS/HIV
human papillomavirus, 142, 178, 184
hydrocele, 164
hyperglycemia, 369
hypersensitivity disease, 256
hypertension. *See* high blood pressure
hyperthyroidism, 355, 374–75
hypoglycemia, 369
hypothalamus, 320, 364